Textbook of Refractive Laser Assisted Cataract Surgery (ReLACS)

Ronald R. Krueger • Jonathan H. Talamo
Richard L. Lindstrom
Editors

Textbook of Refractive Laser Assisted Cataract Surgery (ReLACS)

Springer

Editors
Ronald R. Krueger
Cole Eye Institute, Department of Refractive Surgery
Cleveland Clinic Lerner College of Medicine
Cleveland, OH, USA

Jonathan H. Talamo
Department of Ophthalmology
Harvard Medical School
Talamo Laser Eye Consultants
Waltham, MA, USA

Richard L. Lindstrom
Minnesota Eye Consultants &
Department of Ophthalmology
University of Minnesota, Minneapolis
Minnesota, USA

ISBN 978-1-4614-1009-6 ISBN 978-1-4614-1010-2 (eBook)
DOI 10.1007/978-1-4614-1010-2
Springer New York Heidelberg Dordrecht London

Library of Congress Control Number: 2012951411

Printed on acid-free paper

Springer is part of Springer Science+Business Media (www.springer.com)

To my loving wife, Ivey, who patiently endured the many hours I spent in writing and editing this book, during our engagement and first few months of marriage. I love you, and hope you will enjoy reading this book, and implementing its surgical technology, as we work together under God's plan for our lives in the years ahead!

Ronald R. Krueger, M.D., MSE

To Andrea, Erica and Rachel for their infinite patience, love and support.

Jonathan H. Talamo, M.D.

To my wife Jaci, the joy of my life.

Richard L. Lindstrom, M.D.

Refractive Laser-Assisted Cataract Surgery (ReLACS)

The combination of femtosecond laser technology with cataract surgery is the biggest change in cataract surgery since phacoemulsification was introduced. How well this change is accepted by the ophthalmic community and the general public seeking cataract surgery has yet to be determined, but so far, as of this writing, we have seen more than a hundred U.S. laser placements, and many more worldwide, with a strong penetrance of cases being performed at each center. According to a 2012 Laser Cataract Survey by Lachman Consulting, LLC, the uptake of the use of the laser among many of the U.S. centers acquiring this technology is now 26% of all cases within the first 3 months and up to 33% within the first year.

With this kind of initial uptake of the technology, and the likelihood of continued growth, the procedure of pre-treating the lens and cornea with a femtosecond laser needs a specific name to help facilitate communication among physicians and patients. Much like "LASIK" made refractive surgery a part of everyone's lexicon, we need a similar term for the use of femtosecond lasers with cataract surgery and lens extraction. Recently at the 2012 ASCRS, it was reported that of 30 surveyed practices, 29 different names were used. This broad diversity of names needs to be eliminated, so that communication about this technology can be simplified and improved, for both doctors and patients alike.

Therefore, in this book, we are proposing "ReLACS" (*Re*fractive *L*aser-*A*ssisted *C*ataract *S*urgery) as a useable term that accomplishes this goal. We chose "ReLACS," because the primary focus of this term is "Refractive." In surgically challenging cases, where a therapeutic use of this technology is desired, and where a refractive endpoint is neither essential nor affordable, the term "T-LACS" (*T*herapeutic *L*aser-*A*ssisted *C*ataract *S*urgery) can be used to focus on the "therapeutic" application. These terms are not our own, but belong to John Berdahl, MD and colleagues, who have copyrighted them, so that they can be freely available for use in the ophthalmic community and beyond.

Finally, we feel ReLACS and T-LACS are the most appropriate terms, as there is a clear distinction between cataract surgery as a rehabilitative procedure and cataract surgery as a refractive procedure. The refractive component of cataract surgery requires precise diagnostic and therapeutic approaches that are uncovered services. Hence, we feel the term "refractive" should have a primary role in the acronym to clearly identify the refractive nature of the procedure. The remainder of the acronym (LACS) is fairly straightforward as it describes how the laser assists the surgeon in removing the cataract, but does not do it completely by itself. The term T-LACS refers to the other category, where a therapeutic intervention with the femtosecond laser may be the best option. Although this may or may not be covered with an additional fee by U.S. payors in select cases, such as phacodonesis or Fuchs' endothelial dystrophy, it will likely be embraced outside the U.S.A in countries where governments acknowledge the therapeutic (safety) benefit of using the laser in cataract surgery. Much in the same way that "PRK," (photorefractive keratectomy) and "PTK," (phototherapeutic keratectomy) focus on the refractive and therapeutic aspect of surface laser ablation, so, "ReLACS" and "T-LACS" differentiate the refractive and therapeutic application of laser assisted cataract surgery. We hope that others will embrace this terminology, and therefore we have referred to "ReLACS" as the specific term for the refractive side of this technology throughout this book.

Ronald R. Krueger, MD
Jonathan H Talamo, MD
Richard L. Lindstrom, MD

Foreword

When the femtosecond laser was introduced into the LASIK arena, it changed refractive surgery, but not all at once. Initially, the technology was still somewhat crude, and the costs were high. Yet surgeon acceptance gradually increased, despite the higher costs involved, because of the safety, precision, and improved refractive outcomes in comparison to the manual flap cut of a microkeratome. Certain groups of patients who may not have been eligible candidates for LASIK could now safely undergo the procedure with IntraLase created flaps. And even though complications could not be completely avoided, the degree of damage caused was generally much less and more easily handled by the surgeon. The higher cost to the patient was eventually accepted by most, due to the increase in safety and better results.

In a similar manner, the introduction of the femtosecond laser to cataract surgery is expected to show the same kind of beneficial results as that seen in refractive surgery, with regard to safety, precision, and improved refractive outcomes. From the steps of anterior chamber entry to rhexis, nuclear fragmentation, and astigmatic keratotomy, the goal would be to make cataract surgery less challenging and more complication free to the surgeon. The possibility of creating clear corneal-shaped incisions of varying geometric configurations with precision and safety makes it possible to improve upon the manual 700 μm microphakonit by performing a femtosecond-assisted 700 μm cataract surgery. Well-shaped incisions would decrease the risks of endophthalmitis, wound leak, shallow anterior chamber, and so on. A well-centered rhexis fashioned with an exact size and circular shape would avoid all complications associated with an errant or torn rhexis. It would also, at the same time, make it easier for the surgeon to confidently implant IOLs that are more centration- and capsular-size dependent. Nucleotomy, as a pretreatment, would make it easier to perform the segmentation, chopping, and removal of the nucleus, and finally an astigmatic keratotomy could be performed with great exactitude for astigmatism management.

Cataract surgery today has changed from what it used to be. It essentially began as a therapeutic procedure for elderly people but has now come to encompass people of all ages and expectations. With the baby boomer generation coming of age, there is a large population of cataract surgery candidates, who not only want their cataracts removed but also want it to be done in a faster, better, and smarter manner. Continuous developments have improved phacoemulsification in all aspects, from the surgeon-dependent techniques to the manufactured instruments, machines, and intra-ocular lenses. Newer machines with enhanced software and hardware features, better power modulation, and fluidics are being routinely introduced by our industry. The surgeons have also strived to consistently evolve and improve their techniques, be it from moving to smaller and smaller incisions utilizing biaxial phaco, micro-incisional coaxial phaco, and so on, to incorporating newer techniques to manage complex situations, such as small pupils or subluxated lenses. In spite of all these, there is an element of human error, which is what femtosecond laser-assisted cataract surgery will aim to remove in conjunction with the refractive component it will aim to improve.

The host of newer intra-ocular lenses with varying properties for distance, intermediate, and near vision, as well as astigmatism correction have all contributed to increasing patient expectations. The patient with cataracts desires to regain youthful vision allowing them to see clearer and sharper at all distances without spectacles and leading them to become demanding and informed consumers. These patients who expect refractive precision and fully functional vision from their surgery would more than likely be willing to opt for femtosecond-assisted refractive cataract surgery, despite the higher costs involved.

The cataract surgeon now has a greater responsibility to deliver exacting results and become increasingly aware of the intricacies, potential advantages, and disadvantages of all cataract techniques, devices, and implants. As a refractive cataract surgeon, he or she must be able to offer his or her patients the choice between femtosecond laser-assisted cataract surgery and manual cataract surgery, just as the corneal refractive surgeon has come to offer similar state-of-the-art options to their patients over the past decade. It would certainly increase patient confidence to know the element of human error has been further decreased by incorporation of a new cutting tool that uses a laser instead of a blade. It is here where Drs. Krueger, Talamo, and Lindstrom have stepped in with their wonderful new book *Textbook of Refractive Laser Assisted Cataract Surgery (ReLACS)*, which is exactly what the great number of ophthalmologists have been waiting for, and what the field needs to clarify the facts from the hype about this technology. It describes, in detail, all about this new revolutionary procedure from the laser fundamentals to techniques for using it in cataract surgery to the challenges associated with its use. Different commercially available systems are described, so that the reader can compare the advantages and disadvantages of these commercial products. Finally, the future of femtosecond laser lens-based surgery is discussed to speculate where new potential applications of this technology will head in the future. I would like to congratulate the editors for this excellent resource material, written in a very lucid, clear, and simple style and would like to wish them all success with this book

Chennai, India Amar Agarwal

Foreword

Cataract surgery is the most frequently performed surgical procedure in the world today, approaching 15 million cases each year. It is also one of the oldest surgical procedures. Couching techniques were employed 2000 years before Christ and are still practiced in some remote areas of the developing world.

In the last third of the last century, cataract surgery underwent continuous innovation with incremental improvements in technology, technique, and in all the devices, instruments, and substances used during that surgery. Power modulations led to the utilization of energy levels of approximately one-tenth of one percent of those published in the literature with the use of continuous phacoemulsification and allowed the removal of cataracts of all grades of nuclear densities with appropriate levels of power. Power modulations resulted in decreased invasiveness with less inflammation and a lowered complication rate. The development of micro-pulses of ultrasound energy, which were of shorter duration than the conduction time of heat in tissues, led to cool phacoemulsification and biaxial sleeveless phacoemulsification techniques, with their enormous fluidic advantages. Biaxial techniques are now being employed by many of the initial femtosecond laser cataract surgeons. Innovation in fluidics technology through noncompliant tubing, aspiration-bypass phacoemulsification tips, pump reversal technology, and flow restrictors led to very stable anterior chambers during the surgery. Innovation in surgical instruments, knives, visco devices, pupil expanders, pharmaceuticals, IOLs and implantation devices, technology and technique for IOL power calculations, and imaging systems all led to enhanced outcomes. Clear corneal incisions allowed the surgery to take place through avascular tissues and dramatically reduced the possibility of hemorrhagic complications. Today the procedure is routinely performed on an outpatient basis under topical anesthesia. The patients benefit from fewer systemic contraindications, minimally invasive bloodless surgery, negligible surgically induced astigmatism and for most, an almost immediate visual rehabilitation.

After Kelman's introduction of ultrasound phacoemulsification, 30 years passed before 50 % of the surgeons had adopted the technique. There was a tenfold increase in the cost of the equipment compared to that used in planned extracapsular cataract extraction. Today, cataract and refractive surgery are merging as separate disciplines of the same endeavor and a single technology, the femtosecond laser, is likely to dominate both disciplines. The enormous safety and precision of femtosecond lasers will bring the ideal of the perfect cataract procedure closer to reality. There are cost constraints inherent in the transition from ultrasound to femtosecond lasers with, as before, an almost tenfold increase in the cost of the new equipment. Emerging technology is always very expensive. The first computer installed at the Massachusetts Institute of Technology was built with vacuum tubes prior to the innovation of capacitors and occupied most of a six-story building on that campus. It was vastly more expensive and less capable than an iPhone, which fits into a shirt pocket. There will be enormous, currently unimaginable, improvements in femtosecond technology, techniques, instruments, devices, and substances with a reduction in cost.

Because the technique is less demanding, there will be a more rapid transition to this technology than the transition to ultrasound. In view of this, however, there is some concern that this surgery may become available for use by non-MD health care practitioners. It remains of paramount importance that the procedure be performed by a practitioner with the knowledge, experience, and judgment to customize the surgery to each individual and be prepared to deal with any operative and postoperative complications. This level of expertise can only be achieved through the unique and extensive training of medical doctors.

Textbook of Refractive Laser Assisted Cataract Surgery (ReLACS) is a welcome introduction to the field and an important contribution to the literature. The editors and authors are experts in their fields, and the ophthalmologists are all esteemed surgeons, teachers, and researchers. The book describes the physics and engineering of the femtosecond laser, explains the application of this technology to each of the surgical steps, and gives a description of the systems under investigation or available today. There is also some anticipation of what the future will hold with the utilization of this modality. Baby boomers are less fearful and more desirous of new technology than their parents were. My belief is that they will encourage practitioners to adopt this new technology, making femtosecond cataract refractive surgery the dominant ophthalmic surgical procedure.

This book is of value to all health care practitioners who deal with vision and ophthalmologists at every level of their training.

Eugene, OR, USA I. Howard Fine

Preface

Every so often, a truly disruptive technology comes along that fundamentally changes the practice of medicine. In the subspecialty of ophthalmology, we have been blessed with many such notable advances over the past several decades, each of which has radically improved the ability of the profession to restore and maintain vision. Laser photocoagulation of diabetic retinopathy, scleral buckling, and vitrectomy surgery for retinal detachment, high-resolution OCT for retinal diagnostics and injectable drugs to treat macular degeneration are but several examples. The field of cataract surgery has witnessed remarkable progress through the development of intraocular lenses and small incision phacoemulsification, while the advent of excimer and Femtosecond lasers led to the birth and explosive growth of laser keratorefractive surgery. In the setting of increased awareness of and appreciation for the importance of excellent uncorrected visual acuity after cataract surgery, Presbyopia-correcting and toric IOLs have spawned a new discipline, refractive cataract surgery. The development of image-guided Femtosecond lasers as a precise cutting tool for both the cornea and lens has brought about a further merging of the fields of cataract and refractive surgery, which we refer to throughout this book as Refractive Laser Assisted Cataract Surgery or "ReLACS"

We believe that ReLACS will prove to be a positive, but also "disruptive," advance for cataract surgery, as it will change not only the clinical outcomes but the ergonomics and economics of how cataract surgery is delivered in the twenty-first century. With an unparalleled capability to construct incisions within the cornea and lens, ReLACS has the potential to revolutionize cataract surgical technology and results, making possible a level of surgical precision not achievable by even the most skilled human hands. While all new "disruptive" technologies initially have their critics, the data already available from the early clinical use of ReLACS technology is compelling enough that the greater efficacy and, with time, greater safety benefits of this technology will become evident and widely accepted. Some examples of how ReLACS may change cataract surgery range from small advances like reduced diameter IOL injectors, allowing for smaller incisions, to more accurate refractive outcomes due to improved IOL effective lens position and precise, titratable correction of even small amounts of astigmatism. New IOL designs will become possible, perhaps someday resulting in attainment of the holy grail of cataract surgery, capsular refilling with a truly accommodating artificial lens polymer technology.

When assembling a textbook on a new topic in a fast-moving medical field, one often needs to fill an "information vacuum" that exists. There is inevitably a tension between taking time to compulsively assemble all that is known versus producing a more expedited product in a shorter period of time. While information rapidly emerges both inside and outside the channels of peer-reviewed literature, it can be difficult to find a single source overview that allows an orderly introduction to the subject matter.

It is impossible to remain absolutely current when referencing peer-reviewed publications in a textbook about a new technology that is being actively investigated and iterated: that is not our goal for this book. Nevertheless, we have tried to produce a comprehensively referenced text that summarizes the science behind the development of Femtosecond lasers for cataract surgery, the early results of their clinical use, and what the future may portend for this revolutionary technology. We hope that *Textbook of Refractive Laser Assisted Cataract Surgery (ReLACS)* will serve as a knowledge base that will allow the reader to make informed decisions about the use of lasers for refractive cataract surgery as new information emerges and the technology becomes routinely available to ophthalmic surgeons around the world.

Cleveland, OH, USA — Ronald R. Krueger
Waltham, MA, USA — Jonathan H. Talamo
Minneapolis, MN, USA — Richard L. Lindstrom

Contents

Contributors

Ana P. Canto, M.D. Department of Ophthalmology, Bascom Palmer Eye Institute, Miami, FL, USA

David F. Chang, M.D. Los Altos, CA, USA

Robert Cionni, M.D. The Eye Institute of Utah, Salt Lake City, UT, USA

William W. Culbertson, M.D. Department of Ophthalmology, Bascom Palmer Eye Institute, University of Miami Miller School of Medicine, Miami, FL, USA

Elizabeth A. Davis, M.D., F.A.C.S. Minnesota Eye Laser and Surgery Center, University of Minnesota, Bloomington, IN, USA

Keith H. Edwards, F.C.Optom. Dip.C.L.P. Clinical & Regulatory Affairs, LensAR Inc, Orlando, FL, USA

Mark J. Forchette Optimedica, Santa Clara, CA, USA

Randy Frey LensAR Inc, Orlando, FL, USA

Neil J. Friedman, M.D. Cataract and Lens Surgery, Pacific Vision Institute, Stanford School of Medicine, San Francisco, CA, USA

Christopher Hodge, BAppSc (Orth) Vision Eye Institute Chatswood, Chatswood, NSW, Australia

Kristian Hohla, Ph.D. Technolas Perfect Vision GmbH, Munich, Bavaria, Germany

Krystel R. Huxlin, Ph.D. Flaum Eye Institute, University of Rochester, Rochester, NY, USA

Tibor Juhasz, Ph.D. The Gavin Herbert Eye Institute and Department of Biomedical Engineering, University of California, Irvine, CA, USA

Stephen D. Klyce, Ph.D., FARVO Department of Ophthalmology, Mount Sinai School of Medicine, Port Washington, NY, USA

Wayne H. Knox, Ph.D. The Institute of Optics and Center for Visual Sciences, University of Rochester, Rochester, NY, USA

Douglas D. Koch, M.D. Department of Ophthalmology, Baylor College of Medicine, Cullen Eye Institute, Houston, TX, USA

Ronald R. Krueger, M.D., M.S.E. Cole Eye Institute, Dept of Refractive Surgery, Cleveland Clinic Lerner College of Medicine, Cleveland, OH, USA

Michael A. Lawless, M.B.B.S., FRANZCO, FRACS, FRCOphth Vision Eye Institute Chatswood, Chatswood, NSW, Australia

Richard L. Lindstrom, M.D. Minnesota Eye Consultants & Department of Ophthalmology, University of Minnesota, Minneapolis, Minnesota, USA

James C. Loden, M.D. Loden Vision Centers, Goodlettsville, TN, USA

Holger Lubatschowski, Ph.D. Rowiak GmbH, Hanover, Germany

Shareef Mahdavi SM2 Strategic, Inc, Pleasanton, CA, USA

Zoltan Z. Nagy, M.D., Ph.D., D.Sc. Department of Ophthalmology, Semmelweis University, Budapest, Hungary

Madeleine C. O'Meara, M.S., B.A. Department of Marketing, OptiMedica, Santa Clara, CA, USA

Mark Packer, M.D., F.A.C.S., C.P.I. Casey Eye Institute, Oregon Health and Science University, Eugene, OR, USA

Daniel V. Palanker, Ph.D. Department of Ophthalmology, Stanford University, Stanford, CA, USA

Jean-Marie A. Parel, Ph.D., Ing. ETS-G., FARVO Ophthalmic Biophysics Center, Bascom Palmer Eye Institute, University of Miami School of Medicine, Miami, FL, USA

Prasad Kasu Reddy, M.D. Maxivision Eye Care Centres, Hyderabad, India

Simone Schneider, Ph.D., M.Sc. Clinical Department, LensAR, Orlando, FL, USA

Katrina B. Sheehy, B.S., M.S. OptiMedica, Santa Clara, CA, USA

Stephen G. Slade, M.D., F.A.C.S. Slade & Baker Vision Center, Houston, TX, USA

David Smadja, M.D. Cataract, Cornea & Refractive Surgery Department, Cleveland Clinic, Cole Eye Institute, Cleveland, OH, USA

Anterior Segment Unit & Refractive Surgery, University Center Hospital of Bordeaux, Bordeaux, France

Roger F. Steinert, M.D. Department of Ophthalmology, Gavin Herbert Eye Institute, University of California, Irvine, CA, USA

Jonathan H. Talamo, M.D. Harvard Medical School, Talamo Laser Eye Consultants, Ophthalmology, Waltham, USA

Harvey S. Uy, M.D. Pacific Eye and Laser Institute, Makati City, Manila, The Philippines

Sonia H. Yoo, M.D. Department of Ophthalmology, Bascom Palmer Eye Institute, University of Miami Miller School of Medicine, Miami, FL, USA

Roberto Zaldivar Department of Cataract & Refractive Surgery, Instituto Zaldivar, Mendoza, Argentina

Roger Zaldivar, M.D. Department of Cataract & Refractive Surgery, Instituto Zaldivar, Mendoza, Argentina

Evolution of Cataract Surgery

1

Mark Packer, Richard L. Lindstrom, and
Elizabeth A. Davis

The Ancient Era of Lens Surgery

The word cataract derived from the Latin cataracta, waterfall. The white froth of a waterfall represented the clouding of the lens that occurs with an advanced cortical cataract. The Romans saw suffusion between the pupil and the lens. We now think of cataract as the consequence of natural aging changes [1].

Couching formed the mainstay of cataract surgery until the eighteenth century (see Fig. 1.1) [2]. The surgeon inserted a needle in the eye through the pars plana or cornea and pushed the presumably opaque lens into the vitreous cavity, clearing the visual axis. The resulting aphakic vision could at least restore some independence to the blind. High complication and infection rates appear to have plagued the procedure.

In 1747, the French surgeon Jacques Daviel attempted but failed to couch a lens. Undaunted, he used a knife and scissors to cut open the patient's cornea along the inferior limbus. He then incised the lens capsule and expressed the nucleus from the eye. His publication of a paper about the procedure the same year ushered in the era of lens extraction [3]. Despite high complication rates, lens extraction techniques slowly advanced. The advent of local anesthesia, sterile technique, and specialized instrumentation gradually improved outcomes. Until the middle of the twentieth century, lens extraction remained unchallenged as the standard procedure for treating cataracts. Despite the large incision and the aphakic spectacles, patients generally did well [4, 5] (see Fig. 1.2) [2].

Along with the development of lens extraction there persisted a parallel path of IOL development. The earliest reference to lens implantation is credited to Tadini, an eighteenth century oculist [6–8]. According to his memoirs, Casanova met him in 1766 in Warsaw, where Tadini showed him a box with small spheres that were well polished and suggested that such globes might be placed under the cornea in the place of the crystalline lens. No confirmation is available that Tadini ever actually did perform such an implant operation.

Approximately 30 years later, in 1795, a Dresden ophthalmologist, Casaamata, performed a cataract operation and implanted an artificial lens [6–8]. Apparently, Casaamata performed the procedure by inserting the glass lens through a wound in the cornea. He immediately realized

M. Packer, M.D., F.A.C.S., C.P.I. (✉)
Casey Eye Institute, Oregon Health and Science University, 1550 Oak St., Suite 5, Eugene, OR 97401, USA
e-mail: mpacker@finemd.com

R.L. Lindstrom, M.D. • E.A. Davis, M.D., F.A.C.S.
Minnesota Eye Consultants & Department of Ophthalmology, University of Minnesota, Minneapolis, Minnesota 55431, USA

R.R. Krueger et al. (eds.), *Textbook of Refractive Laser Assisted Cataract Surgery (ReLACS)*,
DOI 10.1007/978-1-4614-1010-2_1, © Springer Science+Business Media, LLC 2013

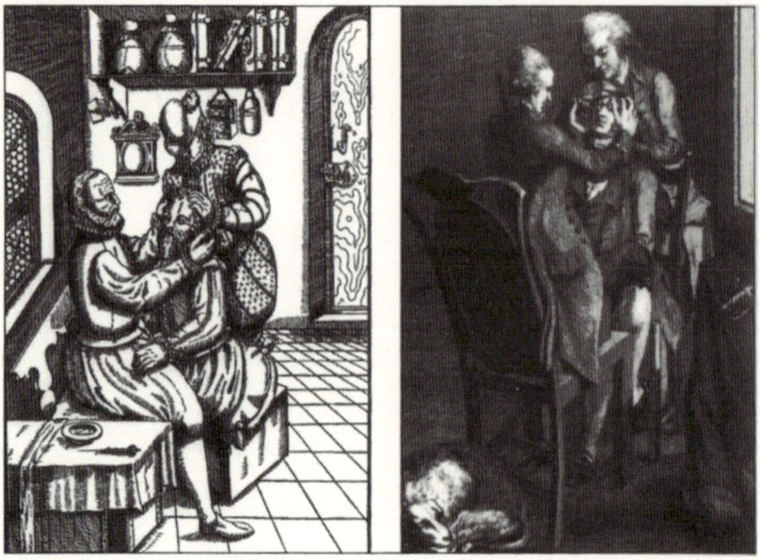

Fig. 1.1 Reprinted with permission from SLACK Incorporated [2]

Fig. 1.2 Reprinted with permission from SLACK Incorporated [2]

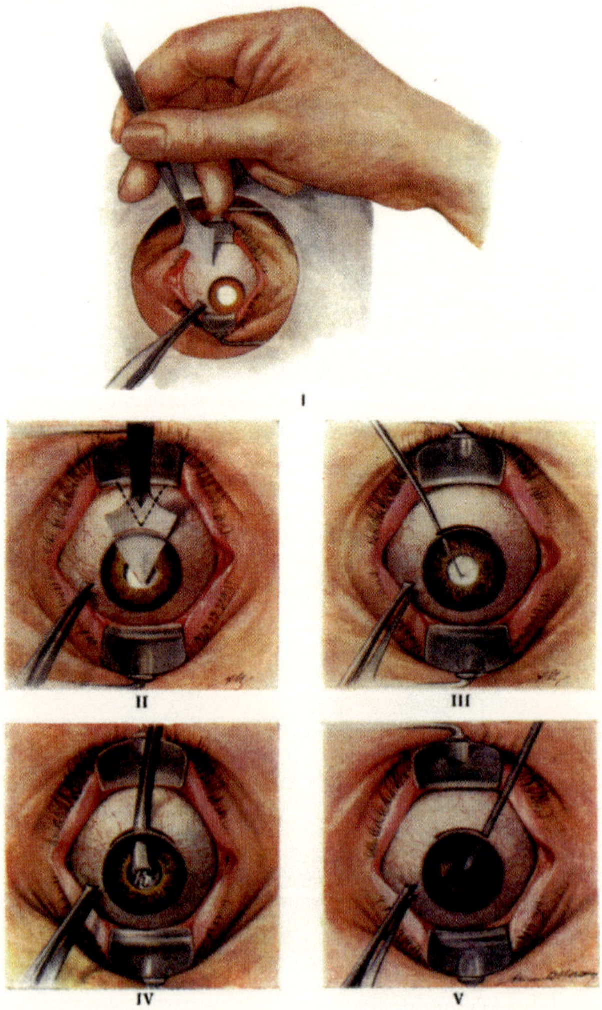

the procedure would not be successful as the glass lens fell deeply into the vitreous. Thus, the first implantation of an IOL as well as the first severe complication, total lens dislocation into the vitreous, appears to belong to Casaamata.

The modern era of lens implantation begins with Harold Ridley of London [9–11]. At the end of a cataract operation in the fall of 1949, Ridley reported he was asked by a medical student why he did not replace the cataractous lens he was removing with a new one. Apparently this gave Ridley the impetus to explore the possibility of lens implantation. During World War II, many ophthalmologists had noted that perforating eye injuries from airplane canopies made from acrylic Perspex plastic often resulted in minimal intraocular irritation secondary to the material itself. It therefore became accepted that acrylic was relatively inert in the eye. This, and the fact that acrylic has a relatively high refractive index of 1.49 and a low specific gravity of 1.19, prompted Harold Ridley to select this material for his initial investigations into lens implantation.

Ridley originally designed his lens to imitate the natural lens (see Figs. 1.3, 1.4, and 1.5). Its diameter was 8.32 mm, and its weight was 112 mg in air and 70.4 mg in water, as compared with a modern intraocular lens, which weighs <4 mg in water. On November 29, 1949, at St. Thomas Hospital in London, Harold Ridley implanted the first posterior chamber lens into the capsular bag after an extracapsular cataract extraction (see Fig. 1.6). It is amazing that his original choice of material, method of cataract extraction, and selection of in-the-bag implantation have been affirmed after more than 40 years of trial-and-error investigation in this field.

The second lens was implanted almost 1 year later, on August 23, 1950. Unfortunately, the initial two patients' postoperative refractive results were significantly myopic, one refracting at −20.0 and one at −15 diopters (D). Ridley then recalculated the basic optics for the lens and began a series

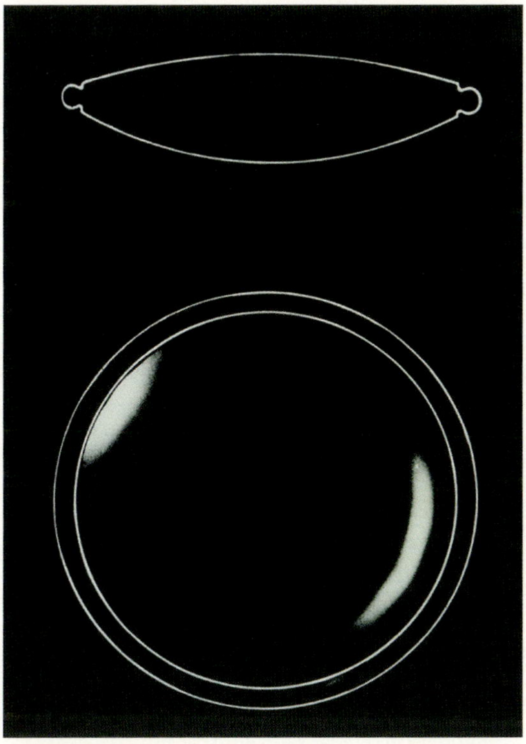

Fig. 1.3 Schematic diagram of original Ridley IOL

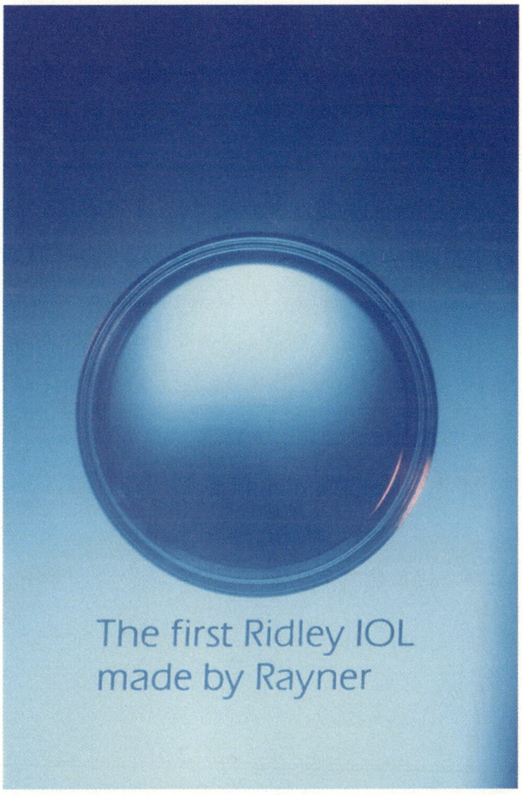

Fig. 1.4 Promotional drawing of Ridley IOL from Rayner, Ltd

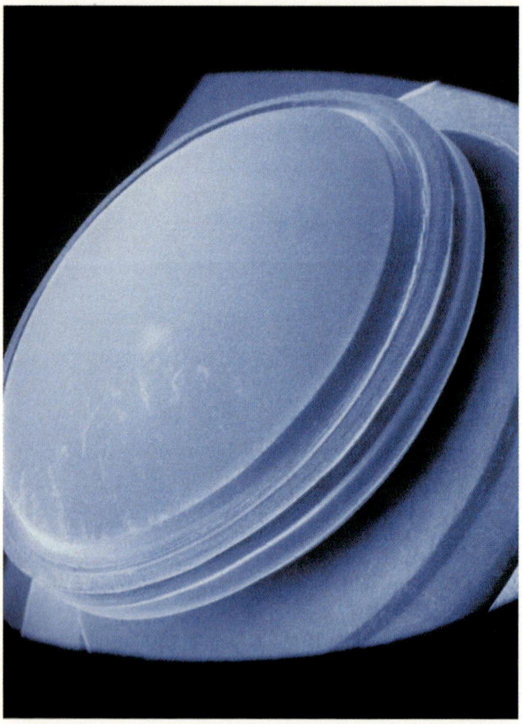

Fig. 1.5 Scanning electron micrograph of Ridley IOL

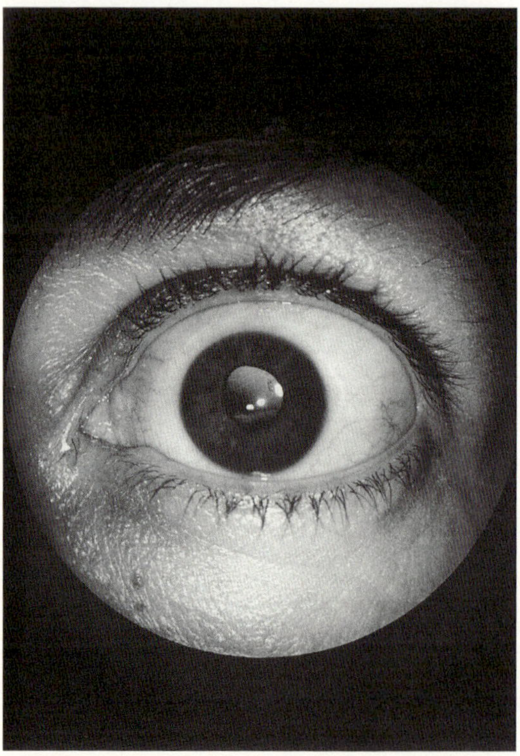

Fig. 1.6 First Ridley IOL implanted in eye

of about 750 implants, which extended to approximately 1959. These early lens implant patients suffered from a significant rate of complication, including severe postoperative inflammation and lens dislocation. Lens dislocation occurred in approximately 13% of the cases, usually into the vitreous. Many patients also developed late secondary glaucoma. Nonetheless, many of these implants performed well for many years.

The Modern Era of Lens Surgery

The introduction and development of phacoemulsification and continuing advances in intraocular lens technology during the second half of the twentieth and the early years of the twenty-first century have revolutionized cataract surgery. Phacoemulsification (phaco) has come to refer to the disassembly and removal of the crystalline lens through a small corneal incision (see Fig. 1.7) [2]. From its introduction in the late 1960s, phaco evolved into a highly effective method of cataract extraction. Incremental advances in surgical technique and the simultaneous redesign and modification of technology permitted increased safety and efficiency. Among the advances that have shaped modern phaco are incision construction, continuous curvilinear capsulorhexis, cortical cleaving hydrodissection and hydrodelineation, and nucleofractis techniques.

United States patent 3,589,363, filed July 25, 1967, lists Anton Banko and Charles D. Kelman as inventors of "an instrument for breaking apart and removal of unwanted material, especially suitable for surgical operations such (as) cataract removal, including a handheld instrument having an operative tip vibrating at a frequency in the ultrasonic range with an amplitude controllable up to several thousandths of an inch" [12].

Even recently, the fundamental mechanisms by which the system known as phacoemulsification operates remained controversial. While some authors described the surgical advantages of a unique type of cavitational energy, others denied any role for cavitational energy in phacoemulsification [13]. Although definitive answers proved elusive, surgeons came to understand the language of physics and engineering.

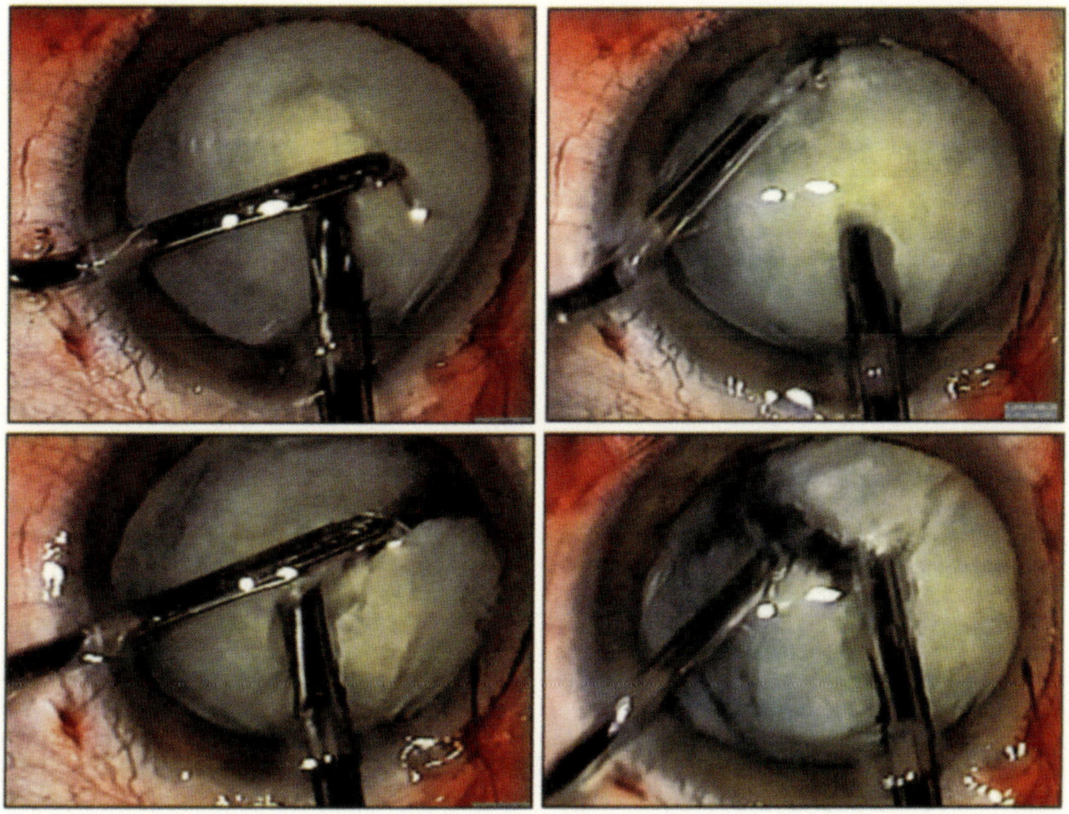

Fig. 1.7 Reprinted with permission from SLACK Incorporated [2]

The principle technical features of state-of-the-art phacoemulsification include the construction of water-tight, self-sealing corneal incisions, the successful completion of an intact, round, centered capsulorhexis with a diameter smaller than that of the intended IOL, gentle, efficient ultrasound power modulation in order to protect the capsule and the cornea, and a resulting perfectly clean capsular bag followed by an uncomplicated IOL insertion. More refined techniques have led to better outcomes, especially with respect to the reduction of postoperative refractive error and the decreasing need for spectacle wear.

Smaller corneal incisions and more precise incision construction have led to a greater predictive outcome for the incisional control of postoperative astigmatism [14]. The further development of technology for intraoperative imaging has permitted improvement in the outcomes associated with peripheral corneal relaxing incisions [15]. The greater consistency in surgically induced astigmatism, the introduction of popular toric IOLs and the added value of spectacle independence has effectively moved the modern day surgeon towards a truly refractive cataract surgery.

In this regard, the perfectly round and centered "rhexis" has remained the prize for the cataract surgeon. It is the most delicate and fun of the procedural steps the cataract surgeon gets to perform. Perfect centration increases consistency in the effective lens position, the primary unknowable variable in IOL power calculation, by insuring that the forces in play during the period of capsular contraction act symmetrically with respect to the intraocular lens in three dimensions. Similar considerations apply when considering accommodative IOLs. Achieving more consistent ELP means a narrower standard deviation around emmetropia [16].

The Femtosecond Future in Lens Surgery

The development of technology for femtosecond (FS) phaco has centered around several industry leaders: LenSx Lasers Inc. (Aliso Viejo, CA; acquired by Alcon Surgical, Ft. Worth, TX), LensAR Inc. (Winter Park, FL), OptiMedica Corp. (Santa Ana, CA), Bausch & Lomb (San Dimas, CA) and Abbott Medical Optics (Santa Ana, CA) [17]. In the winter of 2009/2010, the LenSx technology was highlighted in the first peer-reviewed publication [18] as well as the first US FS laser refractive cataract procedure [19]. The promise of this technology is increased accuracy and safety, beginning with greater reproducibility in the construction of the corneal incisions required to take out a cataract (or a clear lens). The image-guided FS laser aims to correct preexisting and surgically induced astigmatism, precisely opening the anterior capsule and safely disassembling the lens in preparation for aspiration. The future result of this single, rapid application of FS laser energy is an eye fully prepared to disgorge its presbyopic or cataractous crystalline lens and receive a next-generation accommodative intraocular lens or futuristic flexible, injectable polymeric lens replacement.

The clear corneal incision, despite its inherent simplicity, has proven a challenge for cataract surgeons. Doubts about self-sealability [20] and unforgiving construction techniques [21] have led some to return to the cumbersome scleral tunnel [22]. These concerns have sometimes become magnified when consideration is given, for example, to the larger-than-usual incision required for implantation of a dual optic accommodative IOL [23]. However, the FS laser should facilitate predictable construction of custom-designed clear corneal incisions featuring some version of a metaphoric tongue-and-groove design for enhanced sealability. FS technology has already delivered this concept in corneal transplantation surgery [24].

Limbal relaxing incisions for the correction of keratometric astigmatism have been met with a mixed response from the surgical community [25] and a relatively high rate of requisite postoperative excimer laser enhancement [26]. This is due, in part, to common errors in measurement of surgically induced astigmatism and unavoidable inconsistencies in construction technique. The FS guided laser offers the possibility of automated construction of topographically matched incisions and intraoperative enhancements such as we now have only with stand-alone intraoperative aberrometry [27].

The capsulorhexis, an innovation critical to the development of phacoemulsification [28], remains a high hurdle for surgical trainees [29] and accomplished surgeons [30] alike. The FS laser delivers consistent and clean precision construction of a centered, round, custom-designed capsulorhexis in any size of the surgeon's choice. In premium IOL implantation, any error in capsulorhexis construction may mean a significant reduction in patient satisfaction or even elimination of the patient's lens of choice as an option for implantation. Hence, providing consistent capsulorhexis construction reduces the hurdle to adoption of presbyopia-correcting IOLs.

Finally, division and preparation of the lens for emulsification and aspiration is rendered safe and simple by the FS laser. Microphotolysis of lens material effectively eliminates the need for specific mechanical chopping or sculpting techniques, and allows safe aspiration of the contents of the capsular bag.

Cataract surgeons are compelled by their inward drive towards perfection to love the possibilities that FS laser phaco creates. This technology changes everything. The pioneers of phaco, and the surgical techniques they developed that are still in use today, are coming to appear as the devices of medieval artisans relative to the streamlined accuracy of a nascent industrial era. The "craftsman" approach to cataract surgery is ending; the automated, mechanized future is here. Laser precision and improved outcomes will trump the old school manual achievements of our predecessors. Truly, now more than ever, we stand on the shoulders of giants [31].

Conclusion

In the years since Charles Kelman's inspiration in the dentist's chair (while having his teeth ultrasonically cleaned), advances in technology have produced ever-increasing benefits for patients with cataract. The modern procedure simply was not possible even a few years ago, and until the recent era, prolonged hospital stays were common after cataract surgery. The competitive and innovative business environment in concert with the wellspring of surgeons' ingenuity continues to demonstrate synergistic activity in the improvement of surgical technique and technology. Future advances in cataract surgery will continue to benefit our patients as we develop new techniques and technology.

Key Points

1. Cataract surgery has developed from ancient and relatively crude methods to an astonishingly sophisticated and highly technical procedure that offers rapid visual rehabilitations with extraordinarily high levels of safety and effectiveness.
2. Major advances in cataract surgery include the concept of lens extraction, the development of the intraocular lens and phacoemulsification.
3. We stand now on the threshold of a new era of image-guided, highly automated, precision laser cataract surgery. The FS laser represents a disruptive technology with the potential to revolutionize both patient care and surgical practice.

References

1. Fine IH, Packer M, Hoffman RS. Power modulations in new phacoemulsification technology: improved outcomes. J Cataract Refract Surg. 2004;30(5):1014–9.
2. Apple D. Sir Harold Ridley and his fight for sight: he changed the world so that we may better see it. Thorofare, NJ: SLACK Incorporated; 2006.
3. Koelbing HM. Boldness and caution: Jacques Daviel's approach to cataract extraction (1745–1752). Klin Monatsbl Augenheilkd. 1985;186(3):235–8.
4. Packer M, Fine IH, Hoffman RS. Bimanual ultrasound phacoemulsification. In: Fine IH, Packer M, Hoffman RS, editors. Refractive lens surgery. Heidelberg: Springer; 2005. p. 193–8.
5. Zacharias J, Zacharias S. Volume-based characterization of postocclusion surge. J Cataract Refract Surg. 2005;31(10):1976–82.
6. Jaffe NS, Clayman HM, Hirschman H, et al. Pseudophakos. St. Louis, MO: CV Mosby Co.; 1978.
7. Alpar JJ, Fechner PU. Fechner's intraocular lenses. New York, NY: Thieme-Stratton; 1986.
8. Gorin G. History of ophthalmology. Wilmington, DE: Publish or Perish Inc.; 1982.
9. Ridley H. Intraocular acrylic lenses. Trans Ophthalmol Soc UK. 1951;71:617–21.
10. Ridley H. Intraocular acrylic lenses; 10 years' development. Br J Ophthalmol. 1960;44:705–12.
11. Ridley H. Safety requirements for acrylic implants. Br J Ophthalmol. 1957;41:359–67.
12. Banko A, Kelman CD, inventors; Cavitron Corporation assignee. US patent 3,589,363. 25 July 1967.
13. Guttman C, et al. Microbursts of ultrasound increase safety, efficiency. Ophthalmol Times 2003:62–64.
14. Osher RH. Paired transverse relaxing keratotomy: a combined technique for reducing astigmatism. J Cataract Refract Surg. 1989;15(1):32–7.
15. Packer M. Effect of intraoperative aberrometry on the rate of postoperative enhancement: retrospective study. J Cataract Refract Surg. 2010;36(5):747–55.
16. Cekiç O, Batman C. The relationship between capsulorhexis size and anterior chamber depth relation. Ophthalmic Surg Lasers. 1999;30(3):185–90.
17. Slade S. Femtosecond laser cataract surgery. 2011. http://bmctoday.net/crstoday/2009/09/article.asp?f=CRST0909_13.php. Accessed 15 Nov 2011.
18. Nagy Z, Takacs A, Filkorn T, Sarayba M. Initial clinical evaluation of an intraocular femtosecond laser in cataract surgery. J Refract Surg. 2009;25(12):1053–60. doi:10.3928/1081597X-20091117-04.
19. First femtosecond cataract surgeries performed on US patients. 2011. http://www.osnsupersite.com/view.aspx?rid=61811 (Posted on the OSN SuperSite 11 March 2010). Accessed 14 Nov 2011.
20. Vasavada AR, Praveen MR, Pandita D, Gajjar DU, Vasavada VA, Raj SM, Johar K. Effect of stromal hydration of clear corneal incisions: quantifying ingress of trypan blue into the anterior chamber after phacoemulsification. J Cataract Refract Surg. 2007;33(4):623–7.
21. Fine IH. Clear corneal cataract incisions require attention to detail. In: Packer M, Hoffman RS, editors. Cataract Corner. Ophthalmol Times 2003;28(2):12–13.
22. Cooper BA, Holekamp NM, Bohigian G, Thompson PA. Case–control study of endophthalmitis after cataract surgery comparing scleral tunnel and clear corneal wounds. Am J Ophthalmol. 2003;136(2):300–5.
23. Ossma IL, Galvis A, Vargas LG, Trager MJ, Vagefi MR, McLeod SD. Synchrony dual-optic accommodating

intraocular lens. Part 2: Pilot clinical evaluation. J Cataract Refract Surg. 2007;33(1):47–52.
24. Kook D, Derhartunian V, Bug R, Kohnen T. Top-hat shaped corneal trephination for penetrating keratoplasty using the femtosecond laser: a histomorphological study. Cornea. 2009;28(7):795–800.
25. Hill W. Calculating the AcrySof Toric IOL's Power. 2011. http://bmctoday.net/crstoday/pdfs/CRST0506_12.pdf (Cataract & Refractive Surgery Today May 2006). Accessed 15 Nov 2011.
26. Muftuoglu O, Dao L, Cavanagh HD, McCulley JP, Bowman RW. Limbal relaxing incisions at the time of apodized diffractive multifocal intraocular lens implantation to reduce astigmatism with or without subsequent laser in situ keratomileusis. J Cataract Refract Surg. 2010;36(3):456–64.
27. Effect of intraoperative aberrometry on the rate of postoperative enhancement: retrospective study. Packer M. J Cataract Refract Surg, 2010 May;36(5):747–55.
28. Gimbel HV, Neuhann T. Development, advantages, and methods of the continuous circular capsulorhexis technique. J Cataract Refract Surg. 1990; 16(1):31–7.
29. Dooley IJ, O'Brien PD. Subjective difficulty of each stage of phacoemulsification cataract surgery performed by basic surgical trainees. J Cataract Refract Surg. 2006;32(4):604–8.
30. McLeod SD. Optical principles, biomechanics, and initial clinical performance of a dual-optic accommodating intraocular lens (an American Ophthalmological Society thesis). Trans Am Ophthalmol Soc. 2006; 104:437–52.
31. http://en.wikipedia.org/wiki/Standing_on_the_shoulders_of_giants. Accessed 14 Nov 2011.

Current Outcomes with Cataract Surgery: Can We Do Better?

2

David F. Chang

As modern small incision cataract surgery is one of the most successful operations in all of medicine, how much we can hope to further improve results? Adopting a more expensive and time-consuming way to perform the procedure cannot be justified without providing significant benefits to the patient. To contemplate the question of where a new technology might add value, this chapter assesses our current outcomes of cataract surgery from two vantage points—safety and refractive outcomes.

Potential for Improving Safety

Femtosecond (FS) laser cataract technology automates several delicate and critical steps of the cataract procedure. These include the primary and side-port corneal incisions, astigmatic keratotomy, the continuous circular capsulotomy, and nuclear fragmentation and softening. When compared to manual performance of these same functions, we would expect that a FS laser should offer greater precision and reproducibility. As only a handful of peer-reviewed outcome studies are available at this time (Summer, 2011), we are left to ponder what the laser technology's potential impact on safety and complications will be?

D.F. Chang, M.D. (✉)
762 Altos Oaks Drive, Suite 1,
Los Altos, CA, 94024, USA
e-mail: dceye@earthlink.net

Clear Corneal Incisions

A more precise and reproducible incision would improve wound integrity. The possible correlation of an increasing postsurgical endophthalmitis rate since 1992 with increasing utilization of clear corneal incisions was highlighted by Taban and coauthors in 2005 [1]. This observation raised the controversial question of whether clear corneal incisions increased the endophthalmitis risk relative to scleral pocket incisions, because of a higher incidence of subclinical wound leak. Lacking any randomized prospective comparative trials, retrospective studies have provided the only data addressing this question [2, 3]. One compelling study was Wallin and coauthors' 2005 cohort study of 27 consecutive cases of endophthalmitis occurring at a single institution (Utah) [4]. They determined that several factors significantly increased the statistical risk of endophthalmitis at their institution. Failure to use any antibiotic on the same day as surgery increased the endophthalmitis risk five-fold, while zonular or posterior capsular rupture increased the endophthalmitis risk 17-fold. However, the single most dangerous factor was an incision leak, which led to a 44-fold increase in endophthalmitis.

Based on the available evidence, many would agree that clear corneal incisions are less forgiving than scleral pocket incisions with respect to poor wound construction both during and after surgery, and that the risk rises with increasingly wider incisions [5]. Along with astigmatism

R.R. Krueger et al. (eds.), *Textbook of Refractive Laser Assisted Cataract Surgery (ReLACS)*,
DOI 10.1007/978-1-4614-1010-2_2, © Springer Science+Business Media, LLC 2013

Table 2.1 Incidence of anterior capsule tears [11–14]

Study	Date	AC tear (%)	*N*
Muhtaseb	2004	2.8	1,000
Marques	2006	0.8	2,646
Unal	2006	5.0	296
Olali	2007	5.6	358

control, improved incision integrity is one advantage cited by proponents of micro-incisional cataract surgery. Regardless of size, precise and proper wound construction is certainly important for optimizing wound integrity. Newer accommodating IOL technologies will challenge us with the requirement for larger cataract incisions [6]. Sutures and tissue adhesives will allow us to safely increase the size of our clear corneal incisions, and the FS laser may prove to be advantageous in this regard as well.

Continuous Curvilinear Capsulotomy

Long acknowledged by many as the single most important step of our phaco procedure, the capsulorhexis offers many benefits. By allowing us to trap and encapsulate the optic and both haptics, IOL centration is virtually assured [7, 8]. An overlapping capsulorhexis enables the capsular bag to envelope the optic with a shrink wrap effect, by which a sharp posterior optic edge will kink the posterior capsule [9, 10]. This mechanical lens epithelial cell barrier reduces the incidence of secondary membrane formation. One of the most important benefits of a capsulorhexis, however, is that of safety. Like an elastic waistband, the capsulorhexis can stretch without tearing during the multitude of maneuvers to which the capsular bag is subjected during cataract surgery. In contrast, a single radial tear significantly increases the risk of wraparound extension into the posterior capsule [11].

Table 2.1 shows data on the incidence of anterior capsule tears reported from four contemporary studies [11–14]. The lowest published rate of anterior capsular tears comes from Bob Osher's personal series of more than 2,600 consecutive eyes, which was 0.8% [11]. The incidence of tears occurring during the capsulorhexis step was 0.5%. Of note was the fact that 48% of his anterior capsular tears eventually extended into the posterior capsule and 19% of cases with a torn capsulorhexis required an anterior vitrectomy. This study suggests that the rate of anterior capsular tear is reasonably low in the hands of an expert surgeon, but that if it occurs, the risk of significant complications is very high in even the most experienced hands.

At the other end of the spectrum is the resident experience reported by Unal and coauthors [13]. The capsulorhexis is consistently cited by residents as one of the most difficult steps to master [15]. The rate of torn capsulorhexis in the Unal series was 5% and of irregular capsulorhexis was 9%. The overall rate of posterior capsule rupture and vitreous loss was 6.4% [13].

Table 2.2 Published vitreous loss rates—1999–2009 (0.2–4.4%) [16–28]

Author	Published	% Vitreous loss	Study size
Desai	1999	4.4	18,454
Martin	2000	1.3	3,000
Lundstrom	2001	2.2	2,731
Ionides	2001	2.9	1,420
Gimbel	2001	0.2	18,470
Tan	2002	3.6	2,538
Chan	2003	1.1	8,230
Androudi	2004	4.0	543
Hyams	2005	2.0	1,364
Ang	2006	1.1	2,727
Zaidi	2007	1.1	1,000
Mearza	2009	2.7	1,614
Agrawal	2009	1.6	6,564

Posterior Capsule Rupture and Vitreous Loss

Table 2.2 and Fig. 2.1 list 13 studies of vitreous loss rates in non-resident series published during the decade between 1999 and 2009 [16–28]. Excluding Howard Gimbel's exceptionally low rate of 0.2% [20], the vitreous loss rates

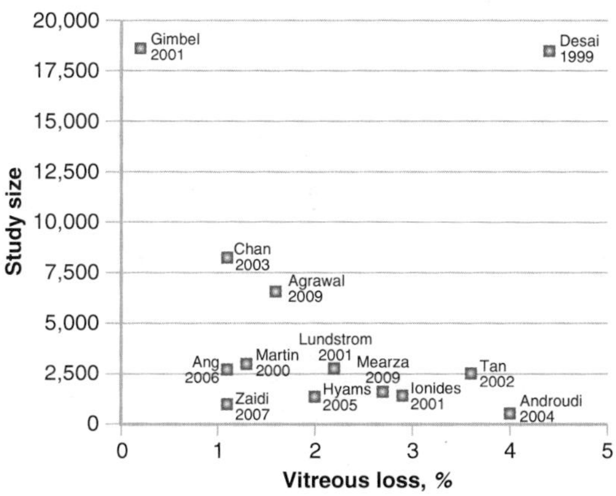

Fig. 2.1 Studies of vitreous loss rates in non-resident series published during the decade between 1999 and 2009 [16–28]

Table 2.3 Published vitreous loss rates residents—2002–2010 (1.3–6.1%) [15, 29–35]

Author	Published	% Vitreous loss	Study size
Blomquist	2002	4.5	1,400
Dooley	2006	4	100
Bhagat	2007	5.4	755
Pot	2008	1.3	982
Rutar	2009	3.1	320
Lee	2009	4.9	226
Carricondo	2010	6.1	261
Blomquist	2010	3.2	1,833

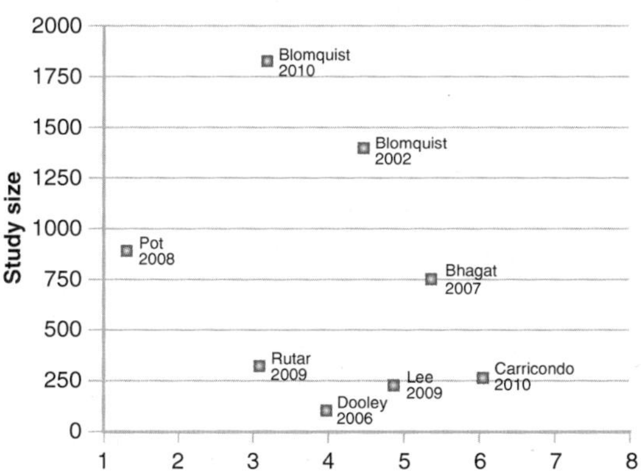

Fig. 2.2 Studies of vitreous loss rates among residency programs that were published from 2002 to 2010 [15, 29–35]

consistently range from 1 to 4%. Table 2.3 and Fig. 2.2 list eight studies of vitreous loss rates among residency programs that were published from 2002 to 2010 [15, 29–35]. With the exception of one study, these rates consistently ranged from 3 to 6%. The best current published data on vitreous loss rates come from two recent studies of large patient populations. Narendran and coauthors' 2009 report on the Cataract National Dataset audit of 55,567 operations from the United Kingdom (UK) reported a 1.9% rate of vitreous loss [36]. Greenberg and coauthors' 2010 published study of cataract surgery in 45,082 US Veterans Administration Hospital cataract surgeries had a vitreous loss rate of 3.5% [37].

Ultrasound Power/Endothelial Cell Loss

A number of studies have shown a reduction in ultrasound energy when employing a phaco chop method compared to divide and conquer [38–41]. The correlation of phaco chop with reduced endothelial cell loss is less consistent in the literature [39, 42, 43]. Part of the variability of the results from these studies undoubtedly relates to the varying density of the nuclei encountered. For example, Park and coauthors compared phaco chop to stop-and-chop in a bilateral eye study involving 51 patients [44]. There was no statistical difference in mean effective phaco time (EPT) for moderately dense nuclei; however, with dense nuclei, there was a statistically significant reduction in mean EPT with chopping ($P<0.01$). The specific comparison of stop and chop to pre-chopping may be more relevant in assessing the FS laser's potential benefit. Pereira and coauthors found that pre-chopping significantly reduced effective phaco time and phaco power in a small prospective trial of 50 eyes [45].

Despite these reported advantages to chopping, the 2010 Leaming survey of ASCRS members reported that only 32% of respondents were performing phaco chop, compared to 62% who were performing divide-and-conquer. The fact

Table 2.4 Hitting emmetropia [54–59]

Author	N	Biometry	% Within 0.50 D	% Within 1.00 D
Landers (2009)	55	IOLMaster	75	93
		Immersion U/S	49	85
Kim (2009)	30	Contact U/S	70	93
Lim (2009)	100	Contact U/S	45	83
Gale (2009)	–	IOLMaster	–	80–87
Eleftheriadis (2003)	100	IOLMaster	–	96
Murphy (2002)	1,676	Contact U/S	45	72
Mean			57	87

that the phaco chop technique is generally more difficult to learn may be an important factor underlying these statistics. Reducing ultrasound time by pre-chopping and softening the nucleus is an important potential benefit of FS laser cataract surgery. The denser the nucleus, the greater the ultrasound reduction should be, and the more likely a clinically significant difference in endothelial cell loss would be found.

Potential for Improving Refractive Outcomes

Spherical Equivalent Accuracy

Many factors must be successfully managed to achieve pseudophakic emmetropia. A major advance has been in the more accurate determination of axial length with non-contact, partial coherence interferometry [47–49]. Two variable IOL power calculation formulae have been successfully used for decades [50–52]. More advanced formulae, such as those developed by Haigis and Holladay, incorporate additional variables in an effort to better predict the effective lens position [53]. Table 2.4 summarizes six published studies that analyze refractive accuracy [49, 54–58]. Some of these series employed contact A-scan biometry, while others employed partial coherence interferometry. Even in the study with the best results, 25% of eyes fail to refract to within 0.5 D of the intended spherical equivalent target postoperatively.

The one important variable that cannot be measured in advance is the final axial resting position of the IOL optic—the so called, effective lens position (ELP). Calculating a surgeon's personalized A-constant is an effort to optimize the ELP prediction based on variables in individual surgical techniques. In addition to capsular bag fixation of the IOL, the primary surgical variable that affects ELP is the diameter and shape of the capsulorhexis [59–61]. The generally accepted surgical objective is a round capsulorhexis that overlaps the optic edge for all 360° of its circumference. This means that as the capsular bag shrinks and contracts postoperatively, the capsular forces are uniformly and symmetrically balanced in all three dimensions. A larger diameter capsulorhexis that is all or partially "off" the optic edge should permit the optic to move slightly anterior to the position of one constrained by a completely overlapping anterior capsular rim.

Accommodating IOL designs may impose additional requirements for capsulorhexis diameter and shape. The ELP of a hinged optic, such as with the Crystalens, would be expected to vary with the capsulorhexis diameter. If one assumes a preferred diameter of 5.0 mm, a smaller diameter capsulorhexis will contract more and may displace the optic more posteriorly. In contrast, a larger diameter capsulorhexis should allow the optic to shift more anteriorly. Studies will be needed to determine whether a FS laser capsulotomy is able to improve refractive outcomes on the basis of greater ELP predictability. Finally, there is one special complication that is unique to premium refractive IOLs—that of a patient receiving a well-positioned monofocal IOL, but not the toric, multifocal, or accommodating IOL that they strongly preferred. For example, with the synchrony dual optic accommodating IOL, the

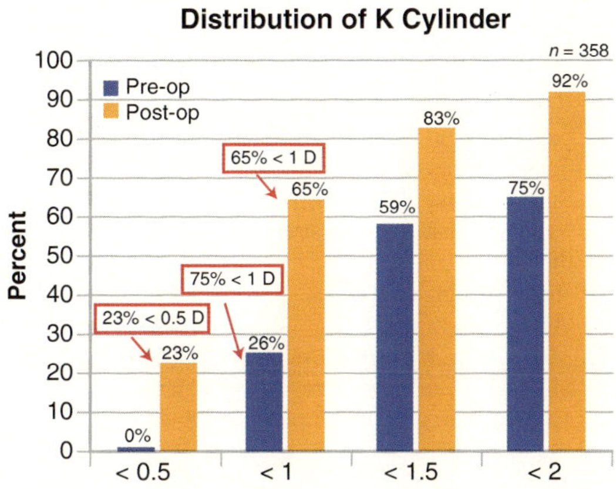

Fig. 2.3 Gills LRI data. $n=358$, Mean pre-op cyl 1.59 D (mild-moderate astigmatism) [68]

anterior optic shifts forward with accommodative effort [6]. If the capsulorhexis does not completely overlap the anterior optic edge, the 5.0 mm diameter anterior optic may partially dislocate out of the bag and into the ciliary sulcus. A capsulorhexis that is too large or eccentric in shape is therefore a contraindication to implanting the synchrony accommodating IOL. A torn capsulorhexis is also a contraindication to using the Crystalens, in my opinion, because of the significant potential for subluxation. A radial capsulorhexis tear also increases the potential for single and three-piece IOL decentration, and may be problematic for a multifocal or toric IOL where proper optical alignment is more critical. Although they might attain excellent corrected visual acuity with an intracapsular monofocal IOL, these aforementioned patients are often emotionally distraught at having permanently lost the opportunity to receive the premium refractive IOL that they had selected preoperatively.

Astigmatism Management

The number of cataract surgical patients with preoperative corneal astigmatism has been determined from several studies. A published study of more than 23,000 eyes found that 8% of patients had at least 2.0 D of corneal astigmatism preoperatively [62]. The percent of eyes with at least 1.0 and 0.5 D of preoperative corneal astigmatism were 36 and 74% respectively. This correlated well with a study of more than 4,500 eyes in which 35% of eyes had at least 1.0 D, and 22% had at least 1.5 D of preoperative corneal astigmatism [63].

Incisional astigmatic keratotomy (AK) is a popular method of simultaneously reducing preoperative corneal astigmatism at the time of cataract surgery [64]. There is a relative dearth of published studies on the efficacy of this method in conjunction with phaco. Carvalho and coauthors found a statistically significant reduction in mean topographic astigmatism from 1.93 ± 0.58 D preoperatively to 1.02 ± 0.60 D postoperatively using limbal relaxing incisions in 25 eyes [65]. Mingo-Botín and coauthors compared toric IOLs to incisional astigmatic keratotomy in 40 eyes undergoing cataract surgery who were randomized to either technique of astigmatism reduction [66]. The mean reduction in keratometric astigmatism was 0.58 D (30% of the preoperative corneal astigmatism) in the 20 eyes receiving AK, and there was with a statistically significant reduction in mean pre-op refractive astigmatism (pre-op -2.17 ± 1.02; post-op -1.32 ± 0.60; $p=0.001$). However, the residual refractive astigmatism was ≤ 1.0 D in only 8/20 eyes (40%) receiving AK, compared to 18/20 eyes (90%) receiving a toric IOL. Poll and coauthors achieved a mean 0.46 D of postoperative astigmatism with astigmatic keratotomy in 115 eyes undergoing cataract surgery, which was comparable to toric IOL results in their series [67].

The largest reported series of eyes undergoing astigmatic keratotomy combined with phaco is from Gills, and is shown in Fig. 2.3 [68]. He analyzed 358 eyes with mild to moderate preoperative astigmatism, of which 74% had more than 1.0 D of astigmatism. The mean preoperative astigmatism of 1.59 D was reduced to a mean of 0.99 D postoperatively. Sixty-five percent of these treated eyes had <1 D of keratometric cylinder postoperatively and only 23% had <0.5 D of astigmatism postoperatively.

In the 2010 Leaming survey, 67% of respondents most often use a toric IOL and 18% of respondents most often use astigmatic keratotomy to treat pre-existing astigmatism in their cataract patients [46]. Astigmatic keratotomy will always be plagued by an unavoidable variable—that of the individual tissue response to the corneal relaxing incision. Nevertheless, it stands to reason that AK results will be more accurate if the depth, curvature, length, diameter and axial orientation of the incisions (upon which the nomograms are developed and based) are made as reproducibly consistent as possible. It will be of great interest to see if FS laser astigmatic keratotomy will fulfill this potential.

Key Points

1. The most recent published cataract surgical studies estimate the rate of vitreous loss to be 2–4%.
2. Thirty-five percent of cataract patients have at least 1 D of corneal astigmatism.

References

1. Taban M, Behrens A, Newcomb RL, et al. Acute endophthalmitis following cataract surgery: a systematic review of the literature. Arch Ophthalmol. 2005; 123:613–20.
2. Cooper BA, Holekamp NM, Bohigian G, Thompson PA. Case–control study of endophthalmitis after cataract surgery comparing scleral tunnel and clear corneal wounds. Am J Ophthalmol. 2003; 136: 300–5.
3. Lertsumitkul S, Myers PC, O'Rourke MT, Chandra J. Endophthalmitis in the western Sydney region: a case–control study. Clin Exp Ophthalmol. 2001;29: 400–5.
4. Wallin T, Parker J, Jin Y, et al. Cohort study of 27 cases of endophthalmitis at a single institution. J Cataract Refract Surg. 2005;31:735–41.
5. Nichamin LD, Chang DF, Johnson SH, et al. American Society of Cataract and Refractive Surgery Cataract Clinical Committee. ASCRS White Paper: what is the association between clear corneal cataract incisions and postoperative endophthalmitis? J Cataract Refract Surg. 2006;32:1556–9.
6. Bohórquez V, Alarcon R. Long-term reading performance in patients with bilateral dual-optic accommodating intraocular lenses. J Cataract Refract Surg. 2010;36:1880–6.
7. Colvard DM, Dunn SA. Intraocular lens centration with continuous tear capsulotomy. J Cataract Refract Surg. 1990;16:312–4.
8. Ram J, Apple DJ, Peng Q, et al. Update on fixation of rigid and foldable posterior chamber intraocular lenses. Part I: Elimination of fixation-induced decentration to achieve precise optical correction and visual rehabilitation. Ophthalmology. 1999;106: 883–90.
9. Ram J, Pandey SK, Apple DJ, et al. Effect of in-the-bag intraocular lens fixation on the prevention of posterior capsule opacification. J Cataract Refract Surg. 2001;27:367–70.
10. Nishi O, Nishi K, Wickstrom K. Preventing lens epithelial cell migration using intraocular lenses with sharp rectangular edges. J Cataract Refract Surg. 2000;26:1543–9.
11. Marques FF, Marques DM, Osher RH, Osher JM. Fate of anterior capsule tears during cataract surgery. J Cataract Refract Surg. 2006;32:1638–42.
12. Muhtaseb M, Kalhoro A, Ionides A. A system for preoperative stratification of cataract patients according to risk of intraoperative complications. Br J Ophthalmol. 2004;88:1242–6.
13. Unal M, Yücel I, Sarici A, et al. Phacoemulsification with topical anesthesia: resident experience. J Cataract Refract Surg. 2006;32:1361–5.
14. Olali CA, Ahmed S, Gupta M. Surgical outcome following breach rhexis. Eur J Ophthalmol. 2007;17:565–70.
15. Dooley IJ, O'Brien PD. Subjective difficulty of each stage of phacoemulsification cataract surgery performed by basic surgical trainees. J Cataract Refract Surg. 2006;32(4):604–8.
16. Desai P, Minassian DC, Reidy A. National cataract surgery survey1997–98: a report of the results of the clinical outcomes. Br J Ophthalmol. 1999;83:1336–40.
17. Martin KR, Burton RL. The phacoemulsification learning curve: per-operative complications in the first 3000 cases of an experienced surgeon. Eye. 2000;14 (Pt 2):190–5.
18. Lundstrom M, Barry P, Leite E, et al. 1998 European Cataract Outcome Study: report from the European Cataract Outcome Study Group. J Cataract Refract Surg. 2001;27:1176–84.
19. Ionides A, Minassian D, Tuft S. Visual outcome following posterior capsule rupture during cataract surgery. Br J Ophthalmol. 2001;85:222–4.
20. Gimbel HV, Sun R, Ferensowicz M, et al. Intraoperative management of posterior capsule tears in phacoemulsification and intraocular lens implantation. Ophthalmology. 2001;108:2186–9 [discussion 2190–2].
21. Tan JHY, Karwatowski WSS. Phacoemulsification cataract surgery and unplanned anterior vitrectomy: is it bad news? Eye. 2002;16:117–20.
22. Chan FM, Mathur R, Ku JJK, et al. Short-term outcomes in eyes with posterior capsule rupture during cataract surgery. J Cataract Refract Surg. 2003;29:537–41.
23. Androudi S, Brazitikos PD, Papadopoulos NT, et al. Posterior capsule rupture and vitreous loss during phacoemulsification with or without the use of an anterior chamber maintainer. J Cataract Refract Surg. 2004;30:449–52.
24. Hyams M, Mathalone N, Herskovitz M, et al. Intraoperative complications of phacoemulsification in eyes with and without pseudoexfoliation. J Cataract Refract Surg. 2005;31:1002–5.

25. Ang GS, Whyte IF. Effect and outcomes of posterior capsule rupture in a district general hospital setting. J Cataract Refract Surg. 2006;32:623–7.
26. Zaidi FH, Corbett M, Burton BJL, Bloom PA. Raising the benchmark for the 21st century—the 1000 cataract operations audit and survey: outcomes, consultant-supervised training and sourcing NHS choice. Br J Ophthalmol. 2007;91:731–6.
27. Mearza AA, Ramanathan S, Bidgood P, Horgan S. Visual outcome in cataract surgery complicated by vitreous loss in a district general hospital. Int Ophthalmol. 2009;29:157–60.
28. Agrawal V, Upadhyay J, Indian Cataract Risk Stratification Study Group. Validation of scoring system for preoperative stratification of intra-operative risks of complications during cataract surgery: Indian multicentric study. Indian J Ophthalmol. 2009;57: 213–5.
29. Blomquist PH, Rugwani RM. Visual outcomes after vitreous loss during cataract surgery performed by residents. J Cataract Refract Surg. 2002;28:847–52.
30. Bhagat N, Nissirios N, Potdevin L, Chung J, Lama P, Zarbin MA, Fechtner R, Guo S, Chu D, Langer P. Complications in resident performed phacoemulsification cataract surgery at New Jersey Medical School. Br J Ophthalmol. 2007;91:1315–7.
31. Pot MC, Stilma JS. Low complication rate with cataract operations carried out by registrars in ophthalmology. Ned Tijdschr Geneeskd. 2008;8(152):563–8.
32. Rutar T, Porco TC, Naseri A. Risk factors for intraoperative complications in resident-performed phacoemul-sification surgery. Ophthalmology. 2009; 116:431–6.
33. Lee J-S, Hou C-H, Yang M-L, Kuo JZ-C, Lin K-K. A different approach to assess resident phacoemulsification learning curve: analysis of both completion and complication rates. Eye. 2009;23:683–7.
34. Carricondo PC, Fortes AC, Mourao Pde C, Hajnal M, Jose NK. Senior resident phacoemulsification learning curve (corrected from cure). Arq Bras Oftalmol. 2010;73:66–9.
35. Blomquist PH, Sargent JW, Winslow HH. Validation of Najjar-Awwad cataract surgery risk score for resident phacoemulsification surgery. J Cataract Refract Surg. 2010;36:1753–7.
36. Narendran N, Jaycock P, Johnston RL, et al. The Cataract National Dataset electronic multicentre audit of 55,567 operations: risk stratification for posterior capsule rupture and vitreous loss. Eye (Lond). 2009;23 (1):31–7.
37. Greenberg PB, Tseng VL, Wu WC, et al. Prevalence and predictors of ocular complications associated with cataract surgery in United States Veterans. Ophthalmology 2010 [Epub ahead of print].
38. DeBry P, Olson RJ, Crandall AS. Comparison of energy required for phaco-chop and divide and conquer phacoemulsification. J Cataract Refract Surg. 1998;24:689–92.
39. Pirazzoli G, D'Eliseo D, Ziosi M, Acciarri R. Effects of phacoemulsification time on the corneal endothelium using phacofracture and phaco chop techniques. J Cataract Refract Surg. 1996;22:967–9.
40. Ram J, Wesendahl TA, Auffarth GU, Apple DJ. Evaluation of in situ fracture versus phaco chop techniques. J Cataract Refract Surg. 1998;24:1464–8.
41. Wong T, Hingorani M, Lee V. Phacoemulsification time and power requirements in phaco chop and divide and conquer nucleofractis techniques. J Cataract Refract Surg. 2000;26:1374–8.
42. Vajpayee RB, Kumar A, Dada T, Titiyal JS, Sharma N, Dada VK. Phaco-chop versus stop-and-chop nucleotomy for phacoemulsification. J Cataract Refract Surg. 2000;26(11):1638–41.
43. Storr-Paulsen A, Norregaard JC, Ahmed S, Storr-Paulsen T, Pedersen TH. Endothelial cell damage after cataract surgery: divide-and-conquer versus phaco-chop technique. J Cataract Refract Surg. 2008; 34:996–1000.
44. Park JH, Lee SM, Kwon JW, et al. Ultrasound energy in phacoemulsification: a comparative analysis of phaco-chop and stop-and-chop techniques according to the degree of nuclear density. Ophthalmic Surg Lasers Imaging. 2010;41:236–41.
45. Pereira AC, Porfirio F, Freitas LL, Belfort R. Ultrasound energy and endothelial cell loss with stop-and-chop and nuclear preslice phacoemulsification. J Cataract Refract Surg. 2006;32:1661–6.
46. 2010 Learning Survey. Accessed at http://www.analeyz.com/AnaleyzASCRS2010.htm
47. Haigis W, Lege B, Miller N, Schneider B. Comparison of immersion ultrasound biometry and partial coherence interferometry for intraocular lens calculation according to Haigis. Graefes Arch Clin Exp Ophthalmol. 2000;238:765–73.
48. Packer M, Fine IH, Hoffman RS, et al. Immersion A-scan compared with partial coherence interferometry: outcomes analysis. J Cataract Refract Surg. 2002; 28:239–42.
49. Landers J, Goggin M. Comparison of refractive outcomes using immersion ultrasound biometry and IOLMaster biometry. Clin Exp Ophthalmol. 2009;37: 566–9.
50. Retzlaff JA, Sanders DR, Kraff MC. Development of the SRK/T intraocular lens implant power calculation formula. J Cataract Refract Surg. 1990;16:333–40.
51. Hoffer KJ. The Hoffer Q formula: a comparison of theoretic and regression formulas. J Cataract Refract Surg. 1993;19:700–12 [Erratum: J Cataract Refract Surg 1994;20:677].
52. Olsen T, Corydon L, Gimbel H. Intraocular lens power calculation with an improved anterior chamber depth prediction algorithm. J Cataract Refract Surg. 1995; 21:313–9.
53. Hoffer KJ. Clinical results using the Holladay 2 intraocular lens power formula. J Cataract Refract Surg. 2000;26:1233–7.
54. Kim SW, Kim EK, Cho BJ, et al. Use of the pentacam true net corneal power for intraocular lens calculation in eyes after refractive corneal surgery. J Refract Surg. 2009;25(3):285–9.
55. Lim LH, Lee SY, Ang CL. Factors affecting the predictability of SRK II in patients with normal

axial length undergoing phacoemulsification surgery. Singapore Med J. 2009;50(2):120–5.
56. Gale RP, Saldana M, Johnston RL, et al. Benchmark standards for refractive outcomes after NHS cataract surgery. Eye. 2009;23(1):149–52.
57. Eleftheriadis H. IOLMaster biometry: refractive results of 100 consecutive cases. Br J Ophthalmol. 2003;87(8):960–3.
58. Murphy C, Tufy SJ, Minassian DC. Refractive error and visual outcome after cataract extraction. J Cataract Refract Surg. 2002;28:62–6.
59. Cekic O, Batman C. The relationship between capsulorhexis size and anterior chamber depth relation. Ophthalmic Surg Lasers. 1999;30:185–90.
60. Norby S. Sources of error in intraocular lens power calculation. J Cataract Refract Surg. 2008;34:368–76.
61. Hill WE. Intraocular lens power calculations: are we stuck in the past? Clin Exp Ophthalmol. 2009; 37:761–2.
62. Hoffmann PC, Hutz WW. Analysis of biometry and prevalence data for corneal astigmatism in 23,239 eyes. J Cataract Refract Surg. 2010;36:1479–85.
63. Ferrer-Blasco T, Montés-Micó R, Peixoto-de-Matos SC, González-Méijome JM, Cerviño A. Prevalence of corneal astigmatism before cataract surgery. J Cataract Refract Surg. 2009;35:70–5.
64. Amesbury EC, Miller KM. Correction of astigmatism at the time of cataract surgery. Curr Opin Ophthalmol. 2009;20:19–24.
65. Carvalho MJ, Suzuki SH, Freitas LL, Branco BC, Shor P, Höffling-Lima AL. Limbal relaxing incisions to correct corneal astigmatism during phacoe-mulsification. J Refract Surg. 2007;23:499–504.
66. Mingo-Botín D, Muñoz-Negrete FJ, Won Kim HR, Morcillo-Laiz R, Rebolleda G, Oblanca N. Comparison of toric intraocular lenses and peripheral corneal relaxing incisions to treat astigmatism during cataract surgery. J Cataract Refract Surg. 2010;36: 1700–8.
67. Poll JT, Wang L, Koch DD, Weikert MP. Correction of astigmatism during cataract surgery: toric intraocular lens compared to peripheral corneal relaxing incisions. J Refract Surg. 2011;27:165–71.
68. Gills JP, Wallace RB, Fine IH, et al. Chapter 7: Reducing pre-existing astigmatism with limbal relaxing incisions. In: Henderson BA, Gills JP, editors. A complete surgical guide for correcting astigmatism. 2nd ed. Thorofare, NJ: Slack; 2011.

Femtosecond Laser Fundamentals

3

Holger Lubatschowski, Ronald R. Krueger, and David Smadja

When reading about a new medical technology, such as femtosecond (FS) lasers for eye surgery, the average clinician is stepping into an unfamiliar world of laser physics and engineering terms that can easily overwhelm his understanding. It may be easy enough to conceptualize how a laser can focus into the lens or cornea in order to achieve a therapeutic effect. But what might be less understood is how the laser works, how it differs from other lasers, how its interaction with the cornea or lens is limited, and how it might lead to unexpected clinical complications, when not set at the proper settings or when deviating from its optimal alignment and performance. In order to truly comprehend this technology and be able to navigate through the subtleties of its clinical use and misuse, the ophthalmologist must get a firm hold of basic laser and femtolaser terminology, the engineering capabilities and limitations of operation and the biophysics of interaction with the diverse presentations in both cornea and lens tissue. In this chapter, we have strived to provide a simplified review of the fundamentals of laser engineering and tissue interaction, as well as the specific details with regard to FS laser physics and its unique clinical use in ocular tissue.

H. Lubatschowski, Ph.D. (✉)
Rowiak GmbH, Garbsener Landstr. 10,
Hanover 30419, Germany
e-mail: H.Lubatschowski@Rowiak.de

R.R. Krueger, M.D., M.S.E.
Cole Eye Institute, Department of Refractive Surgery,
Cleveland Clinic Lerner College of Medicine, Cleveland,
OH 44195, USA

D. Smadja, M.D.
Cleveland Clinic, Cole Eye Institute,
9500 Euclid Avenue, Cleveland, OH 44195, USA

Anterior Segment Unit and Refractive Surgery, University
Center Hospital of Bordeaux, Bordeaux, France

Physical Characteristics of Lasers and How They Work

The uniqueness of laser light in contrast to natural light which is emitted from the sun or from a hot wire in a light bulb arises from only two characteristic properties of laser radiation: (1) monochromatism and (2) coherence. Based on these two features, it is possible to generate light fields with unbelievable short duration, extremely tight focusing, and exorbitant irradiances.

Photonic Energy to Electronic Energy: Light Absorption

To understand how laser light is generated, one has to first get an idea how light is generated. The simple Bohr planetary model of the atom (Fig. 3.1) is adequate to explain the mechanism. Here the electrons move on distinct orbits around the nucleus, which have certain energy levels.

Figure 3.2 shows the population of the electrons of a simple two level system. Under

R.R. Krueger et al. (eds.), *Textbook of Refractive Laser Assisted Cataract Surgery (ReLACS)*,
DOI 10.1007/978-1-4614-1010-2_3, © Springer Science+Business Media, LLC 2013

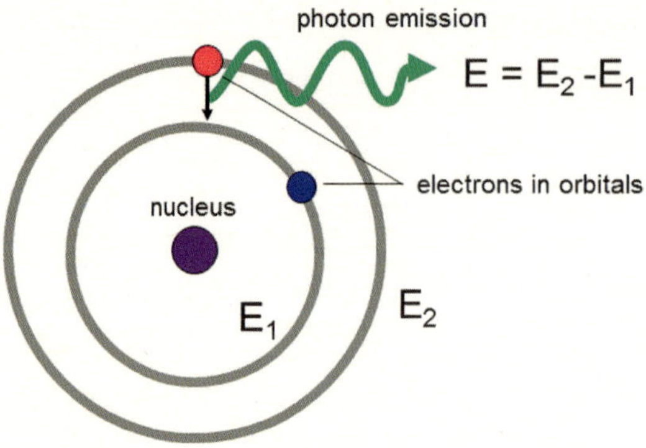

Fig. 3.1 Bohr's planetary model, were the electrons are orbiting around the nucleus. If an electron transfers from von level E_2 to the other level E_1 it emits a photon with energy $E_2 - E_1$

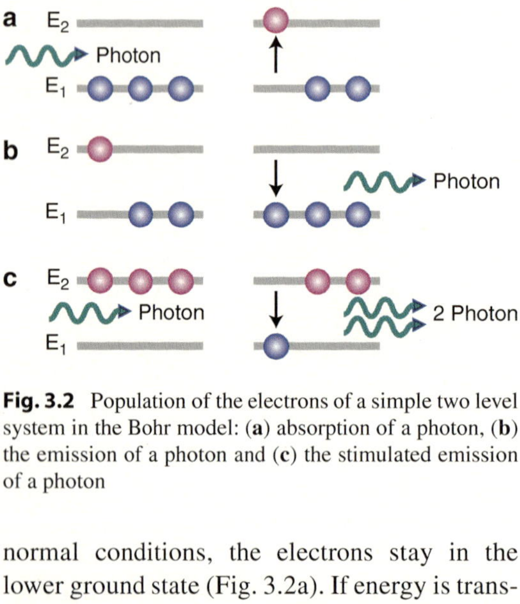

Fig. 3.2 Population of the electrons of a simple two level system in the Bohr model: (**a**) absorption of a photon, (**b**) the emission of a photon and (**c**) the stimulated emission of a photon

normal conditions, the electrons stay in the lower ground state (Fig. 3.2a). If energy is transferred to the atom, the electrons are excited to the upper level. The various ways in which energy can be transferred to the electrons is by (1) the impact of two atoms (heat), (2) the impact of accelerated free electrons (gas discharge), (3) the release of internal energy due to exothermal chemical reactions, or (4) the absorbing an incoming photon. The energy of the photon, which will be absorbed, has to be identical to the energy gap between the upper and lower level of the electron. The frequency ν (or color) of the photon is determined by its energy E. The relationship between energy and frequency of a photon is given by Heisenberg's equation

$$E = h\nu = E_2 - E_1,$$

where h is the so-called Plank constant.

Using $h\nu = c/\lambda$ one can calculate the wavelength λ of the photon as a function of the energy gap:

$$\lambda = \frac{hc}{E_2 - E_1},$$

c is the speed of light.

Electronic Energy to Photonic Energy: Light Emission

In the same way the photon is absorbed by exciting the atom, it can be spontaneously emitted when the electron drops down to the ground state. The emission process is of a statistical nature, which means, the electron relaxes at any time within an average life time, T, and a photon will be emitted in any direction (Fig. 3.2b). The only way to influence this emission process is to send another photon to the atom with an energy corresponding to the energy gap between the ground level and the excited level. In that case, the excited electron will be stimulated to relax down to the ground state and emit an identical photon with the same energy and the same direction (Fig. 3.2c). Moreover, these two photons now have the same phase, which means, the amplitude of the electromagnetic field of both photons, are identical at the same place within the same time. This condition of two or more photons which are in phase is called coherence [1].

Stimulated Emission of Photons

This process of stimulated emission provides the basis for a second important mechanism: the doubling of the number of photons after one stimulated emission. In other words, the process of stimulated emission acts as an amplifier. If a sufficient number of excited atoms exist, an avalanche of coherent photons will be generated.

This process is called *L*ight *A*mplification by *S*timulated *E*mission of *R*adiation (LASER).

However, an important condition to start the amplification process is to have more atoms with their electrons in the excited upper level than in the ground state. This unnatural configuration is called population inversion.

Achieving Population Inversion

Typically, in one atom, the distribution of electrons as a function of energy follows the so-called Bolzmans law of thermodynamic distribution (Fig. 3.3). In this law, the higher the energy level, the lower its population density by electrons. On the other hand, light amplification will take place, only when the upper level has a higher population than the ground state (Fig. 3.2c). This condition, called population inversion, never happens in nature, and this is the reason why no natural light source emits laser radiation. The mechanism which leads to population inversion is called optical pumping. Herein, the energy for excitation can be delivered by the following: (1) an external light source (typical example: Nd:YAG-laser), (2) an electrical excitation due to a gas discharge (typical examples: HeNe-laser, Ar-Ion laser, excimer laser), (3) an electron injection (diode lasers), or (4) a chemical reaction [2].

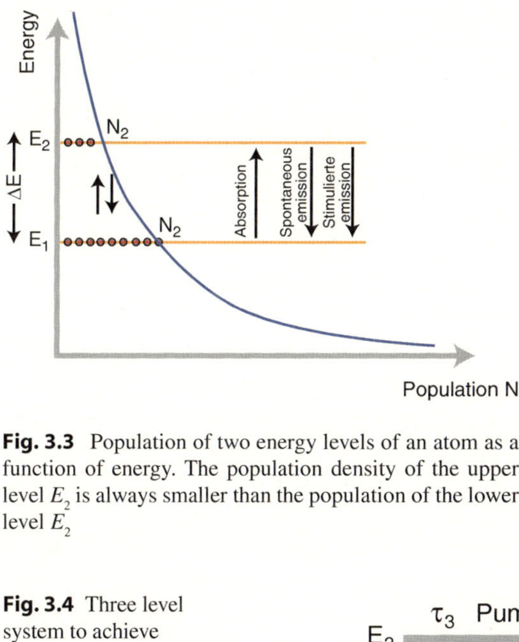

Fig. 3.3 Population of two energy levels of an atom as a function of energy. The population density of the upper level E_2 is always smaller than the population of the lower level E_2

Because the probability of exciting an electron into the upper level (by irradiating light into the active medium) equals the probability of stimulating emission (by forcing an excited electron to the ground state), it is impossible to achieve population inversion on a two level system, regardless of how intense the pumping light happens to be. At the most, an equal population of both levels will exist.

The easiest way to achieve population inversion by optical pumping is to introduce a third energy level (Fig. 3.4). Let us assume we have a ground state, E_1, and an upper pumping level, E_3, where the electrons are excited by absorbing the pumped light. After the natural life time of the upper level, T_3 goes by, the electrons decay into the ground state or they make a transition into the third state which has a little lower energy E_2. If the life time T_2 of this intermediate level E_2 is larger than the life time of the upper level E_3, the electrons which are pumped into E_3 will accumulate in level E_2. Because the pumped light will not lead to stimulated emission into the intermediate state, we will achieve population inversion in E_2 when more than 50 % of the atoms are excited.

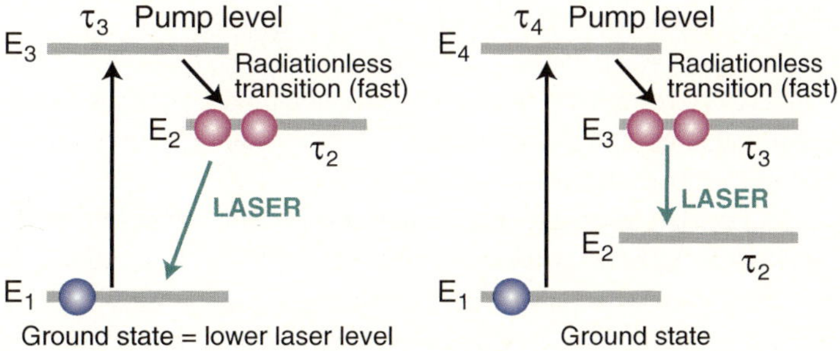

Fig. 3.4 Three level system to achieve population inversion for the laser transition from level E_2 to E_1 (*left*), as well as a four level system, achieving inversion for the laser transition from E_3 to E_2 (*right*)

Fig. 3.5 Schematic drawing of the main components of a laser oscillator

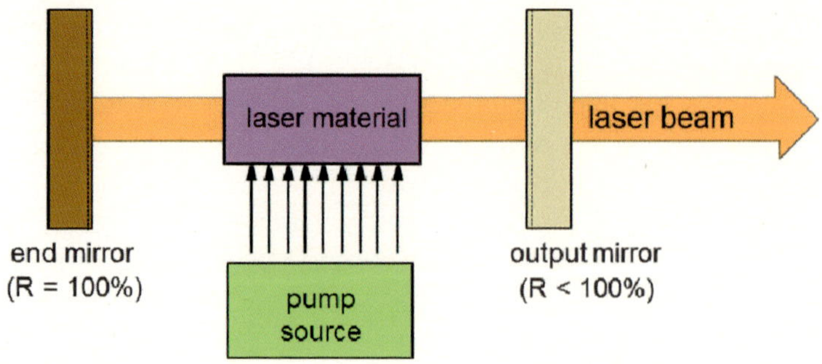

Another, more efficient way to generate population inversion is by introducing a fourth level, which acts as the lower laser level (new E_2). Provided, the life time, T_4 of the upper pumping level (E_4) is much shorter than the life time of the upper laser level (new E_3), and the lower laser level (new E_2) decays quickly into the ground state (new E_1), one can achieve population inversion from the earliest electrons which are excited by the pumped light, and this inversion is independent of the pumping rate. This is the most efficient way to produce laser radiation.

Materials and Modes of Laser Operation

The components, for building a real laser are depicted in Fig. 3.5. We need an active medium, which can be a transparent solid state, a gas, or a liquid. The medium has to be pumped by an external pumping source, which can be, for example, an intense arc lamp or another laser. In order, to direct the stimulated emission process into one direction, we need a feedback mechanism, which is provided by two mirrors, which force the light to oscillate back and forth through the excited laser medium.

Regarding operation time, lasers are divided into continuous wave (cw) and pulsed systems. Continuous wave is usually defined as a period, which lasts longer than 250 ms. The emission time is controlled by and external shutter, or the laser system can be completely turned on and off.

With pulsed laser systems, usually the pumping process, or optical devices inside the oscillator, determines the pulse duration of the laser output. Pulsed lasers are subdivided into so-called free running lasers, q-switched lasers, and mode coupled lasers. In the following section we analyze the different types of pulsed laser systems.

When the laser is pumped by a flash lamp, the laser is running in the so-called, "Free Running-Mode." This means pulse duration is roughly determined by the duration of the pump flash, which is in the range of several hundred microseconds ($1\ \mu s = 10^{-6}$ s) to milliseconds ($1\ ms = 10^{-3}$ s). The characteristic of a free running pulse is its spiking. The emitted pulse consists of many short and intense spikes, each with only a few microseconds duration. This is caused by a nondeterministic interplay of stimulated emission and excitation.

Usually, the duration of a flash lamp pulse cannot be set shorter than a few microseconds. If laser pulse durations in the nanosecond regime ($1\ ns = 10^{-9}$ s) are needed, one has to make use of the so-called "Q-switch" principle [3]. The optical pumping is supported by an optical switch, which reduces the quality (Q) of the resonator. As a consequence, the stimulated emission process is stopped (Fig. 3.6). Only when the optical switch is opened, the highly accumulated inversion will be cleared by a giant laser pulse. The stored pump energy will be released by stimulated emission within several nanoseconds.

Fundamental Components with Femtosecond Lasers

Mode Locking for Femtosecond Lasers

For the generation of picosecond pulses ($1\ ps = 10^{-12}$ s) or even fs pulses ($1\ fs = 10^{-15}$ s), the laser has to be "Mode Locked" [3]. The axial

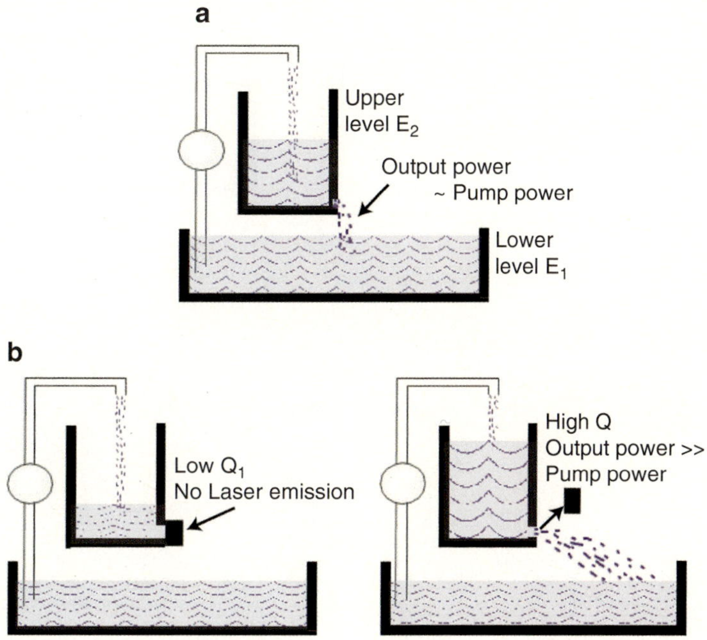

Fig. 3.6 Principle of Q-switching. (**a**) In cw mode the laser output power is proportional to the optical pump power. (**b**) While the quality of the laser resonator is low, the stimulated emission process is stopped and optical pumping leads to high population inversion. Once the upper level is full and the quality of the resonator is high, the accumulated inversion will be cleared by a giant laser pulse within several nanosecond

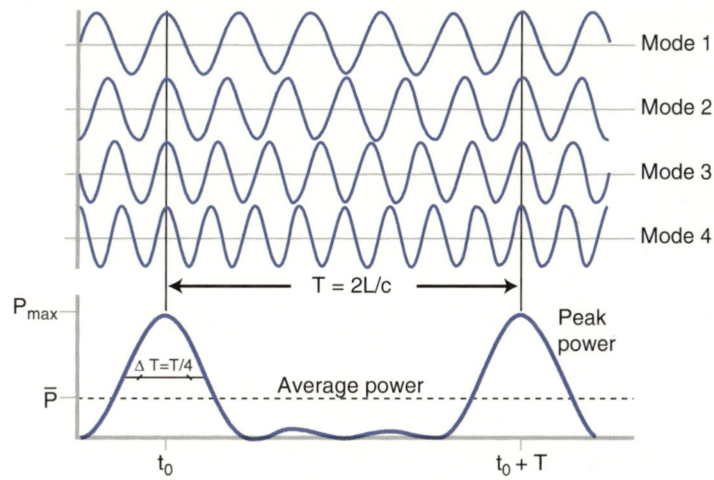

Fig. 3.7 Principle of Mode Locking: Four different modes in a resonator (*top*) and their interference to contribute to either annihilation or higher amplitudes (*bottom*)

laser modes, which are light waves with slightly different frequency or wavelength, have to be synchronized or locked in a fixed phase. When their phases are fixed, they interfere in such a way that their amplitude either adds up or annihilates (Fig. 3.7).

The interference of these modes generates very short, but intense amplitudes. These packages of highly intense waves oscillate inside the resonator and partially leave it at the output mirror (Fig. 3.8).

The duration and the amplitude of these wave packages depend on the number of modes which are generated and locked inside the resonator. The more modes that are locked, the shorter and more intense the pulses are.

The number of modes is limited by the spectral bandwidth of the laser medium. The broader its spectrum (i.e., the broader the laser levels in Fig. 3.4), the more modes can be generated, and the shorter the laser pulse can be. Some laser crystals, for example titanium:sapphire, can

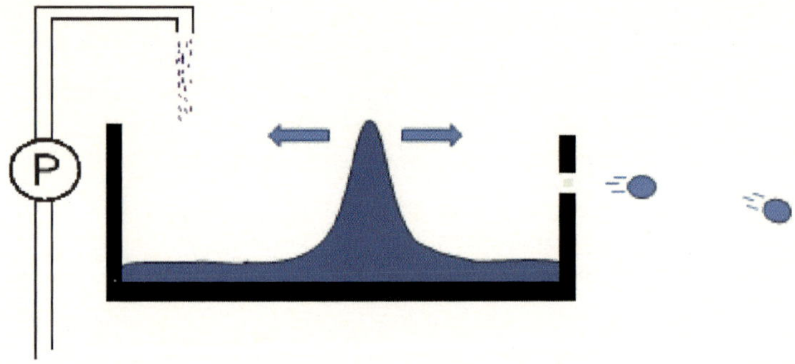

Fig. 3.8 Oscillating wave inside a resonator

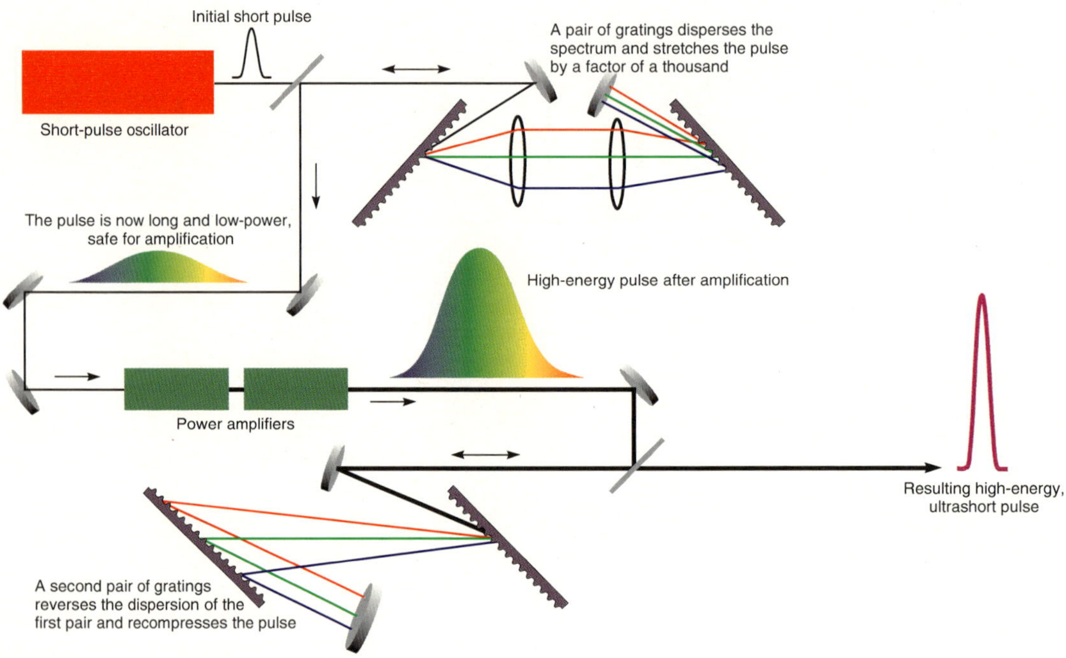

Fig. 3.9 Schematic diagram of an oscillator–amplifier laser system (image courtesy of Lawrence Livermore National Laboratory; used with permission)

stimulate 10,000 modes, which results in pulse widths of only a few femtoseconds. Ytterbium based crystals, which are commonly used in ophthalmic applications at wavelengths around 1,040 nm, are able to generate pulse widths of a few hundred femtoseconds.

Because the wave package oscillates inside the laser resonator with the speed of light, mode locked lasers have very high pulse rates. At a resonator length of typically 2 meters (m) (the resonator usually is folded, so the box of the laser machine can be shorter), the light needs for one full oscillation at 4 m takes only 4/300,000 km/s = 13 ns, which results in a repetition rate of 1/13 ns = 75 MHz.

Need for an Amplifier with Most Femtosecond Lasers

MHz repetition rate pulses cause problems in placing each single pulse to a different place. Common scanner systems are too slow. Moreover, laser oscillators can produce pulse energies up to several hundred nanojoules which is, depending on the focusing optics, too low to reach the threshold of photodisruption.

As a consequence, all commercially available ophthalmic laser systems at the time of this writing, except the LDV from Ziemer, need an amplifier to get enough pulse energy for surgical applications. An example of such an oscillator–amplifier system is sketched in Fig. 3.9.

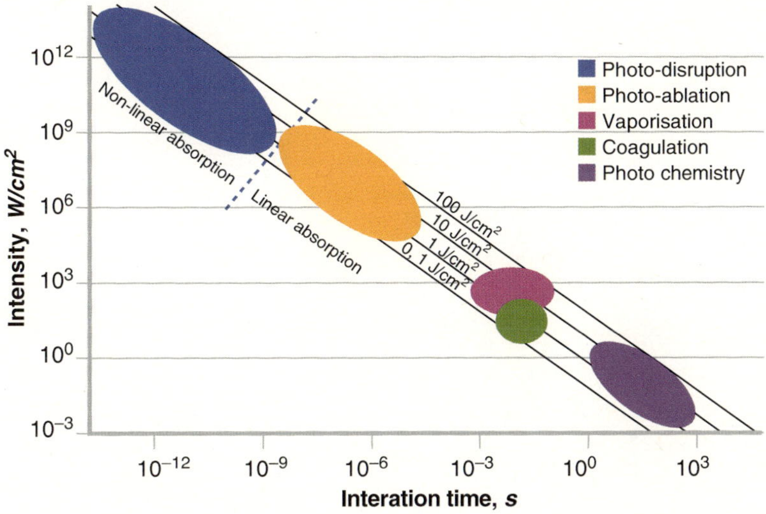

Fig. 3.10 Basic laser–tissue interaction mechanisms

The oscillator, usually a diode pumped solid state or fiber laser, seeds the amplifier with low energy pulses. Because megahertz repetition rate are too high to process, an optical switch (electro-optic modulator (EOM) or acousto-optic modulator (AOM)) selects the pulses and reduces the pulse rate to typically several hundred kilohertz [3]. Moreover, the oscillator pulses are optically stretched to several picoseconds. Making the pulses longer reduces their peak power. If the pulses would be amplified directly, the optical components of the amplifier would be damaged by photodisruption.

The power amplifier consists of a second laser crystal or a laser fiber which is optically pumped by another pump diode. The seed pulses from the oscillator depopulate the inversion by stimulated emission and thus will be amplified by a factor of 100–1,000. Finally, the amplified pulses are compressed by an optical compressor to several hundred femtosecond and pulse energies to several microjoules.

Basics of Laser–Tissue Interaction

Laser–Tissue Interaction Regimes

The nature of the laser–tissue interaction process may be divided into five different regimes, determined primarily by the intensity of the laser beam and its interaction time with the tissue (Fig. 3.10). The physical basis of the first surgical applications of lasers is tissue cutting and removal at relatively high laser-beam intensities with exposure times of milliseconds to seconds, resulting in the rapid deposition of heat and subsequent vaporization or decomposition. These are the processes characteristic of thermal ablation or vaporization. For nanosecond pulses, using high photon energies (ultraviolet wavelengths at 193 nm), single photons can directly break specific chemical bonds, resulting in strong absorption and accurate, nonthermal ablation. Picosecond and shorter pulses can induce nonlinear absorption in biological tissue, providing the capability for localized absorption of laser energy in otherwise transparent tissue such as the eye. Finally, some interactions have been observed at very low laser-intensity levels delivered over minutes or hours. These interactions are strongly coupled to the host tissue response to photochemistry, and remain as yet, poorly understood.

Photocoagulation

With a relatively long exposure time (from 10 to 100 ms) and low irradiance (up to 10 W/cm²), photocoagulation can be achieved. This laser–tissue interaction results from a thermal interaction associated with protein denaturation, due to

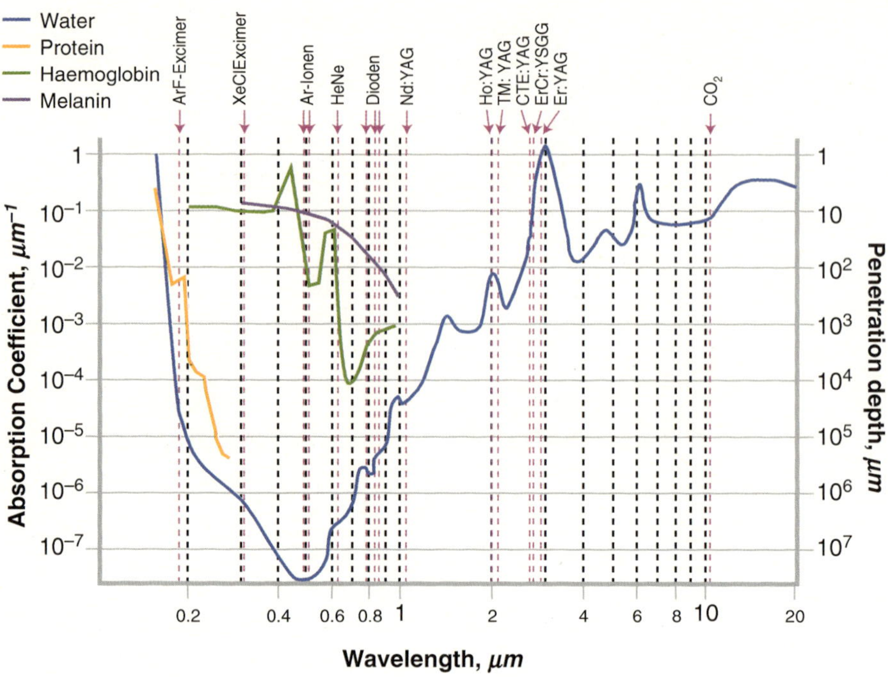

Fig. 3.11 Absorption curves of biological tissue consisting of water, proteins hemoglobin and melanin and typical laser wavelengths use in medical applications

an increased temperature of the tissue. Argon laser is the most common laser source used for such tissue interaction and uses wavelengths of the visible spectrum. Its energy is absorbed by the two main, natural chromophores within the ocular tissue, blood and melanin (Fig. 3.11), allowing the laser to target its effect on ocular structure such as vessels, iris, or deep retinal layer that contain melanin. Argon lasers and recently frequency doubled Nd:YAG lasers as well as green diode lasers have been useful in treating retinal disease and glaucoma.

Photocoagulation of retinal vascular disease has made use of blood as a chromophore whereas laser trabeculoplasty and panretinal photocoagulation have used the absorptivity of melanin to achieve their effects. In the early 1970s [4–6], some studies also reported the use of argon laser pulses to treat certain corneal diseases or conditions that were associated with pigment into the cornea, such as corneal neovascularization, lipid keratopathy, or vitreous adhesion to corneal wound after trauma. Although these studies have shown some efficacy, corneal photocoagulation results in a loss of transparency, and thus limits its indications to the treatment of retinal disease and glaucoma.

Photothermal Shrinkage

One specific form of photocoagulation is photothermal shrinkage. A non-laser form of photothermal shrinkage was first introduced by Lans et al. over 100 years ago as a method for correcting corneal astigmatism [7]. This procedure was abandoned because of the regression of refractive effect over time, even though attempts to refine this method for the correction of hyperopia have been reported over the last 40 years, and are now known as a thermokeratoplasty [8, 9]. The concept is to induce shrinkage of the corneal stromal collagen lamellae by delivering sufficient laser energy in the peripheral cornea, resulting in a circular band of tissue shrinkage with a central corneal steepening. Heating corneal tissue to temperature of 30 °C over the ambient corneal temperature has been shown to shrink corneal collagen lamellae to approximately one third of its original length [10]. Histologically, the surrounding corneal stroma swells immediately after delivering the treatment, losing some of the stromal lamellar pattern before showing a clear shrinkage of the irradiated corneal collagen after 4 weeks. Holmium:YAG laser has been used to induce tissue shrinkage by a noncontact delivery of the laser energy through an eight faceted polyprismatic lens mounted to a slit lamp. In early 1990s, Koch [11] reported a series of 17 eyes treated with a noncontact holmium laser, using a 2,120 nm wavelength and a pulse duration of 250 μs, delivering its energy through an eight-spot pattern at 6–7 mm diameter. By raising the temperature in the collagen to 55 °C, he showed a net steepening effect of the central cornea with relative stability over a 7-month follow up period. Although this demonstrated the short-term viability of this laser interaction for the correction of hyperopia and astigmatism, most of the effect was lost in the long-term, as had been the case with previous methods of thermal shrinkage of corneal collagen.

Photovaporization

Photovaporization is another laser–tissue interaction produced mainly by infrared laser light sources with comparatively high average power. These wavelengths are strongly absorbed by water, allowing vaporization of any water-containing tissue, accompanied by thermal denaturation of the adjacent tissue. While photovaporization is used in conventional surgery, where blood vessels are coagulated and stop bleeding during the cut, this technique is barely used in ophthalmic surgery due to the wide collateral thermal damage.

Infrared Photoablation

Thermal collateral damage due to heat conduction can be minimized when the pulse duration of the laser is equal or shorter than the thermal relaxation time. The thermal relaxation time T_R of a laser heated region of tissue is the time required for the peak temperature to diffuse over the distance of the optical penetration depth δ of the laser light [12].

$$T_R = \frac{\delta^2}{4\kappa},$$

where κ is the thermal diffusivity of the tissue. Typically T_R is in the range of microseconds to milliseconds when the optical penetration depth δ of the laser light is in the range of micrometer to millimeter.

If the pulse duration of the laser pulse is shorter than T_R we call the process photoablation.

The absorption coefficient of the corneal stromal tissue for laser light sources in the 3 μm range, with its corresponding penetration depth δ, allow the production of lesions with greater precision and less thermal damage [13]. The CO_2 laser, Er:YAG laser or hydrogen fluoride laser have been used for their longer infrared wavelengths (in the 3 μm range) to produce precise corneal excision as well as surface ablation and keratectomy [13, 14].

UV-Photoablation

Corneal photoablation using the excimer laser was introduced in 1983 by Trokel and coworkers [15]. In their landmark article, they reported how this UV laser light source could precisely remove corneal tissue without any thermal side effects. This revolutionary finding eventually led to the development of laser vision correction and LASIK as the most frequently performed elective procedure in all of medicine [16].

At that time the unique mechanism of interaction of excimer laser photoablation was understood as a pure photochemical process, where the individual photon energy (6.4 eV) is significantly greater than the energy required to break individual molecular bonds, which is not true of longer laser wavelengths. With photocoagulation, photovaporization, and photothermal shrinkage, there is localized heating of the adjacent collagen tissue as the accumulated laser energy to achieve a therapeutic effect undergoes thermal diffusion. With UV laser corneal ablation, the photon energy is fully absorbed, leading to molecular bond breaking. The subsequent ablation of tissue

a
Absorption

b
Bond
Breaking

c
Ablation

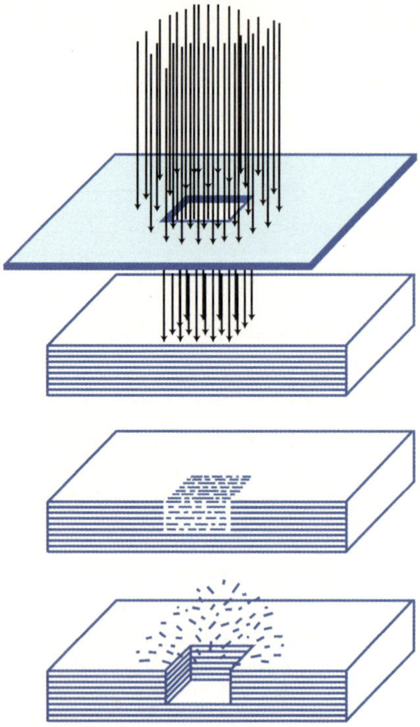

Fig. 3.12 Mechanism of interaction with the excimer laser photoablation: absorption, bond breaking and ablation

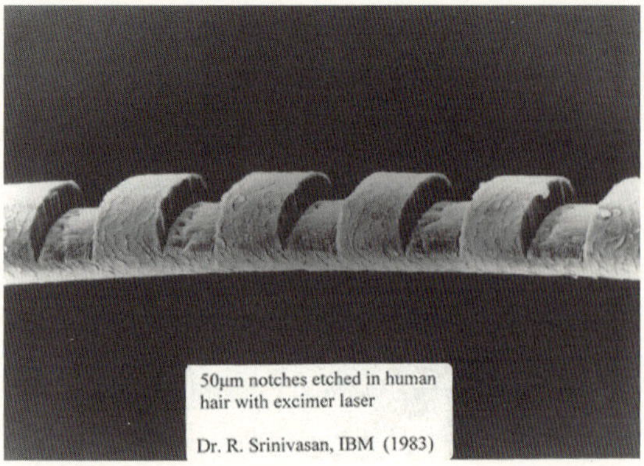

Fig. 3.13 Scanning electron micrograph (SEM) of 193 nm excimer laser photoablation of a human hair, showing detailed etchings with submicron precision (image courtesy of R. Srinivasan. Originally published in R. Srinivasan, "Photophysics and Photochemistry above 6 eV", Ed. F. Lahmani, Elsevier, Amsterdam (1985))

occurs as the fragments are ejected, driven by kinetic energy provided by the energy of the photon in excess of that required for bond breaking (Fig. 3.12) [17].

Today we know that excimer laser photoablation is a mixture of both UV-bond-breaking of the collagen molecules and thermal vaporization of the water [18].

In 1985, Krueger et al., demonstrated the spectrum of UV laser photoablation by comparing the tissue effect produced by different UV wavelengths, using the excimer laser [19]. The argon fluoride (ArF) gas mixture used to generate the 193 nm wavelength achieves the highest level of tissue smoothness and precision in corneal ablation with the lowest amount of thermal damages (Fig. 3.13). The longer UV wavelengths (249, 308, and 351 nm) each showed a progressively higher amount of thermal damage in the adjacent tissue. The 193 nm ArF gas mixture is the current excimer laser source used clinically all over the world to perform refractive surgery in a safe and efficient way.

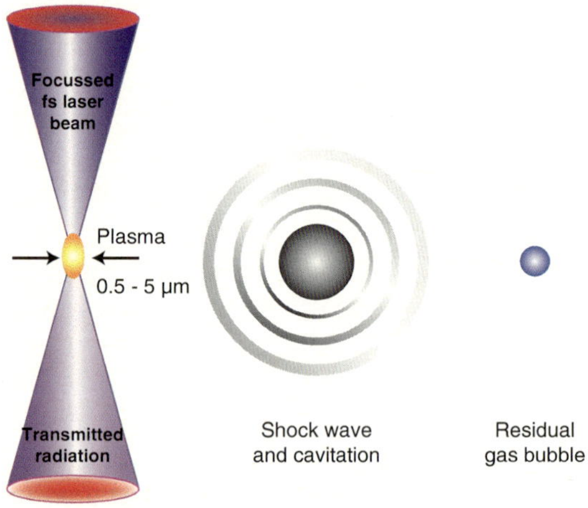

Fig. 3.14 Photodisruption characterized by plasma formation, shock wave generation, cavitation and leaving a residual gas bubble behind

Photodisruption

The mechanism of interaction behind laser photodisruption is best described as plasma-mediated ablation, or optical breakdown. It relies on the nonlinear absorption of laser energy in the target achieved when the material specific radiant expo-

Table 3.1 Typical laser parameters and tissue effects of photodisruption in the nanosecond, picosecond and femtosecond regime

Pulsewidth	Nanosecond (ns)	Picosecond (ps)	Femtosecond (fs)
Intensity (10^{12} W/cm^2)	0.05	0.5–1	5–10
Energy density (J/cm^2)	10–100	2–10	1–3
Pulse energy (μJ)	100–10,000	1–5	0.5–3
Shockwave amplitude at 1 mm (bar)	100–500	10–100	1–5
Cavitation bubble diameter (μm)	1,000–2,000	200–500	<30

sure is exceeded. Fundamentally, optical breakdown is characterized by three successive major events: plasma formation, shock wave generation and cavitation (Fig. 3.14). The plasma is a highly ionized state of matter, and can be generated by laser pulses (from femtosecond to few nanoseconds) of low energy and high peak power. It has been shown that shortening the pulse duration from nanoseconds to femtoseconds decreases the threshold for plasma formation and reduces mechanical effects [20] (Table 3.1).

The process of optical breakdown can be explained by two different but equivalent models. On the one hand, we can regard the laser focus as an extremely strong electromagnetic field. Under the action of this field, electrons are stripped from their atoms and accelerated by the electric field to high kinetic energy. The accelerated electrons in turn can collide with further atoms and ionize them. This process which leads to plasma formation is called "cascade ionization."

Another way to explain the process of ionization is with the photonic model. A free electron can be generated when the energy absorbed by a photon is higher than the energy necessary to excite the electron to the outermost energy level. Typically this energy is 6–10 eV. However, the photon energy at wavelengths within the range of 1.06 μm, is only 1.17 eV. Thus, at this wavelength, which is typical for clinical lasers in transparent media, an extra 6–10 photons would be necessary to promote an electron to leave its atom. Optical breakdown occurs when the irradiance is sufficient to produce a critical density of photons so that the probability of a simultaneous absorption of six or more electrons is considerably high.

After the laser pulse ends, the free electrons transfer their energy to the tissue by locally elevating the temperature that stays confined in the focal volume. The thermal diffusion is too slow to dissipate the laser energy by heat conduction. So, the created plasma first expands at supersonic velocity emitting a shock wave due to its high temperature and pressure, and then slows down to the speed of the sound,. The elevation of the temperature creates a highly localized tensile stress which exceeds the critical tension for mechanical breakdown, resulting in tissue disruption and cavitation bubble formation. Mass spectroscopy analysis of the residual gas bubbles reveals a mixture of CO, CO_2, methane, CH_4, together with some fragments of CH_3, CH_2, and water vapor [21, 22]. Photodisruption with ultrashort pulses enables one to achieve a fine and highly localized cutting without collateral thermal effects, but also has the benefit of tissue cleaving, due to the presence of rapidly expanding cavitation bubbles, which help to separate the tissue. As a result, the sequential placement of tissue cutting pulses is a function of pulses energy. Using very low pulse energies in the range of some nanojoules, the cutting process is confined by the focal spot size of the laser pulse. As a consequence, more pulses are needed to cut the same area. To keep the total operation time at the same level, higher pulse repetition rates of some megahertz are required (Fig. 3.15, left).

At comparatively high pulse energies, the cutting process is driven by mechanical forces which are applied by the expanding bubbles, disrupting the tissue. This cutting process is very efficient because the radius of disrupted tissue is larger than the laser spot size (Fig. 3.15, right). Hence,

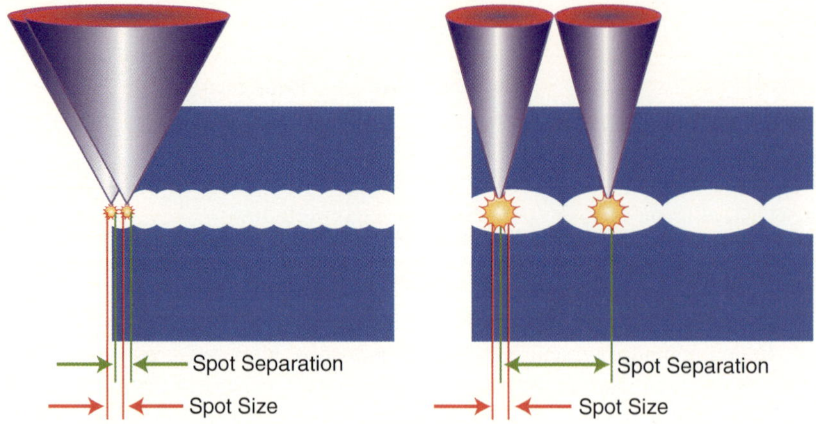

Fig. 3.15 Sequential FS laser pulses separate the tissue in part by cutting at lower pulse energies (*left*) or by cleaving due to the presence of rapidly expanding cavitation bubbles

the spot separation of the scanned laser pulses can be larger than the spot diameter.

To summarize, the physical mechanisms ruling the laser–tissue interaction differ strongly depending on the laser operation regime, thus allowing a broad variety of surgical applications. The interplay between wavelength, laser beam intensity and exposure time determine the laser–tissue interaction and can induce mechanical, thermal and/or chemical modifications, that result in either hemostatic effects, molecular denaturation (photocoagulation and vaporization), structural changes (photothermal shrinkage), tissue removal (photoablation), or cutting (photodisruption).

Detailed Physics of Femtosecond Laser Interaction

Femtosecond Laser Interaction

As explained in the previous chapter, the... interaction process of FS laser pulses is based on non linear absorption and consecutive disruption of the tissue accompanied with cavitation and a remaining gas bubble. Non linear absorption means that usually the corneal tissue is transparent for the infrared laser radiation at moderate intensities and no absorption takes place. Only at very high intensities, which can be achieved by compressing the laser pulse in time ("ultrashort") and in space (strongly focused), several infrared photons act as one UV photon and are absorbed by the tissue.

Due to the Gaussian intensity profile in time and space, the threshold for multiphoton photodisruption can be reached both before and behind the focal point of the laser beam. Moreover, the lateral narrowness of the region of photodisruption depends on the degree to which the beam is strongly focused and is never, in practice, a single point in space.

The multi photon absorption process ionizes the tissue and thus generates free electrons. Depending on the pulse duration and the pulse intensity, many more free electrons will be generated as an avalanche process. The number of free electrons characterizes the following disruption process. At low pulse intensities, only a so-called low density plasma is produced. The cutting process is dominated by photochemically induced decomposition of the tissue and thermoelastic disruption. At higher pulse intensities, a luminescent plasma is generated. This process is called plasma mediated ablation, due to the explosive expansion of the plasma. Mechanical rupture and transient cavitation, as well as remaining gas bubbles, are typical side effects for this process.

In order to achieve maximum precision of the cut and minimize the collateral damage, one has to minimize the energy threshold for optical breakdown by shortening the pulse duration and minimizing the focal spot volume (Fig. 3.16).

Pulse Duration

Shortening the duration of a laser pulse leads to a basic physical problem, which is related to the spectral bandwidth of the laser medium. For a given spectral width, there is a lower limit for the pulse duration. This limit has its origin by the uncertainty principle and is called the time bandwidth product. Titanium sapphire lasers, for example, have the broadest spectrum and the shortest (<100 fs) pulses; however, they are very complex in their setup and relatively expensive. Yb-doped fiber lasers or solid state lasers which emit around 1,000 nm wavelength are today the most reliable systems and also the easiest way to produce ultrashort pulses. Their pulse duration is typically around 200–800 fs. High levels of surgical precision can already be achieved with 200 fs pulses. From that standpoint, there is no need to further shorten the pulses. Moreover, the beam delivery gets very expensive when laser pulses are shorter than 100 fs. The shorter the pulse, the broader its spectrum; however, if the optical spectrum is very broad, the different wavelengths have significantly different velocities due to dispersion, which elongates the beam in time while it passes through the media.

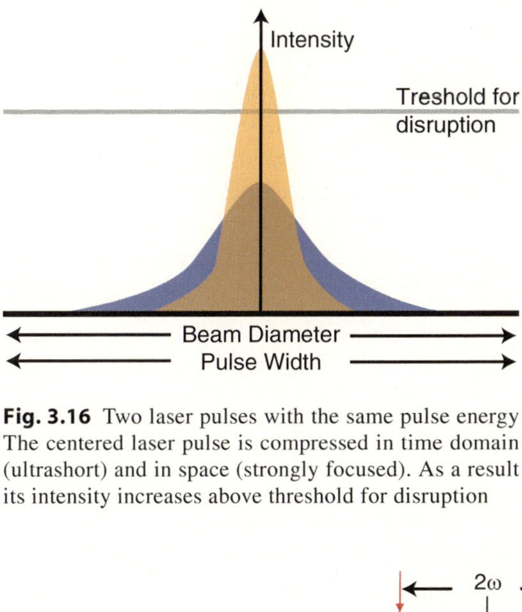

Fig. 3.16 Two laser pulses with the same pulse energy The centered laser pulse is compressed in time domain (ultrashort) and in space (strongly focused). As a result its intensity increases above threshold for disruption

Numerical Aperture

The second way to decrease the energy threshold is to minimize the focal volume of the laser spot. The focal volume V_f of a Gaussian laser beam is dependent on the axial extension, the so-called Rayleigh length [3] ($z = \pi\omega_0^2/\lambda$) and the lateral extension which is the beam waist $\omega_0 = f\lambda/\pi\omega_L$, where f is the focal length of the lens and ω_L the radius of the beam at the focusing lens:

$$V_f \sim z \cdot \omega_0^2 = \frac{\lambda^3 f^4}{\pi^3 \omega_L^4} = \frac{\lambda^3}{\pi^3} \cdot \frac{1}{NA^4}.$$

In other words, the focal volume varies inversely with the power of four of the numerical aperture $NA = \omega_L/f$ of the focusing optics. The larger the NA, the smaller the focal spot and finally, the smaller the energy threshold (Fig. 3.17).

According to its definition, there are two ways to increase the NA. One possibility is to increase

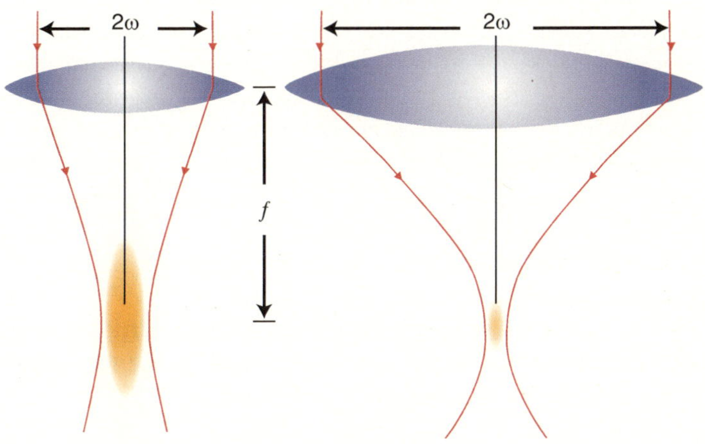

Fig. 3.17 The focal volume of a Gaussian laser beam scales with the numerical aperture NA of the focusing lens. The larger the NA, the smaller is the focal spot volume

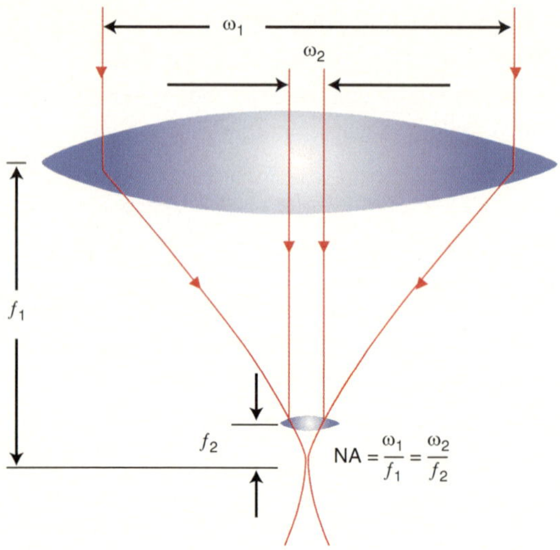

Fig. 3.18 Certain focal diameter of the laser beam can be achieved at constant numerical aperture NA either by using broad lenses and long working distances or by smaller lenses with shorter working distances

the beam diameter at the focusing optics, which requires large and expensive optical components. As an alternative, one can also decrease the focal length of the focusing objective, which on the other hand reduces the working distance of the laser system (Fig. 3.18).

Self-focusing and Streak Formation

Very intense electromagnetic radiation can change the refractive index of transparent material [23]. Depending on the type of material and on the intensity of the radiation, several mechanisms produce variations in the refractive index, which result in a self-focusing of the laser beam. The main effect which produces self-focusing is the so-called optical Kerr-effect, which induces a variation of the refractive index n as described by the formula $n=n_0+n_2I$, where n_0 and n_2 are the linear and nonlinear components of the refractive index, and I is the intensity of the radiation. Because n_2 is positive in materials like cornea or water, the refractive index becomes larger in the areas where the intensity is higher. Thus, the spatial beam profile of a high-intensity laser beam leads to a spatial variation in the index of refraction of the medium, in which the laser is propagating. In the case of a Gaussian beam profile, the central part along the beam axis has a higher index of refraction than its wings. As a result, the light will be focused as is known from graded-index devices [24].

Self-focusing occurs if the radiation power P is greater than the critical power P_{cr}

$$P_{cr} = \frac{\alpha\lambda^2}{4\pi n_0 n_2},$$

where λ is the radiation wavelength and α is a constant which depends on the initial spatial distribution of the beam [25]. For a Gaussian beam $\alpha \approx 1.8962$. Typical numbers for P_{cr} in water is in the range of 4 MW [26] corresponding to a pulse energy of about 3 μJ at 800 fs.

Self-focusing probably plays a major role in filamentation of the laser beam near to its focal point. Due to inhomogeneities in the beam profile ("hot spots"), scattered locations with higher intensity occur, which lead to filamentation by self-focusing [27]. The nature of the filaments might be a change in the structure of the medium by local melting and solidification or due to the interaction of the free electrons, which are generated by multi photon ionization (Fig. 3.19).

Similar streaks were created inside the corneal tissue when using small numerical apertures and high pulse energies of 2 μJ (Fig. 3.20).

In TEM, the streaks can be seen as a dark staining, crossing the picture in the vertical direction (Fig. 3.21). The diameters of the streaks were estimated to be in the range of 200–500 nm, which is below the diffraction limit of the focused laser beam. The distance between two single streaks is equal to the separation of the laser pulses, which is 3.5 μm. It is assumed that due to the high intensity, a significant number of free electrons is produced which do not reach plasma density. However, the free electrons might have induced radical reactions that damage the collagen and lead to the streak formation.

Unique Engineering Requirements for Femtosecond Laser Cataract Surgery

Although the FS laser devices for corneal surgery are in principle the same as the systems for

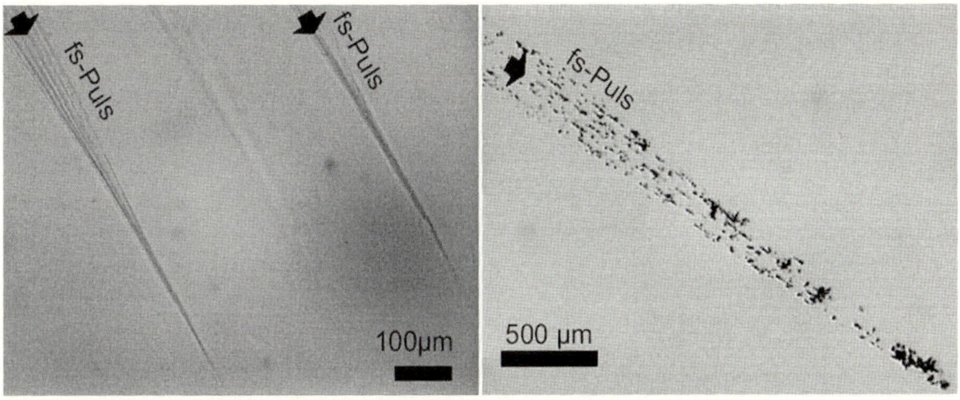

Fig. 3.19 Filamentation of a focusing FS laser beam in gelatine (*left*). The laser pulse energy was 500 µJ and 100 pulses were applied. Similar structures can be found in PMMA (*right*). At pulse energies of 300 µJ various locations of cracks, generated by optical breakdown, can be observed (images from: F. Dausinger, F. Lichtner, H. Lubatschowski (Eds.): Femtosecond Technology for Technical and Medical Applications, Topics Appl. Phys. 96 (2004), Springer Page 99)

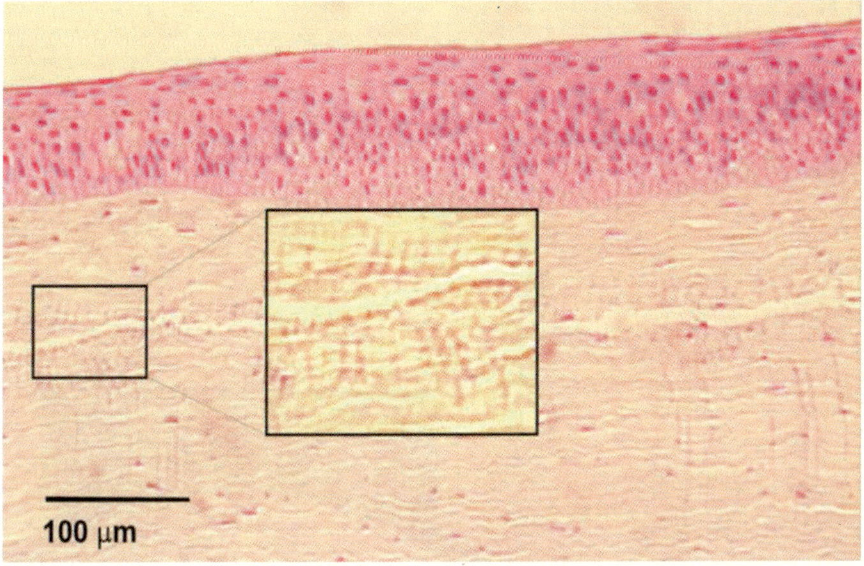

Fig. 3.20 Histological section (HE staining) of a porcine cornea, irradiated with 160 fs laser pulses at a pulse energy of 2 µJ. Streaks were created inside the corneal tissue that represent each single laser pulse. The corneal flap was opened and closed for better demonstration of the cutting line (images from: F. Dausinger, F. Lichtner, H. Lubatschowski (Eds.): Femtosecond Technology for Technical and Medical Applications, Topics Appl. Phys. 96 (2004), Springer Page 196)

cataract surgery, the engineering requirements between the two differ in several specific ways.

Laser systems for corneal refractive surgery are optimized to cut a smooth and precise area of approximately 10 mm width. For lens surgery, one has to target a *volume* of 7 mm diameter and 4 mm depth, which is also located significantly deeper inside the eye, passing through a number of refractive surfaces with different indices of refraction (Fig. 3.22).

If a large volume has to be addressed by the laser focus, it is much simpler to do this with

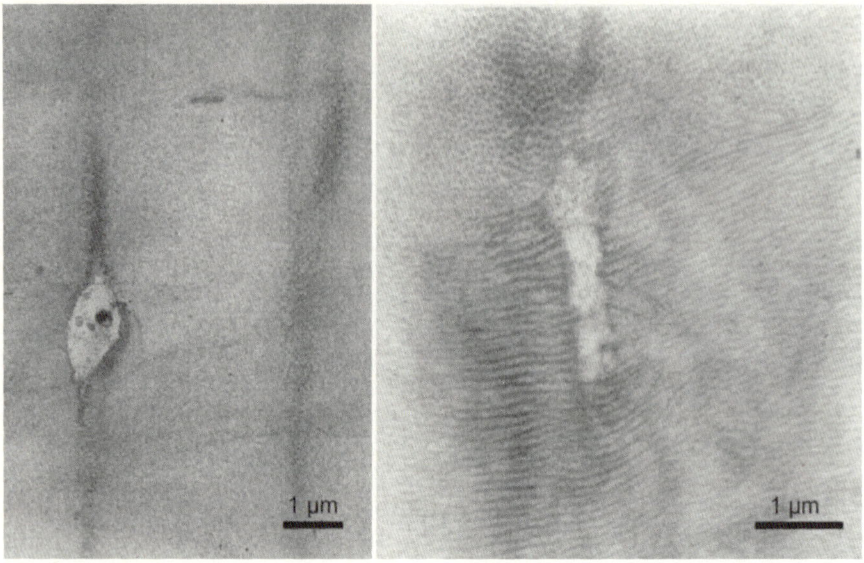

Fig. 3.21 In TEM, the streaks can be seen as a dark staining, crossing the picture in the vertical direction. The diameters of the streaks are in the range of 200–500 nm, which is below the diffraction limit of the focused laser beam. The distance between two single streaks is equal to the separation of the laser pulses, which is 3.5 µm. The left micrograph shows two streaks within the focusing plane of the cornea. On the left streak, optical breakdown occurred, which is indicated by the bubble. On the right streak, obviously no optical breakdown took place. The right micrograph shows the collagen fibrils around an optical breakdown (image from: F. Dausinger, F. Lichtner, H. Lubatschowski (Eds.): Femtosecond Technology for Technical and Medical Applications, Topics Appl. Phys. 96 (2004), Springer Page 197)

Fig. 3.22 Beam parameters for corneal and lens application

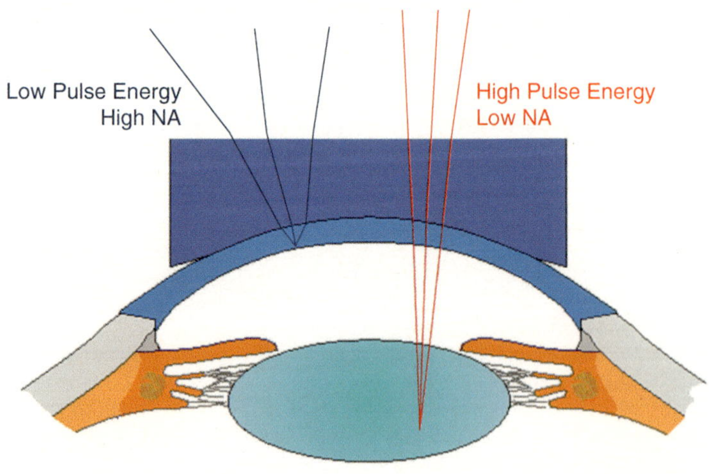

optics of low numerical aperture (Fig. 3.17). As a consequence, the required pulse energy will be higher, and the focal spot size will be larger, both laterally and, even more so, axially. Where this would be unacceptable for corneal surgery, it is sufficiently adequate for lens based cataract surgery, since the required precision for lens fragmentation is not as demanding.

Not only must the pulse energy in the lens be higher due the larger spot size, it must also be further increased because of strong scattering losses inside the sclerotic crystalline lens. As a

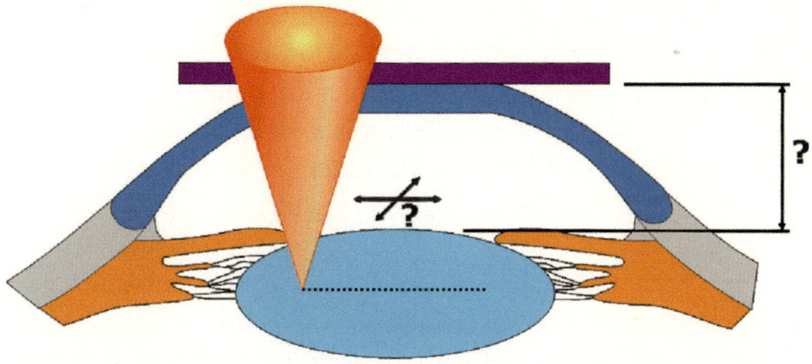

Fig. 3.23 The clinical diversity of eyes with differing anterior chamber depth and lens geometry, make image guided surgery an essential for refractive laser assisted cataract surgery

result, a factor of 5–10 greater pulse energy is required for photodisruptive lens surgery than what is currently being implemented for photodisruptive corneal surgery.

Finally, beyond the differences of laser beam delivery and pulse energy in cataract surgery, the precise localization of laser pulses must be navigated between the posterior and anterior lens capsule in keeping an adequate safety margin, especially with respect to the posterior capsule (Fig. 3.23).

Fortunately, since the laser beam incorporates 3D scanning delivery, and the essential imaging also requires 3D scanning for intraocular localization, the two components can be used synchronously within the laser system. As a result, the target tissue can be both imaged and treated very easily without making room for additional scanning mirrors and lenses. OCT imaging can be coupled along the laser beam path, and the target tissue can be easily localized before surgery to navigate the laser pulse delivery [28].

While OCT imaging is implemented in most of the first generation FS laser cataract surgery systems, other techniques, such as confocal structured illumination imaging or confocal imaging can also be implemented into the beam delivery system.

Overview of Femtosecond Lasers in Clinical Ophthalmology

Pre-femtosecond Laser Photodisruption

In the early 1970s, Krasnov first showed the feasibility of laser-induced optical breakdown and plasma formation of transparent media by a high-powered pulsed ruby laser [29]. Few years later, Dr. Aron-Rosa and her coworkers, reported the first clinical use of the Nd:YAG laser pulse energy for performing posterior capsulotomy [30]. These findings led to the widespread use of the Nd:YAG laser in ophthalmology, and have established the framework for the future uses of ocular tissue photodisruption for a broad range of anterior segment laser procedures.

In the early 1990s, photodisruption with the Nd:YAG laser was already a well-established tool for intraocular surgery, being used in posterior capsulotomy, but also for iridotomy, vitreolysis, and pupillary membranectomy. However, laser delivery with a pulsewidth in the nanosecond range, and pulse energy in the millijoule range, left the spectrum of clinical applications limited, due to the large potential for collateral damage to the surrounding tissue. In 1994, Vogel et al. [31] demonstrated the use of single shot picosecond laser pulses with energies in the microjoule range. He showed how they could significantly increase the surgical precision of intraocular Nd:YAG laser surgery and reduce disruptive side effects.

Within the next year, a quasicontinuous pulse train of picosecond laser pulses was introduced by intelligent surgical lasers (ISL) with a proposal to perform intrastromal photorefractive kertectomy (isPRK). Unfortunately, the picosecond laser was ineffective in removing corneal collagen from within the stroma, but rather was more effective in separating and cutting the corneal fibers [32]. This eventually led to the next generation of FS lasers, and the proposed use for flap cutting in lieu of using a microkeratome.

Femtosecond Laser LASIK

With faster visual recovery, less discomfort, milder wound healing and less risk for corneal haze, LASIK offers several advantages over photorefractive keratectomy (PRK). However, the flap creation remains the most critical step in a successful LASIK procedure as an incomplete flap, irregular flap, partial flap, decentration, or unexpected flap thickness can lead to significant complications.

It has been 10 years since the IntraLase FS laser for flap creation was introduced, and this technology has considerably improved the safety of the procedure. What started out as an expensive cutting tool has now become a standard of care with nearly 70 % of all LASIK surgery in the USA using a FS laser for flap creation. When compared to mechanical microkeratomes, FS laser flaps present several advantages: Regarding flap shape and thickness, it has been shown that FS flaps are more uniform compared to the so-called "meniscus shape" flap of the microkeratome. The thicker periphery leads to greater biomechanical variability and aberrations, but also could be associated with more extreme mechanical complications, such as a buttonhole flap or excessively thick flap [33]. FS flap thickness has also been found to be highly predictable and reproducible, thus further increasing the safety of flap formation [34]. Flap diameter and centration tend also to be more predictable with the FS laser than micokeratome, since FS laser flaps are not dependant on corneal curvature or diameter, allowing for the creation of larger or smaller flap diameters, which can be centration adjusted toward the center of the entrance pupil. Regarding the smoothness of the stromal bed, studies have reported at least comparable if not better smoothness of the flap interface. There is also less induction of high order aberrations (HOAs) when using the FS laser rather than a microkeratome during LASIK [35]. This is believed to be due to the tendency for a meniscus flap shape. These aberrations are due to biomechanical changes in the cornea, which also poses a risk for post LASIK ectasia. The residual stromal bed, and thus, the predictability of the flap thickness remains a key factor in LASIK safety. In summary, FS laser flaps demonstrate a clear advantage over microkeratome flaps in term of reproducibility and predictability of the flap thickness.

Femtosecond Lenticular Extraction: Flex and Smile Procedure

FS lenticule extraction is a treatment for myopia using a FS laser, but without an excimer laser, and is a new refractive procedure available when using the Zeiss VisuMax system. A corneal stromal lenticule is first cut with the FS laser, and then extracted either by creating and lifting a flap that exposes the lenticule to be removed (FLEx) or by creating a second layer that is externalized through a single small incision without a flap (SmILE) [36]. The theoretical advantage over a standard LASIK procedure is that there is no need for two different lasers to be involved, reducing the cost and increasing the ergonomics, time and energy efficiency. In addition, the SmILE procedure is believe to induce less dry eye symptoms, biomechanical shifts, and hydration changes in the cornea, since the flap is not lifted [37].

Femtosecond Laser Therapeutic Keratotomy

Other corneal surgery procedures such as keratoplasty, intracorneal ring channels, or astigmatic keratotomy have greatly benefited from the introduction and technological improvements of FS lasers over the last decades. Manual dissection techniques for penetrating and/or lamellar keratoplasty involve critical steps which strongly depend upon the precise alignment and matching shape of donor and recipient tissue, as well as the depth and uniformity of the lamellar dissection. FS lasers ensure cutting with accuracy, reproducibility, and geometric shape matching between the donor and host corneas. Furthermore, current commercially available FS lasers offer a wide variety of cutting patterns such as top hat, mushroom, or Z-shapes, which may favor wound healing [38]. Several different surgical techniques involving the use of FS lasers to cut the donor cornea or both, donor and recipient, have been proposed to improve the biomechanical stability and allow for rapid healing. Deep lamellar anterior keratoplasty (DALK) combined with a zigzag cutting pattern, or FS laser endothelial keratoplasty (FLEK) are of particular interest and currently under investigation [39].

The correction of astigmatism has also been a hot topic in the past few years, and FS laser assisted astigmatic keratotomy (FS-AK) has been shown to be effective, especially for high postkeratoplasty astigmatism [40]. FS-AK has the advantage of being more precise in depth, length and curvature than manual astigmatic keratotomy with a diamond knife, although an optimal nomogram for a more accurate correction is still needed to potentiate the high precision offered by FS laser technology [41].

The implantation of intracorneal rings segments (ICRS) is another corneal procedure that has been improved by the introduction of the FS laser. It has been used for the treatment of keratoconus, pellucid marginal degeneration, or post-LASIK ectasia [42, 43]. In comparison to the traditional manual method, the FS laser has allowed for the creation of channels inside the cornea in a faster and more reproducible way [44]. The depth, diameter, and width of the channels have been shown to be more precise, and the rate of complications such as epithelial defect, perforation, displacement, or decentration has been lowered by using FS laser [45].

Biomechanical Modification of the Central Cornea with Intrastromal Femtosecond Lasers (INTRACOR)

In addition to the clinical benefits of FS laser flap creation, lenticular extraction, astigmatic keratotomy, and therapeutic keratectomy, the cornea can also be altered biomechanically for presbyopia correction by central intrastromal delivery (INTRACOR). This procedure, introduced by Dr. Luis Ruiz in 2009, is among the most recently investigated, and is currently only available with the Technolas Femtec system [46]. It aims to induce biomechanical changes in the cornea by performing deep intrastromal incisions along a cylindrical shaped pattern with five concentric rings centered on the center of the entrance pupil (line of sight). These biomechanical changes lead to a hyperprolate, aspheric corneal shape with an induction of both negative spherical aberration and positive secondary spherical aberration to enhance the depth of focus for near vision. The first clinical results seem to improve the uncorrected near visual acuity in most patients with few side effects [46, 47], but further studies are still needed to evaluate the long-term stability of the procedure.

Femtosecond Laser Assisted Cataract Surgery

Moving beyond the cornea, ultrashort FS laser pulses of low energy (<10 μJ/pulse) can be tightly focused inside the natural crystalline lens to enable cutting without damage to surrounding structures. With the introduction of FS laser assisted refractive cataract surgery, improvements in safety and refractive predictability are expected during the various critical steps of the cataract procedure in a manner similar to the improvement seen during FS laser LASIK flap creation. Currently, four companies (LensAR, LenSx, OptiMedica, and Technolas) are developing FS lasers for making the primary incision and paracentesis [48], capsulotomy [49], lens fragmentation [50, 51], and limbal-relaxing incisions. The use of image guided FS laser delivery in performing these various crucial steps is the subject of this book, as presented in the subsequent chapters.

Key Points

1. Lasers operate when sufficiently exited electrons of the laser material are stimulated to emit photons in phase (coherence). The stimulated emission is amplified in a resonating cavity to produce light amplification by the stimulated emission of radiation (LASER).
2. Optical Q-switching is one method of pulsing in the nanosecond range, but mode-locking is necessary to achieve picosecond or FS laser pulses. The more (laser) modes locked in phase, the shorter the pulse width and higher the pulse intensity.

3. Photocoagulation uses low irradiance, long exposure pulsing to achieve a wavelength-dependent tissue absorption. With photoablation, the highly absorbed photons in the UV or in the mid infrared cleave molecular bonds (UV) or vaporize the water of the tissue (IR) and set particles in motion, ejecting them away from the tissue surface. Pulse duration has to be in the micro or nanosecond range in order not to deposit thermal energy into the tissue by heat diffusion. Photodisruption uses a sufficiently high density of ultrashort laser pulses of low energy and high peak power to create ionized material (plasma) by optical breakdown, which locally disrupts internal tissues with a subsequent shock wave and expanding cavitation bubble, separating these tissues.
4. With FS laser photodisruption, maximal precision of the cut with minimal collateral damage can be achieved by lowering the threshold energy for optical breakdown by minimizing the pulse width and focal spot volume.
5. The pulse width can only practically be reduced to several hundred femtoseconds, while the focal spot volume can be reduced by increasing the numerical aperture. Numerical aperture (NA) is increased by enlarging the beam diameter at the focusing optic or by shorting the focal length, which reduces the working distance.
6. A low energy and high NA is ideal for precision corneal cutting. However, deeper cutting within the crystalline lens needs a higher energy and lower NA, which expands the focal range of treatment, but compromises on the precision of cutting.

References

1. Hecht E, Zajac A. Optics. 4th ed. Amsterdam: Addison-Wesley Longman; 2003 (International edn.).
2. Csele M. Fundamentals of light sources and lasers. Hoboken, NJ: Wiley; 2004.
3. Iffländer R. Solid-state lasers for materials processing: fundamental relations and technical realizations. Berlin: Springer; 2001.
4. Cherry P, Faulkner J, Shaver R. Argon laser treatment of corneal neovascularization. Ann Ophthalmol. 1973;5(8):911–20.
5. Marsh R, Marshall J. Treatment of lipid keratopathy with the argon laser. Br J Ophthalmol. 1982;66(2): 127–35.
6. Bahn C, Vine A, Wolter J. Argon laser photocoagulation of a vitreo-corneal adhesion after trauma. Ophthalmic Surg. 1982;13(1):53–5.
7. Lans L. Experimentelle Untersuchungen ueber Entstehung von Astigmatismus durch nicht perforierende Corneawunden. Graefes Arch Clin Exp Ophthalmol. 1889;44:117–52.
8. Gruenberg P, Manning W, Miller D. Increase in rabbit corneal curvature by heated ring application. Ann Ophthalmol. 1981;13(1):67–70.
9. Horn G, Spears K, Lopez O. New refractive method for laser thermal keratoplasty with Co:MgF2 laser. J Cataract Refract Surg. 1990;16(5):611–6.
10. Shaw E, Gasset A. Thermokeratoplasty temperature profile. Invest Ophthalmol Vis Sci. 1974;13(1):181–6.
11. Koch DD, Abarca A, Villarreal R, Menefee R, Kohnen T, Vassiliadis A, Berry M. Hyperopia correction by noncontact holmium YAG laser thermal keratoplasty. Clinical study with two-years follow-up. Ophthalmology. 1996;103(5):731–40.
12. Boulnois JL. Photophysical processes in recent medical laser developments: a review. Lasers Med Sci. 1986;1(1):47–66. doi:10.1007/BF02030737.
13. Wolbarsht M, Foulks G, Esterowitz L. Corneal surgery with an Er:YAG laser at 2.94 μm. Invest Ophthalmol Vis Sci. 1986;27(suppl):93.
14. Peyman G, Badaro R, Khoobehi B. Corneal ablation in rabbits using an infrared (2.9 μm) Er:YAG laser. Ophthalmology. 1989;96(8):1160–70.
15. Trokel S, Srinivasan R, Braren B. Excimer laser surgery of the cornea. Am J Ophthalmol. 1983;96(6):710–5.
16. Solomon KD, Fernandez de Castro LE, Sandoval HP, et al. Joint LASIK Study Task Force. LASIK world literature review: quality of life and patient satisfaction. Ophthalmology. 2009;116(4):691–701.
17. Srinivasan R. Kinetics of the ablative photodecomposition of organic polymers in the far UV (193 nm). J Vac Sci Technol B. 1983;1(4):923–6.
18. Staveteig PT, Walsh Jr JT. Dynamic 193-nm optical properties of water. Appl Opt. 1996;35(19):3392–403.
19. Krueger RR, Trokel S, Schubert H. Interaction of ultraviolet laser light with the cornea. Invest Ophthalmol Vis Sci. 1985;26:1455–64.
20. Stuart BC, Feit MD, Herman S, Rubenchik AM, Shore BW, Perry MD. Nanosecond-to-femtosecond laser-induced breakdown in dielectrics. Phys Rev B Condens Matter. 1996;53(4):1749–61.
21. Kaiser R, Habib M, Speaker M. Mass spectrometry analysis of cavitation bubbles generated by intrastromal ablation with the Nd:YLF picosecond laser. Invest Ophthalmol Vis Sci. 1994;35(suppl):2026.
22. Heisterkamp A, Ripken T, Mamom T, Drommer W, Welling H, Ertmer W, Lubatschowski H. Nonlinear side effects of fs-pulses inside corneal tissue during photodisruption. Appl Phys B. 2002;74:1–7.
23. Mourou GA, et al. Optics in the relativistic regime. Rev Mod Phys. 2006;78:309.

24. Gaeta AL. Catastrophic collapse of ultrashort pulses. Phys Rev Lett. 2000;84:3582.
25. Fibich G, Gaeta AL. Critical power for self-focusing in bulk media and in hollow waveguides. Opt Lett. 2000;25:335.
26. Wilkes ZW, Varma S, Chen YH, Milchberg HM, Jones TG, Ting A. Direct measurements of the nonlinear index of refraction of water at 815 and 407 nm using single-shot supercontinuum spectral interferometry. Appl Phys Lett. 2009;94:211102.
27. Yamada K, Watanabe W, Toma T, Itoh K. In situ observation of photoinduced refractive-index changes in filaments formed in glasses by femtosecond laser pulses. Opt Lett. 2001;26:19–21.
28. Palanker DV, Blumenkranz MS, Anderson D, et al. Femtosecond laser-assisted cataract surgery with integrated optical coherence tomography. Sci Trans Med. 2010;2:58ra85.
29. Krasnov M. Laser phakopuncture in the treatment of soft cataracts. Br J Ophthalmol. 1975;59(2):96–8.
30. Aron-Rosa D, Aron J, Griesemann M, Thyzel R. Use of the neodymium-YAG laser to open the posterior capsule after lens implant surgery: a preliminary report. J Am Intraocul Implant Soc. 1980;6(4):352–4.
31. Vogel A, Busch S, Jungnickel K, Birngruber R. Mechanisms of intraocular photodisruption with picosecond and nanosecond laser pulses. Lasers Surg Med. 1994;15(1):32–43.
32. Ito M, Quantock AJ, Malhan S, Schanzlin DJ, Krueger RR. Picosecond laser-in-situ keratomileusis with 1057-nm Nd:YLF laser. J Refract Surg. 1996;12(6):721–8.
33. Netto M, Mohan RR, Medeiros FW, et al. Femtosecond laser and microkeratome corneal flaps: comparison of stromal wound healing and inflammation. J Refract Surg. 2007;23(7):667–76.
34. Binder PS. One thousand consecutive IntraLase laser in situ keratomileusis flaps. J Cataract Refract Surg. 2006;32(6):962–9.
35. Tran DB, Sarayba MA, Bor Z, et al. Randomized prospective clinical study comparing induced aberrations with IntraLase and Hansatome flap creation in fellow eyes. J Cataract Refract Surg. 2005;31(1):97–105.
36. Shah R, Shah S, Sengupta S. Results of small incision lenticule extraction: all-in-one femtosecond laser refractive surgery. J Cataract Refract Surg. 2011;37(1): 127–37.
37. Sekundo W, Kunert KS, Blum M. Small incision corneal refractive surgery using the small incision lenticule extraction (SMILE) procedure for the correction of myopia and myopic astigmatism: results of a 6 month prospective study. Br J Ophthalmol. 2011;95(3):335–9.
38. Farid M. Femtosecond laser-assisted corneal surgery. Curr Opin Ophthalmol. 2010;21(4):288–92.
39. Farid M, Steinert R. Deep anterior lamellar keratoplasty performed with the femtosecond laser zigzag incision for the treatment of stromal corneal pathology and ecstatic disease. J Cataract Refract Surg. 2009;35(5):809–13.
40. Kymionis G, Yoo S, Ide T, Culbertson W. Femtosecond-assisted astigmatic keratotomy for post-keratoplasty irregular astigmatism. J Cataract Refract Surg. 2009; 35(1):11–3.
41. Kim P, Sutton GL, Rootman DS. Applications of the femtosecond laser in corneal refractive surgery. Curr Opin Ophthalmol. 2011;22(4):238–44.
42. Alio JL, Shabayek MH, Belda JI, Correas P, Feijoo ED. Analysis of results related to good and bad outcomes of Intacs implantation for keratoconus correction. J Cataract Refract Surg. 2006;32(5):756–61.
43. Pinero D, Alio J, Uceda-Montanes A, El-Kady B, Pascual I. Intracorneal ring segment implantation in corneas with post-laser in situ keratomileusis keratectasia. Ophthalmology. 2009;116(9):1665–74.
44. Kubaloglu A, Cinar Y, Sari E, Ozdemir B, Ozerturk Y. Comparison of 2 intrastromal corneal ring segment models in the management of keratoconus. J Cataract Refract Surg. 2010;36(6):978–85.
45. Kanellopoulos AJ, Pe LH, Perry HD, Donnenfeld ED. Modified intracorneal ring segment implantations (Intacs) for the management of moderate to advanced keratoconus; efficiency and complications. Cornea. 2006;25(1):29–33.
46. Ruiz LA, Cepeda LM, Fuentes VC. Intrastromal correction of presbyopia using a femtosecond laser system. J Refract Surg. 2009;25(10):847–54.
47. Holzer MP, Mannsfeld A, Elmer A, Auffarth GU. Early outcomes of INTRACOR femtosecond laser treatment for presbyopia. J Refract Surg. 2009;25 (10):855–61.
48. Masket S, Sarayba M, Ignacio T, Fram N. Femtosecond laser-assisted cataract incisions: architectural stability and reproducibility. J Cataract Refract Surg. 2010;36 (6):1048–9.
49. Friedman NJ, Palanker DV, Schuele G, et al. Femtosecond laser capsulotomy. J Cataract Refract Surg. 2011;37(7):1189–98.
50. Naranjo-Tackman R. How a femtosecond laser increases safety and precision in cataract surgery? Curr Opin Ophthalmol. 2011;22(1):53–7.
51. Nagy Z, Takacs A, Filkorn T, Sarayba M. Initial clinical evaluation of an intraocular femtosecond laser in cataract surgery. J Refract Surg. 2009;25(12):1053–60.

Challenges of Femtosecond Laser Technologies for Cataract Surgery

4

Tibor Juhasz

Introduction

The ability to transmit light energy to almost any ocular structure, as well as the functional importance of vision, has continued to make the eye a favored target for laser surgery. Not surprisingly, newly developed laser technologies such as femtosecond (FS) lasers have undergone rapid development for ophthalmic surgery. FS lasers utilize photodisruption to mediate their surgical effects. Photodisruption is a complex, nonlinear process based on ionization in transparent tissue. As in inorganic materials, tissue photodisruption begins with laser induced optical breakdown (LIOB), when a strongly focused, short duration laser pulse generates a high intensity electric field, leading to the formation of a mixture of free electrons and ions that constitutes the plasma state [1]. The optically generated hot plasma expands with supersonic velocity, displacing surrounding tissue [1–5]. As the plasma expansion slows, the supersonic displacement front propagates through the tissue as a shock wave. The shock wave loses energy and velocity as it propagates, relaxing to an ordinary acoustic wave that dissipates harmlessly [6]. Adiabatic expansion of the plasma occurs on a time scale that is short in comparison to the local thermal diffusion time constant, thereby confining thermal damage. The cooling plasma vaporizes a small volume of tissue, eventually forming a cavitation bubble. The cavitation bubble consists mainly of CO_2, N_2, and H_2O, which can diffuse out from the tissue via normal mechanisms [7].

Photodisruption with the nanosecond-pulsed Nd:YAG laser was already well established clinically in the early 1980s for procedures such as posterior capsulotomy and internal sclerostomy [8]. These procedures were associated with relatively large collateral tissue damage zones due to the high energy threshold associated with the nanosecond pulse durations. Laser–tissue interaction studies have shown that the photodisruption threshold (and therefore the amount of laser energy deposited in the tissue) can be markedly decreased when the pulse duration is shortened to the hundred femtosecond range [9]. The decreased laser pulse energy results in smaller shock waves and cavitation bubbles, resulting in more precise tissue effects and minimized collateral tissue damage. Additionally, the development of compact diode-pumped FS laser technologies, such as Nd:glass and ytterbium (Yb) based laser crystals has further enabled commercial developments of FS laser technologies for ophthalmic surgery [10].

Although this book focuses on FS laser cataract surgery, it is useful first to review building blocks and operating principles for the corneal FS lasers that were developed a decade earlier.

T. Juhasz, Ph.D. (✉)
The Gavin Herbert Eye Institute
Department of Biomedical Engineering,
University of California, 118 Med Surge I,
Irvine, CA 92697-4375, USA
e-mail: tjuhasz@uci.edu; tjuhasz@lensxlasers.com

R.R. Krueger et al. (eds.), *Textbook of Refractive Laser Assisted Cataract Surgery (ReLACS)*,
DOI 10.1007/978-1-4614-1010-2_4, © Springer Science+Business Media, LLC 2013

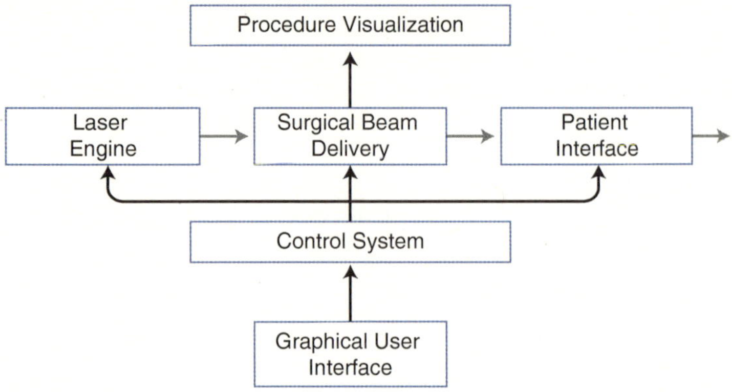

Fig. 4.1 The schematics of a corneal FS laser. The *vertical arrows* describe the information flow in order to control the system. The *horizontal arrows* describe the propagation of the laser beam

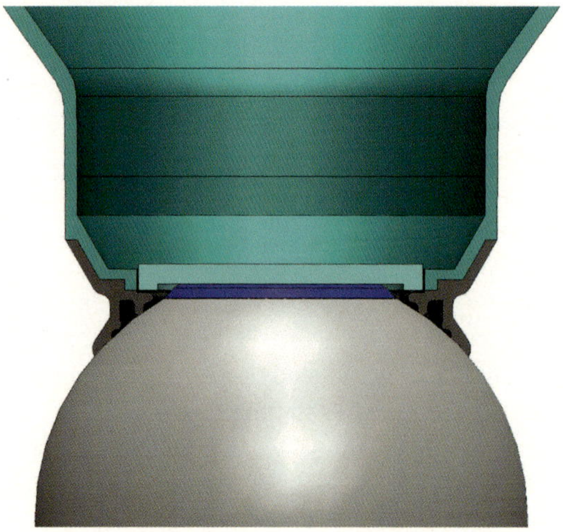

Fig. 4.2 The schematics of a flat applanating PI

Challenges of Femtosecond Laser Technologies for Corneal Surgery

The cornea presents an attractive initial target for FS laser surgical applications because it is easily accessible and lacks blood vessels. Only 500–600 μm thick centrally, the cornea allows delivery of femtosecond pulses with negligible nonlinear effects. The cornea is highly transparent in the near infrared region, up to 1.2 μm wavelength, allowing the use of the near infrared FS lasers without any restrictions.

The block diagram of a corneal FS laser is shown in Fig. 4.1. The most important building blocks are the laser source (or engine), the delivery system, the patient interface (PI), and the control system. A more detailed schematic of a flat applanating PI is shown in Fig. 4.2.

Since high precision cutting of the cornea requires the generation of cavitation bubbles that are <10 μm in diameter, the use of low energy laser pulses is necessary. This requirement puts a strong limitation on the pulse duration of the laser. Earlier investigations on the photodisruptive damage threshold on the surface of corneal tissue indicated that a considerable decrease of the damage threshold can be obtained as the pulse duration decreased from the nanosecond range to the hundred femtosecond pulse duration range [10]. Accordingly, the pulse duration of commercially available FS lasers ranges from 200 to 800 fs.

To minimize collateral tissue effects, the pulse energy of corneal FS lasers is best set as close as possible to the photodisruption breakdown threshold. While the first commercial lasers were introduced with pulse energies from 1 to 3 μJ, more recently corneal systems operate in the sub-microjoule energy range.

Since creation of a corneal flap requires many millions of laser pulses and since the shortest possible procedure time is desired, the repetition rate of corneal FS lasers must be very high. In fact, the pulse repetition rate has been the key technology driver during the development of corneal FS lasers. While the first FS laser had a repetition rate of 15 kHz at introduction (Intralase Inc., Irvine, CA), all systems now are marketed with much higher repetition rates, from 150 kHz up to the megahertz range (Ziemer AG, Port, Switzerland). While repetition rate is

Table 4.1 Summary of requirements and corresponding design parameters for corneal FS laser systems

Corneal laser requirement	Design parameter
Pinpoint accuracy	Small spot size, low laser pulse energy
Minimal collateral damage	Short pulse duration, high repetition rate
Consistent cutting quality in cornea	Homogeneous spot size distribution throughout cutting zone
Short distance to tissue	Short focal length, (high NA) optics
Need for globe stabilization and thin flaps	Mandating suction ring/ applanation PI device
Visualization needs	Surgical/video microscope

an important parameter, the procedure time is not necessarily inversely proportional with this value. Since lasers with higher repetition rates also utilize lower energy pulses that are placed closer to each other, a greater number of total pulses are required than lower repetition lasers, somewhat limiting the potential reduction in procedure time. While the procedure time for the first Intralase laser was approximately 1 min, most currently marketed lasers create flaps in approximately 10 s.

Although the FS laser source is the technologically most advanced building block of a corneal laser system, the beam delivery device is equally important and expensive. The most important property of the beam delivery device is the numerical aperture of the focusing objective that determines the spot size of the system. Achieving smaller spot size allows the system to use smaller laser pulse energies and provides higher flap depth precision. Therefore, the designers of all commercially available corneal FS laser systems try to achieve the smallest possible spot size allowed by the geometry of the human head. It is difficult to compare spot sizes of the different corneal lasers, since numerous definitions of the spot size are used in the literature, but most companies are quoting their system's spot size in the 2–3 μm diameter range. One of the most challenging difficulties of the beam delivery system design is achieving a homogeneous and distortion free spot size in the entire cylinder shaped scanning volume with usual dimensions of 10 mm in diameter and 1 mm in height. The beam is scanned within this volume using a three dimensional scanning system, with depth scanning (usually referred to as *Z* directional scanning) achieved by a moving lens, and lateral (*X–Y* scanning) achieved by angular movement of small mirrors attached to fast scanning motors. The numerical aperture (NA) of the FS laser pulse delivery, which depends on the focal distance and diameter of the last focusing lens, must be within a range of 0.1–0.3 in order to achieve the appropriate laser spot size for corneal applications.

The spatially confined surgical effect of the FS laser, together with the fine spatial control of the focal spot with respect to the corneal surface, allows the execution of highly precise cuts in the cornea. To accomplish this, all corneal procedures also utilize a suction ring and a contact lens (flat or curved) located at the tip of the laser delivery system. The suction ring fixates the eye, allowing the corneal anterior surface to temporarily assume the curvature of the contact glass (see Fig. 4.2). The depth of the cut is calibrated relative to the lower surface of the contact glass, which provides a reference surface for the calibration of the laser, achieving depth precision of <10 μm [11]. A flap is created by scanning a spiral or raster pattern of laser pulses at the desired depth to create a resection plane parallel to the applanated corneal surface. An arc is then scanned with progressive movement closer to the surface to create a hinged side-cut. Following creation of the flap, the suction ring is released and the applanating contact lens removed. The flap is then elevated to facilitate excimer laser treatment. The design parameters for the corneal FS laser technology are outlined in Table 4.1.

Clinical studies indicate that reproducible 100 μm thick corneal flaps can be created for laser in situ keratomileusis (LASIK) surgery [11]. The accuracy and reproducibility of FS laser flaps generally surpasses those created with traditional mechanical microkeratomes, thereby enabling more consistent outcomes and safety [11, 12].

Since 2001, several corneal FS laser systems have been introduced, primarily for LASIK flap

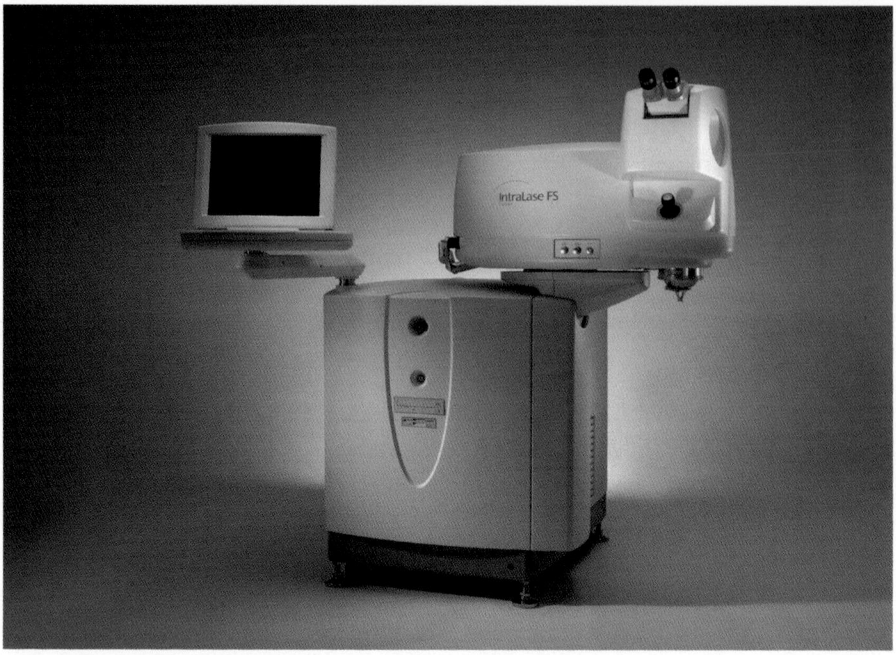

Fig. 4.3 The photograph of the IFS FS Laser. This device performed the highest number of corneal flap cutting procedures in LASIK surgery

creation [12]. Although there are several new devices available on the market today, the majority of flap cutting procedures are still performed by one of the various generations of the Intralase device (Abbott Medical Optics, Santa Ana, CA). The newest version of this technology, the IFS FS Laser is shown in Fig. 4.3.

While flap creation is the most common application of the corneal FS lasers, several stand-alone refractive procedures that use only the FS laser are under clinical investigations. These include removal of laser-cut lenticules [13], as well as the combination of direct volumetric tissue destruction and corneal biomechanical changes induced by selective FS laser treatment [14].

In addition to refractive corneal procedures, corneal FS laser technology has also been evaluated for a variety of corneal transplantation procedures. Faster visual rehabilitation and improved refractive outcomes have been reported when FS laser cuts were used to create self sealing corneal cuts in full thickness corneal transplantation surgery [15].

Technical Challenges of Femtosecond Laser Development for Cataract Surgery

Cataract surgery with intraocular lens implantation is the most common ophthalmic surgical procedure worldwide. It is also the most common surgery that corrects refractive error, performed over five times more frequently than that of corneal refractive surgery [16]. Phacoemulsification is the dominant form of cataract surgery in developed countries, accounting for over 90% of procedures. [17, 18]. While there have been a number of recent developments in intraocular lens technology, the basic phacoemulsification procedure has remained largely unchanged over the past 20 years, involving a series of individual steps including corneal incision creation, capsulorrhexis, and phacofragmentation.

Although highly successful, each of these manual steps presents an opportunity for improvement in both safety and effectiveness. For example, in experienced hands (rates for resident surgeons are much higher—see Chap. 2

for a detailed discussion), manual capsulorrhexis results in capsular tears in approximately 1% of cases, and limitations in the accuracy of size and shape can affect intraocular lens centration, postoperative anterior chamber depth, and posterior capsular opacification rates [19–22]. Separately, the surgical challenges posed by nuclear chopping techniques have hindered widespread adoption, despite evidence that they reduce ultrasound requirements relative to traditional phacoemulsification [23].

The precision of FS lasers can potentially be directed towards the various steps in cataract surgery [9, 24–27]. In the next few paragraphs, we summarize the technical challenges of FS laser cataract surgery and discuss differences between cornea-only and cataract FS laser surgical systems.

Among the several important differences between corneal and cataract laser surgical systems, the most important is the difference in the targeted tissue. By definition, corneal lasers target only corneal tissue, while cataract lasers have three tissue targets: the crystalline lens, the anterior lens capsule, and the cornea. This obviously drives major differences in technical requirements, since corneal systems deliver laser energy only to approximately 150 μm depth, while cataract systems are required to cut tissue located as deep as 8 mm from the corneal surface. Since laser energy needs to be delivered much deeper into the eye, any loss of power that occurs during beam propagation must be compensated by the laser source. Due to limitations in the focusing cone angle when the crystalline lens or the lens capsule is targeted, the achievable laser spot size is also larger in the lens than in the cornea, further contributing to the need for larger laser energy for cuts in the crystalline lens. Although decreases in the required laser energy may occur as delivery system technology improves, currently the use of pulse energies in the 10 μJ range are required in the lens (versus 1 mJ in the cornea) [28].

While corneal cuts can be performed with the same spot size the system produces in the lens, a smaller spot size in the corneal cuts using smaller laser pulse energies is desirable, which we know from our corneal laser experience. Therefore, the development of a delivery system that can deliver a variable focusing cone angle may be desirable, though this introduces considerable additional complexity for the surgical beam delivery system.

Since the anterior chamber depth and the lens thickness vary from patient to patient, there is a clear necessity for an accurate ranging device that locates the exact position of the surgical target. To date, all FS laser cataract surgery systems have incorporated a ranging device in some form of optical imaging. Three companies (Alcon LenSx Inc., Aliso Viejo, CA; OptiMedica Corp., Santa Clara, CA; and Technolas Perfect Vision AG, Munich, Germany) use optical coherence tomography (OCT) technology, while one company (LensAR Inc., Winter Park, FL) uses a confocal laser imaging device, called 3-D Confocal Structured Illumination (CSI) to locate the targeted tissue. After obtaining the image of the anterior segment of the eye, some level of image processing is necessary in order to locate and visualize the targeted tissue. Thus, the block diagram of a cataract surgical laser, shown in Fig. 4.4, is more complex than that of the corneal laser, with the addition of a high precision 3D imaging system coupled to the beam delivery device and an image processing and visualization unit that provides information to the user and feeds back to the control system. While accurate cross calibration in between the imaging and the beam scanning devices is important, the resolution requirement of the 3D imaging device is determined by the surgical beam delivery device. Since the depth of focus of the surgical beam focusing objective is approximately 10 μm, the imaging resolution requirement need not be any greater than this value.

The markedly increased beam delivery range and the addition of the 3D imaging device increase the complexity of the cataract laser beam delivery system. Clearly, the most complex building block of the cataract laser is the beam delivery device and its development represents a major challenge to optical engineers.

The higher pulse energy requirement increases the average power of the laser source to several

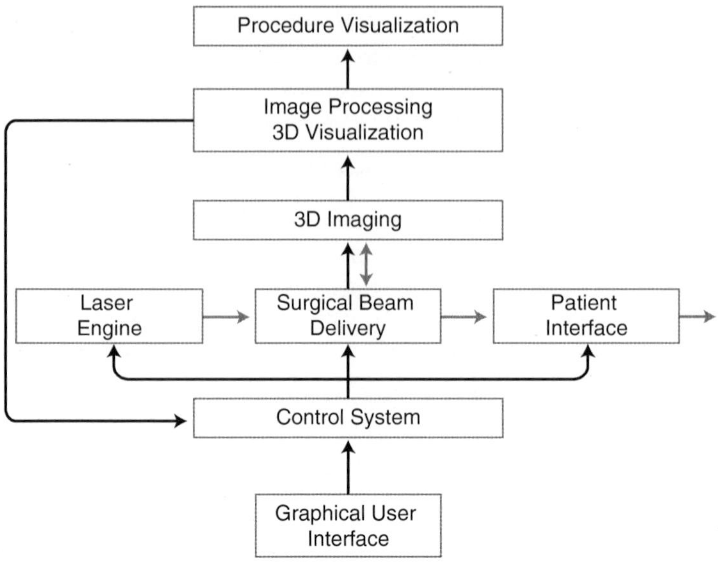

Fig. 4.4 The schematics of a cataract FS laser. The *blue arrows* describe the information flow in order to control the system. The *brown arrows* describe the propagation of the laser and measurement beams

Table 4.2 Summary of requirements and corresponding design parameters for cataract FS laser systems

Cataract laser requirement	Design parameter
Deeper treatment	Longer focal length (lower NA) optics, larger spot size
Higher ablation energy, more tissue volume to treat	More powerful laser
Corneal and LRI incisions	Large field of view for beam delivery
Locating lens and lens capsule	Need for high precision 3D imaging
Proximity of delicate structures	Establishment of safety zones
Visualization needs	Surgical/video microscope, 3D imaging device

times higher than that of a corneal laser engine. The development of higher power, compact laser sources represents another major challenge for development engineers. Since the maximum average power generated by the a specific laser material is limited by available pump power and the thermal characteristics of the laser material, cataract lasers operate at lower repetition rates than corneal systems. To date, repetition rates from 50 kHz up to 80 kHz have been reported for cataract surgery laser systems. The design parameters for the cataract FS laser technology are outlined in Table 4.2.

Since procedure times for cataract surgery are somewhat longer than that for corneal flap cutting and since cataract patients are generally older, any increase in intraocular pressure should be minimized during the laser procedure. This requirement precludes the use of a flat applanating PI. Some commercially available cataract surgery devices now use a curved applanating surface. Although the radius of curvature of the PI is selected to be close to that of the cornea, the inherent mismatch may produce slight corneal wrinkles at the posterior surface of the cornea. Initial experience with the LenSx system indicates however that these corneal wrinkles do not significantly influence beam focusing and/or the cutting quality of the surgical beam. This can be easily understood since the index of refraction difference between the aqueous humor and the cornea is small, and thus, the corneal wrinkles do not introduce large changes in the wave front of the surgical beam. Additionally, the diameter of the surgical beam at the corneal plane is relatively large when the laser is focused onto the lens, and thus, the occasional corneal wrinkle interacts only with a small portion of the surgical beam.

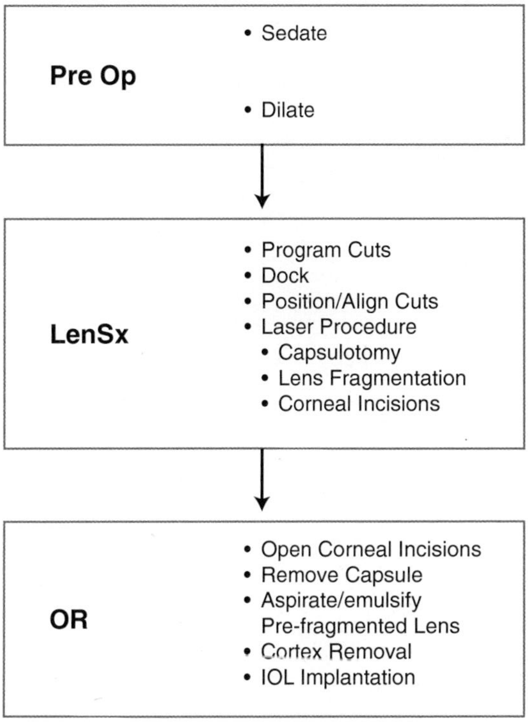

Fig. 4.5 The flow diagram of the FS laser cataract surgery

In order to eliminate corneal wrinkles competing companies (LensAR and OptiMedica) have promoted the use of a PI that is filled with an index matching liquid. The liquid PI fills the gap between the eye and the delivery optics with a liquid, leaving the cornea close to its native shape and avoiding corneal wrinkles. While there is a heated discussion among competing companies about the two interface designs, there will be the responsibility of the community of cataract surgeons to decide which PI works better for the patient.

Once the eye is docked to the beam delivery device and the globe is stabilized by applying suction to the PI, the position of the corneal surfaces and the posterior and anterior lens capsule is determined using the 3D imaging device. Once scanning of the eye with the imaging device is completed, image recognition software can be used to determine the position of the corneal surfaces, anterior and posterior lens capsule. Different cross sectional images of the eye can also be displayed, with the planned surgical cuts visualized on the images. The user can approve the position of the cuts or change their locations using a graphical user interface. If significant tilt exists in the position of the lens relative to the cornea, the docking of the interface can be released and reattempted in order to improve the alignment. Some systems use software to compensate for angle of tilt in the pattern of laser delivery.

Once the positions of the cuts are accepted by the surgeon, the laser procedure is initiated by pressing the footswitch. Capsulorrhexis, lens fragmentation, and corneal cuts are performed by the scanning system while the user observes the procedures through a video or optical microscope. The flow diagram of the FS laser cataract surgery is shown in Fig. 4.5.

Safety margins to prevent damage to the lens capsule are implemented for cuts performed inside the crystalline lens. Unlike the large shock and acoustic waves generated by ultrasonic phacoemulsification devices, that can be associated with capsular and endothelial cell damage [29–32], those generated by FS photodisruption dissipate within approximately 30 μm of the targeted lens tissue [33]. The laser wavelength is also not absorbed by the cornea, and the maximum fluence at the level of the retina is approximately five times less than the multiple shot damage threshold determined by Schumacher [34]. These findings are consistent with the safety record established by FS laser corneal surgery systems with several million procedures being performed during the past decade.

Figure 4.6 displays images of the first commercial FS lasers introduced specifically for cataract surgery. Figure 4.6a is the LenSx Laser from Alcon LenSx, Fig. 4.6b is the LensAR laser and Fig. 4.6c is the OptiMedica Catalys laser system. Comparing these images to that of the corneal laser (Fig. 4.3), the addition of the image visualization screen is apparent. A comparison of Figs. 4.1 and 4.4 reveals additional differences in the building blocks of the systems, with corneal FS lasers not yet having incorporated imaging and image processing components. The differences in key design parameters for corneal and cataract FS lasers are detailed in Table 4.3.

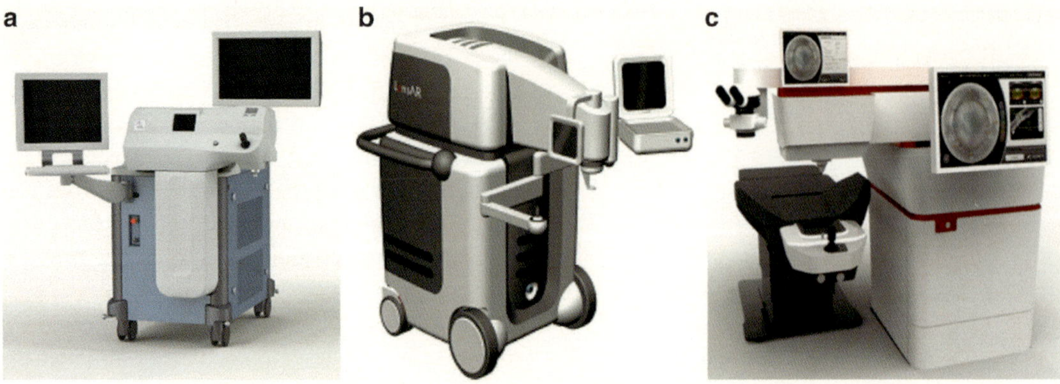

Fig. 4.6 The photograph of three publicly revealed cataract FS lasers. (**a**) The LenSx FS Laser System, (**b**) the LensAR FS Laser System, (**c**) the OptiMedica FS Laser System

Table 4.3 Comparison of basic design characteristics of corneal and cataract FS laser technologies

	Cornea lasers	Cataract lasers
Wavelength	1,030–1,060 nm	1,030–1,060 nm
Pulse duration	200–800 fs	600–800 fs
Pulse energy	1 μJ or less	8–15 μJ
Repetition rate	60–250 kHz	33–80 kHz
Scanning range	10 mm diameter	12 mm in diameter
	1 mm in depth	8 mm in depth
3D imaging	No	Yes

For example, the laser engine of the corneal laser produces laser pulses with sub-microjoule energies but at very high repetition rates, while the laser source of the cataract laser produces pulses in the 10 μJ energy range which is currently possible only at moderate repetition rates. Similarly, there are major differences in the performance of the delivery system, with corneal lasers delivering pulses usually to a depth of 100–150 μm, while the cataract lasers deliver laser energy as deep as 8 mm.

While the complexity of FS laser technology for cataract surgery is high and, therefore, represents a major barrier to market entry, the high initial market response to laser cataract surgery has led several companies to develop competing technologies. The ophthalmic community will benefit from this diversity, which will drive continued development of FS laser cataract technologies in the years to come.

Challenges for Cataract Femtosecond Laser Technology Users

While technology advances continue to benefit patients, it is important to remember that surgeons are still the key requirement for excellent surgical outcomes. Surgeons must decide when and how to apply FS laser technology. Unlike LASIK surgery, where cases could be aborted prior to flap elevation, cataract surgery must be completed following laser application. For this reason, patients should be treated only as they are about to enter, or are already in, the operating room. Due to limitations in ocular anatomy and/or pupil dilation status, successful delivery of laser pulses may not always be possible for all procedure steps in all patients. Surgeons must be ready and able to complete surgical procedures manually, with the same level of skill that they now use during traditional cataract surgery. Surgeons must also be open to changes in technique that best take advantage of laser-performed steps or avoid potential problems. It is likely that the surgical techniques surrounding laser cataract surgery will evolve at an even faster pace than the technology itself.

Key Points

1. Cataract FS lasers are advanced surgical laser technologies capable of performing high precision incisions in the crystalline lens, lens capsule, and cornea.
2. Well known characteristics of FS laser technology are high precision and minimized collateral tissue damage.
3. A major advance in the last few years is high resolution 3D imaging technology to aid the surgeon with incision placement and ensure safety.
4. It is likely that rapid development of the technology and surgical techniques related to the technology will strongly benefit the ophthalmic community and cataract surgery patients in the years to come.

References

1. Bloembergen N. Laser-induced electric breakdown in solids. IEEE JQE. 1974;10:375–86.
2. Fujimoto JG, Lin WZ, Ippen EP, Puliafito CA, Steinert RF. Time-resolved studies of Nd:YAG laser-induced breakdown. Invest Ophthalmol Vis Sci. 1985;26:1771–7.
3. Zysset B, Fujimoto JG, Puliafito CA, Birngruber R, Deutsch TF. Picosecond optical breakdown: tissue effects and reduction of collateral damage. Lasers Surg Med. 1989;9:193–204.
4. Vogel A, Hentschel W, Holzfuss J, Lauterborn W. Cavitation bubble dynamics and acoustic transient generation in ocular surgery with pulsed neodymium:YAG laser. Ophthalmology. 1986;93:1259–69.
5. Glezer EN, Scaffer CB, Nishimura N, Mazur E. Minimally disruptive laser induced breakdown in water. Opt Lett. 1997;23:1817.
6. Voegel A, Schweiger P, Freiser A, Asio MN, Birngruber R. Intraocular Nd:YAG laser surgery: light–tissue interactions, damage-range and reduction of collateral effects. IEEE J Quant Electron. 1990;26:2240–60.
7. Habib MS, Speaker MG, Shnatter WF. Mass spectrometry analysis of the byproducts of intrastromal photorefractive keratectomy. Ophthalmic Surg Lasers. 1995; 26:481–3.
8. Steinert RF, Puliafito CA. The Nd:YAG laser in ophthalmology. Philadelphia, PA: Saunders; 1985.
9. Loesel FH, Niemz MH, Bille JF, Juhasz T. Laser-induced optical breakdown on hard and soft tissues and its dependence on the pulse duration. IEEE J Quant Electron. 1996;32:1717–22.
10. Juhasz T, Loesel FH, Kurtz RM, Horvath C, Bille JF, Mourou G. Corneal refractive surgery with femtosecond lasers. IEEE J Select Top Quant Electron. 1999;5:902–10.
11. Slade SG, Durrie DS, Binder PS. A prospective, contralateral eye study comparing thin-flap LASIK (sub-Bowman keratomileusis) with photorefractive keratectomy. Ophthalmology. 2009;116(6):1075–82.
12. Sutton G, Hodge C. Accuracy and precision of LASIK flap thickness using the IntraLase femtosecond laser in 1000 consecutive cases. J Refract Surg. 2008;24:802–6.
13. Sekundo W, Kunert K, Russmann C, Gille A, Bissmann W, Stobrawa G, Sticker M, Bischoff M, Blum M. First efficacy and safety study of femtosecond lenticule extraction for the correction of myopia: six-month results. J Cataract Refract Surg. 2008;34(9):1513–20.
14. Ruiz LA, Cepeda LM, Fuentes VC. Intrastromal correction of presbyopia using a femtosecond laser system. J Refract Surg. 2009;25(10):847–54.
15. Steinert RF, Ignacio TS, Sarayba MA. "Top hat"-shaped penetrating keratoplasty using the femtosecond laser. Am J Ophthalmol. 2007;143(4):689–91.
16. Comprehensive report on global single-use ophthalmic surgical product market. Market Scope; 2009.
17. Leaming DV. Practices styles and preferences of ASCRS members—2003 survey. J Cataract Refract Surg. 2004;30:892–900.
18. Leaming DV. Practices styles and preferences of ASCRS members—2001 survey. J Cataract Refract Surg. 2002;28:1681–8.
19. Marques FF, Marques MV, Osher RH, Osher JM. Fate of anterior capsule tears during cataract surgery. J Cataract Refract Surg. 2006;32:1638–42.
20. Dick HB, Pena-Aceves A, Mannis A, Krummeanauer F. New technology for sizing the continuous curvilinear capsulorhexis: prospective trial. J Cataract Refract Surg. 2008;34:1136–44.
21. Norrby S. Sources of error in intraocular lens power calculation. J Cataract Refract Surg. 2008;34:368–76.
22. Hollick EJ, Spalton DJ, Meacock WR. The effect of capsulorhexis size on posterior capsular opacification: one-year results of a randomized prospective trial. Am J Ophthalmol. 1999;128(3):271–9.
23. Can I, Takmaz T, Cakici F, Ozgül M. Comparison of Nagahara phaco-chop and stop-and-chop phacoemulsification nucleotomy techniques. J Cataract Refract Surg. 2004;30:663–8.

24. Vogel A, Schweiger P, Frieser A, Asiyo MN, Birngruber R. Intraocular Nd:YAG laser surgery: light–tissue interaction, damage range, and reduced collateral effects. J Quant Electron. 1990;26:2240–60.
25. Juhasz T, Kastis G, Suárez C, Turi L, Bor Z, Bron WE. Shockwave and cavitation bubble dynamics during photodisruption in ocular media and their dependence on the pulse duration. In: Jacques SL, editor. Laser–tissue interactions. VIIth ed. Proc SPIE 1996;2681:428–36.
26. Kurtz RM, Liu X, Elner VM, Squier JA, Du D, Mourou G. Photodisruption in the human cornea as a function of laser pulse width. J Cataract Refract Surg. 1997;13:653–8.
27. Seitz B, Langenbucher A, Homann-Rummelt C, Schlötzer-Schrehardt U, Naumann GOH. Non-mechanical posterior lamellar keratoplasty using the femtosecond laser (femto-PLAK) for corneal endothelial decompensation. Am J Ophthalmol. 2003;136:769–72.
28. Nagy Z, Takacs A, Filkorn T, Sarayba M. Initial clinical evaluation of an intraocular femtosecond laser in cataract surgery. J Refract Surg 2009; 25(12):1053–60.
29. Shin YJ, Nishi Y, Engler C, Kang J, Hashmi S, Jun AS, Gehlbach PL, Chuck RS. The effect of phacoemulsification energy on the redox state of cultured human corneal endothelial cells. Arch Ophthalmol. 2009;127(4):435–41.
30. Murano N, Ishizaki M, Sato S, Fukuda Y, Takahashi H. Corneal endothelial cell damage by free radicals associated with ultrasound oscillation. Arch Ophthalmol. 2008;126(6):816–21.
31. Storr-Paulsen A, Norregaard JC, Ahmed S, Storr-Paulsen T, Pedersen TH. Endothelial cell damage after cataract surgery: divide-and-conquer versus phaco-chop technique. J Cataract Refract Surg. 2008;34(6):996–1000.
32. Richard J, Hoffart L, Chavane F, Ridings B, Conrath J. Corneal endothelial cell loss after cataract extraction by using ultrasound phacoemulsification versus a fluid-based system. Cornea. 2008;27(1):17–21.
33. Juhasz T, Kastis GA, Suarez C, Bor Z, Bron WE. Time-resolved observations of shock waves and cavitation bubbles generated by femtosecond laser pulses in corneal tissue and water. Lasers Surg Med. 1996;19:23–31.
34. Schumacher S, Sander M, Stolte A, Doepke C, Baumgaertner W, Lubatschowski H. Investigation of possible fs-LASIK induced retinal damage. In: Södergerg PG, Ho A, Manns F, editors. Ophthalmic technologies. XVI ed. Proc SPIE 2006;6138:61381I-1–61381I-9.

5 Imaging Systems and Image-Guided Surgery

Stephen D. Klyce, Daniel V. Palanker,
Keith H. Edwards, and Ronald R. Krueger

Major advances have been made in applied imaging techniques in ocular diagnostics and surgery. While traditional slit lamp biomicroscopy still forms the mainstay of the ocular examination, approaches have been developed to determine the shape of the cornea (topography), to determine the total eye aberrations (wavefront aberrometry), and to refine retinal imaging resolution with adaptive optics. Further refinements in optical coherence tomography (OCT) have transitioned this technology from the time domain to the spectral or Fourier domain, an approach now standard of care for retinal diagnostics. Furthermore, its success in the posterior segment is now making its way to the anterior segment, so that OCT is becoming a standard three-dimensional imaging technique. At the same time, Scheimpflug imaging with the high depth of field it provides has been instrumental to extend corneal pachymetry from 1–3 dimensions. Similarly, confocal microscopy has enhanced the resolution of slit examination so that single cell morphology can be observed and corneal infections routinely identified.

The introduction of the femtosecond (FS) laser to ocular surgery has added precision, speed, and safety to LASIK flap creation. With the current efforts to apply the FS laser to cataract surgery, new imaging strategies have been developed to meet the challenge.

Background

In order to use the FS laser for cataract surgery, precise imaging of the anterior and posterior lens capsule surfaces is necessary along with accurate range determination to locate the position of these structures within the eye. This requires accurate determination of the anterior lens capsule position, as well as the greater challenge of finding the posterior capsule location behind the light scattering of the dense nuclear sclerotic, sometimes brunescent, cataract. Delivering laser energy to the posterior capsule can cause its rupture with the potential for vitreous loss and lens nucleus drop. Short pulse (FS) lasers can provide precise photodisruption without significant collateral damage and the utilization of this precision is therefore dependent on the ability to image and locate the target structures accurately.

S.D. Klyce, Ph.D., F.A.R.V.O. (✉)
Department of Ophthalmology, Mount Sinai School of Medicine, 5 North Court, Port Washington, NY 11050, USA
e-mail: sklyce@klyce.com

D.V. Palanker, Ph.D.
Department of Ophthalmology, Stanford University, 452 Lomita Mall, Stanford, CA 84305, USA

K.H. Edwards, F.C.Optom., Dip.C.L.P.
Clinical & Regulatory Affairs, LensAR Inc., 2800 Discovery Drive, Orlando, FL 32826, USA

R.R. Krueger, M.D., M.S.E.
Cole Eye Institute, Department of Refractive Surgery, Cleveland Clinic Lerner College of Medicine, Cleveland, OH 44106, USA

R.R. Krueger et al. (eds.), *Textbook of Refractive Laser Assisted Cataract Surgery (ReLACS)*,
DOI 10.1007/978-1-4614-1010-2_5,

In optical imaging technologies, resolution is often limited by the numerical aperture (NA, or angle of convergence) of the imaging optics. Therefore, imaging deep inside the eye, which usually requires lower NA, often implies lower resolution. In OCT, however, axial resolution does not depend on NA, but is rather determined by the coherence of the beam and spectral resolution of the interferometer. This provides an opportunity for optical imaging deep inside the eye and with high axial resolution. However, the axial range of imaging in the Frequency Domain OCT is limited by the spectral width of the radiation.

For cataract surgery, a clear view must be obtained from the corneal surface (the reference plane from which distances are measured) to beyond the posterior capsule. Equally important is the specification of the field of view. For imaging during cataract surgery, the field of view must be at least as wide as the diameter of the dilated pupil. However, if relaxing incisions are also contemplated, the field of view must encompass from limbus to limbus. These requirements can present significant challenges for the imaging system, particularly as mentioned above through a cataractous lens of varying opacification. Current optical systems have an adequate field of view, but a sufficiently long depth of field, to be able to image from anterior cornea to posterior lens, can be challenging. One method to achieve the requisite imaged volume is to "stitch" multiple scans together to produce a mosaic of the required width and depth of image, but resolution and positional accuracy may be compromised even with significant image processing. With spectral domain OCT, recent advances suggest that scan depths of over 7 mm may be achieved with an axial resolution of 6 μm in an experimental system [1]. This can also be extended further with improvement of the light sources. The axial distance between the corneal surface and the posterior capsule is close to 7 mm, which can make this approach viable for ReLACS. It is particularly important for any system developed for this application to achieve high contrast with high signal to noise ratio to allow the landmark structures to be identified while retaining relevant detail within the structures being imaged.

Imaging Requirements

The anterior surface of the cornea is normally used as the biometric reference plane from which distances to the lens surfaces are measured. Its structure and dimensions are also important if surgical and keratotomy incisions are to be made with the laser. Imaging the whole of the anterior chamber in detail will require inclusion of the cornea which varies in thickness on average from approximately 515 μm centrally to 600 μm or more in the periphery [2]. Anterior chamber depth measurements from clinical cataract studies have shown that a cataract population of 880 eyes had a mean (±SD) anterior chamber depth of 3.08 (±0.056) mm [3]. Lens thickness is known to vary with age, but in 932 eyes of cataract patients, the lens thickness was 4.52 (±0.57) mm [3]. The human lens capsule has a minimum thickness of between 8 and 10 μm at the anterior apex and approximately 4-μm minimum thickness at the posterior apex [4, 5]. At other locations the capsule is thicker and there is an age-dependent thickening except for the posterior apex which remains fairly constant [5].

For the focal laser energy shots to be placed safely within the lens without penetrating the posterior capsule, while at the same time precisely creating an intended anterior capsulotomy, the imaging system must be capable of simultaneously identifying the surfaces of the structures in question. In order for this to be achieved automatically, robust image feature recognition algorithms must developed. If the imaging system is poor and fails to determine the interfaces with sufficient reliability, the minimum safety margin that is required to protect the capsule from the impact of the laser generated bubbles and acoustic waves will need to be increased substantially to ensure safety, and the effectiveness of the treatment will consequently be decreased. The same considerations apply to making full or partial thickness corneal incisions where precision of the incisions placement will depend on the quality of the metrics acquired by the imaging system.

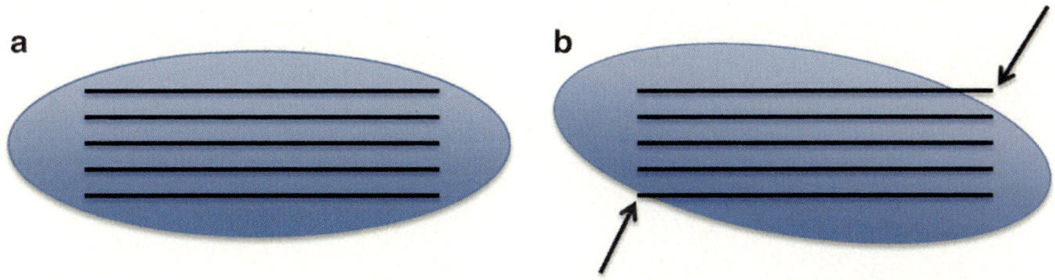

Fig. 5.1 Effect of lens tilt on treatment placement. (**a**) Untilted lens. Treatment pattern represented by *horizontal lines* fits within the capsular bag without encroachment on the capsule. (**b**) Tilted lens of the same dimensions. Treatment pattern of the same dimensions now encroaches on the anterior and posterior capsule due to the tilt (*arrows*). Image courtesy of Keith Edwards

One major challenge to anterior segment imaging systems and to the laser cataract treatment is the iris behind which light-based imaging is blind. Even with a dilated pupil, a significant part of the lens remains un-imaged and assumptions have to be made about the anatomy of the lens behind the iris. Furthermore, treatment can only be conducted within the dilated pupillary area. High frequency ultrasound is the only currently known technology that can image through ocular tissues such as the iris, but this has not currently been adapted to ReLACS.

Lens tilt can be a significant issue for the treatment, if the cutting patterns are not properly aligned. Some imaging and laser systems use a reference surface within the laser interface to determine the relative location of structures in space. If the laser patterns are horizontal this may cause issues when the lens is tilted relative to the plane of the cornea or the laser reference plane. Figure 5.1a shows how a treatment of standard dimensions, when placed in an untilted lens, maintains the prescribed capsular clearance. In Fig. 5.1b, the capsular bag and treatment pattern are of the same standard dimensions, but the tilt of the lens results in the pattern breaking through both anterior and posterior capsules. It is therefore critical that the imaging system can detect lens tilt and allow the modification of the treatment pattern orientation and its dimensions to maintain the safety margins around the lens capsule. Without proper compensation for lens tilt, the minimum separation distance between the apparent lens capsule and the laser shot will need to be increased substantially to ensure safety in the presence of an indeterminate amount of lens tilt. Decreasing the depth of laser treatment will reduce the treatment effectiveness. For lens tilt to be determined, an image of sufficient quality must be created that allows the apex and curvature of the surfaces to be determined so that the system can model the lens in its entirety.

If the outlines of the lens anterior and posterior apices can be determined with high resolution, then the optical axis of the lens can also be identified, which then gives the surgeon additional information regarding the placement of the capsulotomy center. Currently, surgeons tend to center the capsulotomy over the center of the dilated pupil, since its boundary is the most convenient guidance line during surgery. Since the center of the physiologic constricted pupil may not be coincident with that of a dilated one, shifting by as much as 0.6 mm nasally [6], additional landmarks may be needed for proper capsulotomy and lens centration. One strategy would be to identify the optical axis of the lens, and then center the capsulotomy over this lens optical axis in order to closely align the IOL to the same location as the optical axis of the crystalline lens that was removed. Alternatively, the capsulotomy and IOL may be centered beneath the center of the physiologic constricted pupil, which is especially important for symmetry and alignment of the multiple diffraction fringes in multifocal IOLs. With either strategy, the most important aspect is to optimize the IOL centration and effective lens position, so as to enhance the predictability of early outcomes, and minimize the long-term shifting of the lens with capsular fibrosis by the symmetry of centration and circularity the capsulotomy. Although the best centration strategy is

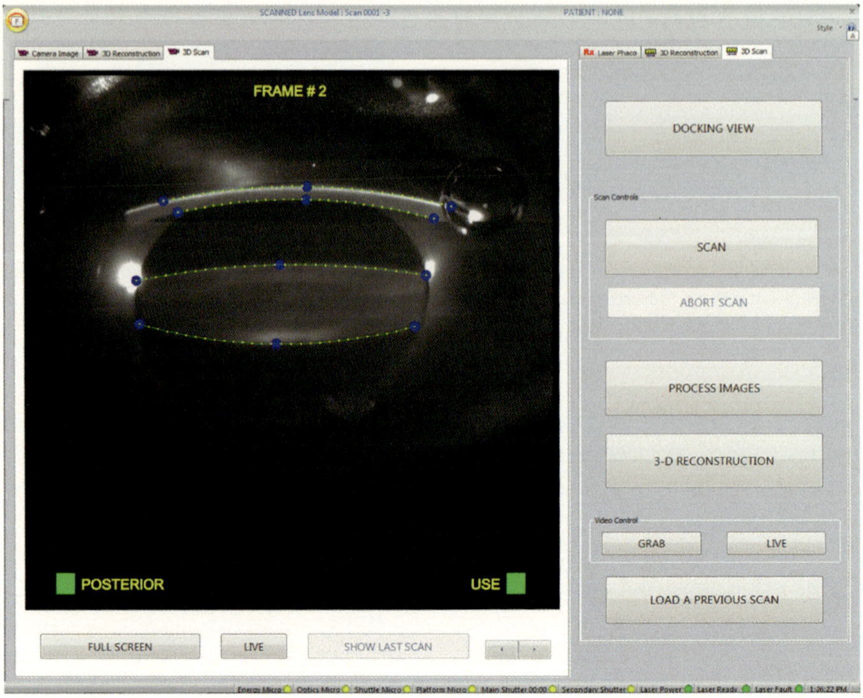

Fig. 5.2 Single video frame of a LensAR 3D-CSI scan with corneal and lens surfaces automatically located. Image courtesy of Keith Edwards

not known at this time, for the first time this technology should provide the means to examine and to resolve this issue.

Imaging Technology

The imaging systems available for use in laser cataract surgery applications are optical. Both OCT and a combined optical approach described below as 3D confocal structured illumination have proven viable solutions to the imaging challenges posed by ReLACS.

The combined optical method of 3D-CSI is being implemented by LensAR Inc. (Winter Park, FL) under the trade name "Augmented Reality". The phrase "augmented reality" is described in Wikipedia as "a live view of a physical, real-world environment whose elements are augmented by computer generated sensory input". This well describes 3D-CSI, where a super luminescent diode (SLD) is used to create the infrared light that illuminates the eye. By scanning the illumination beam across the surfaces, different scan rates can be applied to surfaces of different reflectances to maintain good exposure across the area of interest. A high-speed, wide field of view video camera records the image employing the Scheimpflug principle to maintain an in-focus image from anterior cornea to posterior lens. A single optical section of the eye is captured on a single video frame (see Fig. 5.2). Several images are taken at different angles to the illumination beam to detect differences in surfaces across the various meridia. Using the principle of structured illumination with patterned light to enhance resolution, the LensAR system creates multiple images that are used to construct a 3D model of the anterior segment and lens (see Fig. 5.3). By combining the imaging and laser treatment into a single optical pathway, this confocality assures that shots are delivered accurately to the precise spot that is imaged.

The LenSx and the OptiMedica cataract lasers utilize OCT to determine the locations of the lens surfaces. There are many variations and recent advances in optical coherence tomography, but the basic principles all rely on interferometry.

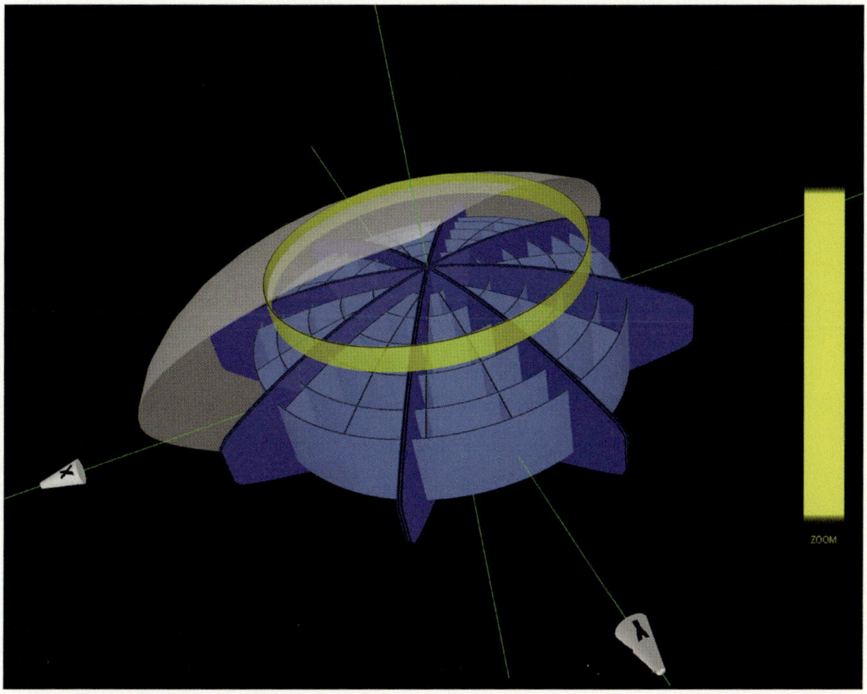

Fig. 5.3 Multiple slice images of the anterior segment are combined to form a 3D model of the anterior segment (LensAR system). Image courtesy of Keith Edwards

Interference fringes are obtained when the axial distance, the distance to and from the tissue being imaged, matches that of a reference beam. In time-domain OCT, the reference arm is scanned to provide mapping along an axial line (A-scan) while two-dimensional images (B-scans) can be created by scanning the beam laterally across the tissue, acquiring an axial scan at every location and combining this into a single image.

Time domain OCT is relatively slow and requires scanning of the reference arm in time. Frequency domain (FD) OCT obtains an axial map of the tissue scattering from the spectrum of the interferogram. Thereby the information of the full A scan can be acquired within a single exposure. In a swept source OCT, the wavelength of the illumination light is rapidly changing with time (time-encoded frequency), which eliminates the need of a spectrometer. FD OCT significantly improves imaging speed and signal to noise ratio, but may limit the scanning range or resolution.

The OptiMedica system integrates the novel FD OCT, the video microscope and the FS laser to enable image-guided cataract surgery [7, 8]. The axial resolution of the FD OCT in OptiMedica's system is 11 μm. After the OCT image is acquired, the system automatically delineates the surfaces of the cornea and lens, as shown in Fig. 5.4. On a cross-sectional image of the anterior chamber, the system also depicts the safety zones (approximately 0.5 mm from posterior capsule and iris) where laser pulses will not be placed. Treatment patterns for anterior capsulotomy, lens segmentation and nucleus softening are then displayed for surgeons' review and approval. In addition, system provides a live frontal view of the eye via video camera, to allow lateral alignment of the laser patterns.

The LenSx system also uses a novel OCT, video microscope, and FS laser to enable image-guided cataract surgery. The system provides real-time cross-sectional images of the anterior segment, extending from the corneal epithelium to beyond the posterior lens capsule (see Fig. 5.5). The cross-sectional view of the lens is taken along the cylindrical surface of a circular scan of OCT, and "unwrapped" to show a flat representation of it on the display.

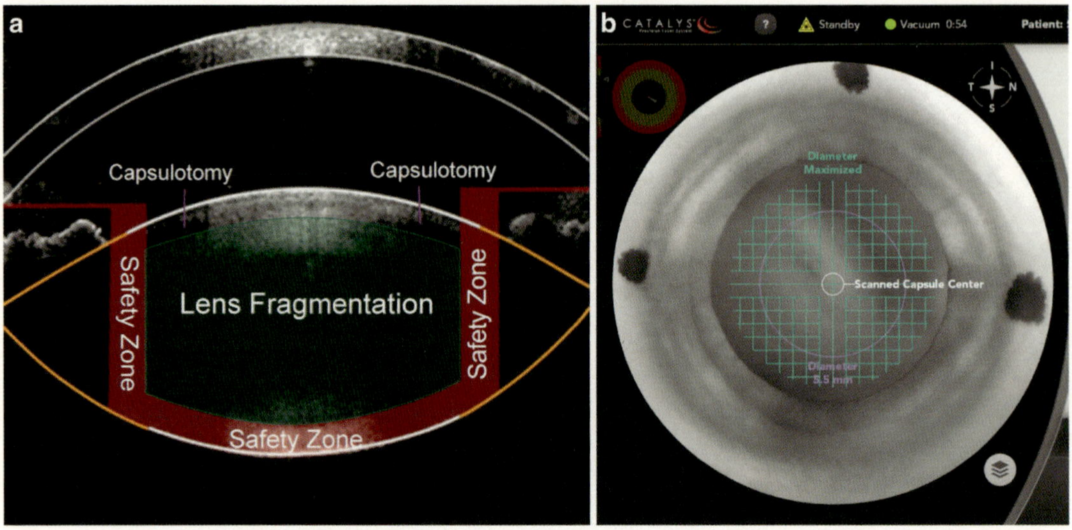

Fig. 5.4 (**a**) Cross-sectional view of the anterior segment and lens obtained with OptiMedica Catalys™ system. Boundaries of the lens and cornea in OCT image are automatically identified and delineated. A safety zone (*red*) is applied approximately 0.5 mm from the posterior capsule and the iris. Image courtesy of Daniel Palanker. (**b**) Frontal view of the patient's eye with overlayed patterns for capsulotomy (*magenta*) and lens segmentation (*green*). On the same view patterns for corneal incisions can be displayed. Image courtesy of Daniel Palanker

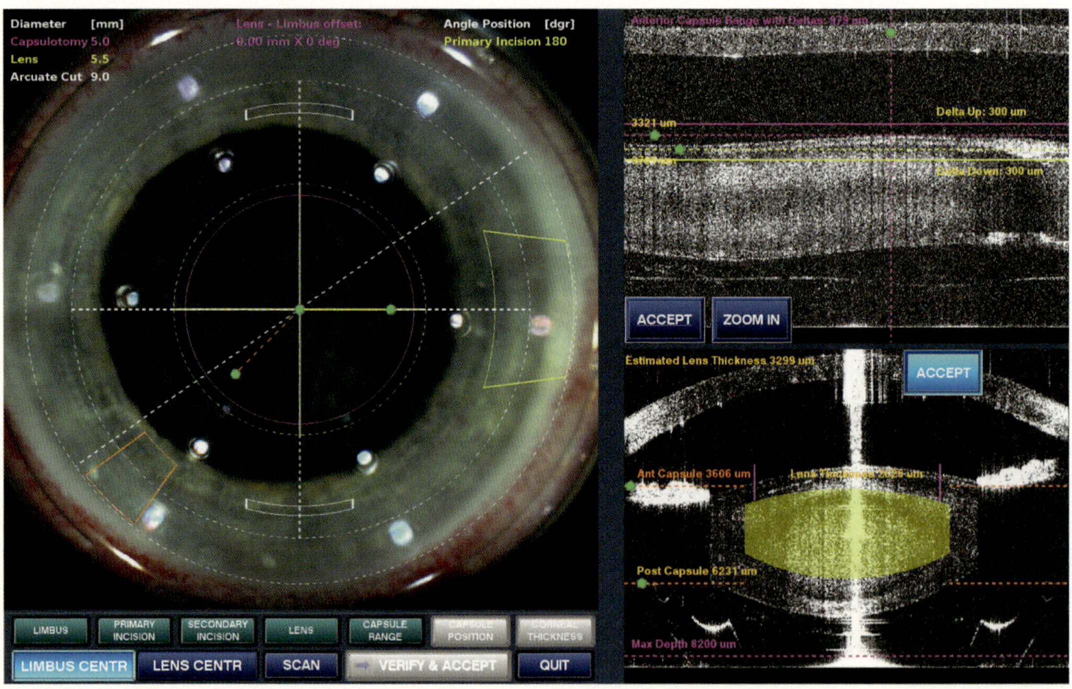

Fig. 5.5 With the LenSx system, live images from the video microscope and OCT are used to align the patient's eye with the system during docking. The laser treatment patterns are then positioned onto the high resolution OCT video images in three dimensions. Image courtesy of Eric Weinberg, Alcon LenSx Lasers, Inc.

It is very important to maintain a high quality optical interface between the optical system and patient's cornea. This is accomplished by the patient interface (PI) device, and is discussed in great detail in Chap. 6. Typically, this interface includes a flat or spherical applanation lens and a suction ring along its edge. Since corneal curvature varies from patient to patient, even a curved optical interface often introduces folds on the posterior surface of the cornea. These folds may distort the laser beam and affect the quality of the imaging and laser cutting and should be taken into account in the system designs. Such distortions can be avoided using a liquid optical interface, where the cornea does not touch any hard surface, but rather is immersed in a thin layer of fluid. This technique is implemented in both the LensAR and OptiMedica Catalys™ systems.

Image Enhancement

In order to obtain the appropriate images of suitable quality for intraocular dimensional analysis, some image enhancement is often required. Conflicting requirements can make the acquisition of a suitable image difficult.

When attempting to increase the range of OCT to reach the posterior surface of the lens, the necessary increase in depth of field may sacrifice quality by increasing the signal to noise ratio. Loss of image quality makes the accurate localization of surfaces more difficult. Image enhancement techniques may improve the quality of the image, but the estimated position of the posterior capsule may lose accuracy due to the particular method of contrast enhancement. Commonly, the algorithms used to sharpen or enhance the contrast of images involve averaging of neighboring pixel intensities that generally degrade resolution, and must take this issue into account to maintain accuracy. Additionally, for OCT images having detectors with a wide dynamic range such as the anterior segment of the eye, the brightness of the corneal surface and points of specular reflection on the ocular axis can be reduced to improve visibility of the other surfaces.

One of the greatest imaging challenges is detecting the posterior capsule through a fairly dense cataract. Grade 3 and 4 cataractous lenses scatter a significant amount of light and ordinary slit imaging is inadequate to view the whole lens. A popular solution to this challenge is the use of near-IR illumination light for OCT or other imaging modalities, since scattering greatly decreases with increasing wavelength ($1/\lambda^4$ for Rayleigh scattering).

Another method that has been used to "see through" translucent tissues with light is confocal microscopy. With this scheme, a narrow pin hole or slit is placed in front of the detector, in the conjugated plane of the illumination spot on the object. This rejects light scattered from outside of the focal plane, thereby significantly reducing the amount of glare from the scattering object.

A further challenge to lens imaging is the fact that the various interfaces of the anterior segment have varying contrast and reflectance. Hence, methods must be found to create an adequate image exposure for the highly reflective and bright corneal surfaces as well as the low reflective surfaces of the anterior and posterior lens capsule. One solution used in laser cataract systems is a scanning imaging source that reduces the illumination intensity for brightly reflective surfaces and increases it for the lower reflective surfaces. This method, which is the "structured illumination" of 3D confocal structured illumination (3D CSI), allows a single video frame to show a uniformly exposed image of the anterior segment without image enhancement.

Image Processing

Once images of the anterior ocular structures have been captured, it is necessary to delineate the tissue surfaces and assign treatment zones for placement of various laser patterns. It is important to provide sufficiently detailed imaging in order to properly detect the lens shape and orientation in space, such as a tilt or a shift. For the Scheimpflug methods of capture in 3D CSI imaging, several images obtained from different meridia must be registered to form a 3D reconstruction. The detection and identification of the various interfaces, including the anterior and posterior corneal surfaces and the anterior and posterior capsule, can be achieved manually or automated. Manual identification can be performed by placing a series of cursors on the corneal and lens surfaces, which are then connected to obtain the curvature of the surface. In the OptiMedica and LensAR systems this identification is performed automatically. In the LenSx system, the laser patterns are pre-positioned automatically as well, with added flexibility that the user can still make any desired adjustments. A 3D model of the anterior segment can be generated using the imaging data and the preoperative biometric data, such as the anterior and posterior radii of curvature for cornea and lens, the corneal and lens axial thicknesses and the anterior chamber depth. Care should be taken when considering the use of imaging data prior to docking since the eye may be significantly deformed by the suction ring and/or applanation interface of the surgical system.

If, in the strategy of laser pulsing, the photodisruption is commenced within a closed capsule (i.e., if lens fragmentation is executed before the capsulotomy), the position of the capsule will have to be reestablished prior to cutting the capsulotomy, since the gas generated from photodisruption will distend the capsule. If the capsulotomy is conducted first, this is not an issue, since the minute quantity of gas generated during the capsulotomy does not significantly displace the lens orientation within the eye.

Laser Placement and Energy Requirements

The ideal system will use image-guided laser treatment so that the laser shots are directly placed according to the 3D model obtained from the imaging system. For this to be most effective, the imaging and treatment systems should be properly co-registered. One way of achieving this capability is having the imaging and cutting beams coaxial and confocal. This is accomplished by using the same optical pathway and having a common focus, so that there are no systematic errors between the imaging and laser placement systems.

The laser energy, pulse repetition frequency and shot spacing will need to be tailored to the specific laser being used and the tissue being treated. One may need to have a range of alternative parameters in order to deal with the vast range of tissue properties of crystalline lenses of different degrees of hardness. The laser energy delivered must be above the threshold of dielectric breakdown (plasma formation) in order to create the necessary cleaving of tissue. However, excess energy may be counter-productive, due to the increased roughness of the cut edge, especially in capsulotomy [8]. Since the threshold of dielectric breakdown increases with pulse duration [9], laser systems with longer pulse widths use higher energy, which may affect the quality of the tissue cutting, due to an increased zone of rupture by larger photodisruption bursts and expanding cavitation bubbles.

In the OptiMedica system, pulses from 3 to 10 μJ are typically applied with lateral spacing, varying from 5 to 10 μm, and axial spacing, from 10 to 20 μm in different ocular tissues [7, 8]. In general, the FS laser patterns typically include a spiral for capsulotomy, and various multiplanar cross patterns for lens segmentation to facilitate a chop technique. In addition, nucleus fragmentation patterns typically involve a denser mesh, with spacing of the vertical and horizontal cutting planes on the order of 1 mm to fragment the lens into pieces small enough to be aspirated during the cataract surgery. This is with the ultimate goal of reducing or eliminating the need for phacoemulsification.

The need for ocular safety limits the average laser power for tissue cutting, due to cumulative heating. This ultimately limits the pulse repetition rate [7]. Since dense placement of the laser pulses is required for continuous cutting, care should be taken to properly design the tissue segmentation patterns that on one hand, allow for greater ease in removing segmented tissues, but on the other hand, are able to accomplish the segmentation within a reasonably short amount of time. For example, with a pulse repetition rate of 50 kHz, the nucleus fragmentation pattern is composed of rectangles of 1 mm in width, and includes ~360,000 spots that require about 7 s for delivery [7].

Image-Guided Safety Zones

In addition to the safety limits of laser power and pulse repetition rate, there are also safety zones, beyond which laser spots cannot be applied; these need to be established with each laser system. The two main safety zones that are required for image-guided cataract surgery are (1) the margin within the iris pupillary border and (2) the safety zone anterior to the posterior lens capsule (see Fig. 5.4a). The former margin is necessary for defining the maximum safe capsulotomy diameter and most peripheral extent of nucleus fragmentation, while the latter defines the maximum depth of laser pulses within the crystalline lens to maintain a safe zone from the posterior capsule.

When establishing a safe zone, the individual parameters of the laser and resolution of the imaging system must be considered in order to maintain safety, while maximizing therapeutic benefit. For both the clearance zone from the iris/pupillary border and the posterior capsule, a minimum distance of 0.5 mm is generally targeted. In general, the FS laser software may be customized to create a thicker posterior epinuclear plate or "safety zone" of 0.75 mm or more that protects the posterior capsule from inadvertent puncture by instruments or sharp nuclear fragments in brunescent cataracts. It is only with the precision of image-guided surgery that one can define the target tissues and direct the laser pulses along these subtle margins. In the future, as more surgeons become familiar with the technology, further strategies and techniques for optimizing safety and efficacy during the steps of capsulotomy and nucleus fragmentation will be developed to take full advantage of the versatility of FS laser assisted refractive cataract surgery.

Summary

For refractive laser assisted cataract surgery to meet its full potential, it is crucial to have the proper imaging system that determines where the laser pulses will be placed. High quality, high contrast images with high signal to noise ratios are a prerequisite for determining the precise location of the target (lens, cornea, and/or other ocular structure). Optical methods must cope with the wide range of focusing depth required, as well as with the need to record the image, despite variations in light scatter and the broad reflectance range of the differing ocular structures. In particular, imaging systems should have the capability to "see" through brunescent cataracts in order to be useful for the range of patients normally encountered. Accurate image analysis is crucial to the outcome, with identification of anterior segment structures relying on either manual placement of measurement cursors on surfaces or automatic determination through feature recognition algorithms.

The image-guided optical system must cope with factors such as lens tilt, and provide sufficient information to allow for extrapolating the lens shape and position behind the iris, through which the existing systems cannot penetrate. Sophisticated ray tracing algorithms must be implemented in order to properly take into account refractive index variations within the anterior segment.

Laser assisted cataract surgery has emerged as a major technological step forward to enhance the safety and efficacy of cataract removal, intraocular lens placement, wound construction, and astigmatism management. This technology relies heavily on state of the art imaging techniques for accurate placement of the laser treatment shots. This technology can provide multiple benefits for cataract surgery. It allows for exact placement and sizing of the capsulotomy. It should prove to reduce substantially the higher risk of the procedure in elastic pediatric capsules or in elderly patients with soft zonules. The continuous sharp-edged capsular cuts will reduce the likelihood of radial nicks or tears, or zonular dehiscence.

Improved strength of the capsule after laser capsulotomy could reduce the risk of its rupture during phacoemulsification and IOL insertion. Lens segmentation and nucleus fragmentation simplify its emulsification and reduce the phaco energy, especially with dense cataracts. In addition, the multiplanar self-sealing cataract incision and exact placement of the limbal relaxing incisions have the potential to bring cataract surgery to the precision and reproducibility previously attainable thus far only in refractive corneal laser surgery. It is up to ophthalmic surgeons to embrace this advance for the benefit to our patients.

Key Points

1. Accurate placement of laser shots depends upon high resolution imaging of the anterior segment from the corneal surface to the posterior capsule of the lens.
2. Current FS lasers developed for cataract surgery achieve high resolution imaging through advanced OCT technology or with a novel three dimensional confocal structured illumination approach.
3. Accurate imaging of potential lens tilt is essential to prevent inadvertent encroachment of the capsular bag.
4. Clear imaging of the posterior capsule through brunescent cataracts is a requisite for safe fragmentation to provide an accurate clearance zone.

Acknowledgements This work was supported in part by an unrestricted grant from Research to Prevent Blindness Inc., New York, NY (SDK, RRK).

References

1. Shen M, Wang MR, Yuan Y, Chen F, Karp CL, Yoo SH, Wang J. SD-OCT with prolonged scan depth for imaging the anterior segment of the eye. Ophthalmic Surg Lasers Imaging. 2010;41(Suppl):S65–9.
2. Prospero Ponce CM, Rocha KM, Smith SD, Krueger RR. Central and peripheral corneal thickness measured with optical coherence tomography, Scheimpflug imaging, and ultrasound pachymetry in normal, keratoconus-suspect, and post-laser in situ keratomileusis eyes. J Cataract Refract Surg. 2009; 35(6):1055–62.
3. LensAR clinical study data—on file (data were collected using an applanation ultrasound method from older cataract patients in a predominantly Asian eye population).
4. Ziebath NM, Manns F, Uhlhorn SR, Venkatraman AS, Parel J-P. Noncontact optical measurement of lens capsule thickness in human, monkey and rabbit postmortem eyes. Invest Ophthalmol Vis Sci. 2005;46(5): 1690–7.
5. Barraaquer RI, Michael R, Abreu R, Lamarca J, Tresserra F. Human lens capsule thickness as a function of age and location along the sagittal lens perimeter. Invest Ophthalmol Vis Sci. 2006;47(5):2053–60.
6. Wilson MA, Campbell MC, Simonet P. The Julius F Neumueller award in optics, 1989: change of pupil centration with change of illumination and pupil size. Optom Vis Sci. 1992;69(2):129–36.
7. Palanker DV, Blumenkranz MS, Andersen D, Wiltberger M, Marcellino G, Gooding P, Angeley D, Schuele G, Woodley B, Simoneau M, Friedman NJ, Seibel B, Batlle J, Feliz R, Talamo J, Culbertson W. Femtosecond laser-assisted cataract surgery with integrated optical coherence tomography. Sci Transl Med. 2010;2:58ra85.
8. Friedman NJ, Palanker DV, Schuele G, Andersen D, Marcellino G, Seibel BS, Batlle J, Feliz R, Talamo JH, Blumenkranz MS, Culbertson WW. Femtosecond laser capsulotomy. J Cataract Refract Surg. 2011;37(7): 1189–98.
9. Vogel A, Venugopalan V. Mechanisms of pulsed laser ablation of biological tissues. Chem Rev. 2003;103:577 [Erratum: Chem Rev 2003;103:2079].

The Patient Interface: Setting the Stage for Treatment

6

Katrina Bell Sheehy and Jonathan H. Talamo

The Definition and Significance of Patient Interfaces for Femtosecond Laser Assisted Cataract Surgery

> An interface is a surface that forms a common boundary between two things. In the case of laser eye surgery, the patient interface (PI) is the location where surgical laser technology couples to and interacts with the eye (target tissue).

In laser cataract surgery, a PI allows the optical laser system to couple to the eye for image-guided treatments. "Docking" has been described in laser-assisted in situ keratomileusis (LASIK) flap creation as the process of moving an applanation cone connected to a femtosecond (FS) laser down into the suction ring stabilizing the globe, where the cone can then applanate the cornea and allow precise focusing of laser energy within the corneal stroma. For the purposes of this text, docking is the process by which the eye and laser system are prepared and coupled prior to treatment. In corneal FS laser applications, docking is critical because a bad, poorly centered, or incomplete flap can lead to complicated surgery. *Docking is* equally *critical for laser assisted cataract surgery: it is the first surgical "point of touch" between the surgeon and patient*, and one that is not part of traditional lens removal and intraocular lens insertion. Mastery of the docking procedure can quickly set the tone for the rest of the surgery. The design of the PI can enhance both the ease of use for docking and accuracy of laser treatment.

The objectives of this chapter are to:

- Provide a historical overview of the use of PIs in ophthalmology as a paradigm for the evolution of current FS laser cataract technology.
- Define important attributes of PIs for laser cataract surgical applications.
- Describe and compare PIs of commercially available laser cataract platforms.
- Provide clinical considerations and guidance for docking from early experience with laser cataract systems.

K.B. Sheehy, B.S., M.S. (✉)
Product Marketing, OptiMedica,
3100 Coronado Dr., Santa Clara, CA 95054, USA
e-mail: ksheehy@optimedica.com

J.H. Talamo, M.D.
Harvard Medical School, Talamo Laser Eye Consultants,
Reservoir Place, Suite 184, 1601 Trapelo Rd., Waltham,
MA 02451, USA

R.R. Krueger et al. (eds.), *Textbook of Refractive Laser Assisted Cataract Surgery (ReLACS)*,
DOI 10.1007/978-1-4614-1010-2_6,

Historical Uses and Purposes of Patient Interfaces in Ophthalmology

Diagnostic and Therapeutic Uses of Patient Interfaces

There is a long history of PI usage in ophthalmology to stabilize, magnify, and position the eye for diagnostic and therapeutic applications, including indirect ophthalmoscopy, gonioscopy, retinal photocoagulation, iridotomy, capsulotomy, and trabeculoplasty, to name a few.

PIs have been used for diagnostic analysis of ocular tissues in both posterior and anterior segments of the eye. Retinal diagnostics started with indirect ophthalmoscopes to neutralize the power of the cornea in order to visualize the back of the eye. PIs for gonioscopy evolved over the twentieth century to provide better views of internal structures and more convenient exam techniques [1]. In 1915, Maximillian Salzmann found that a highly convex lens could be used to overcome total internal reflection to view the iridocorneal angle [2]. Direct gonioscopy was difficult due to patient positioning and slit lamp requirements so in 1938, Goldmann introduced the mirrored contact lens for indirect gonioscopy [3]. To improve ease of use, the Allen-Thorpe gonioprism included flanges to hold the lens in place so as to free the hands of the examiner [4].

PIs for most therapeutic ophthalmic laser applications have been used in conjunction with the slit lamp. Retinal photocoagulation introduced new PI requirements: not only to keep the eyelids open but to steady the eye, and avoid exposing the optic nerve and fovea to laser energy. Contact lenses for laser photocoagulation were developed to match the average corneal radius of curvature, provide a good fit and stabilize the eye. Coupling directly to the eye with the contact lens caused irritation of the corneal epithelium and patient discomfort, so topical gel and anesthetic drops were introduced as part of the early evolution of PIs. Optic coatings and manufacturing techniques were developed for PIs to reduce reflections and improve both transmission and focusing for laser therapeutic applications. With the emergence of the Q-switched YAG laser, contact lens interfaces were used to hold the eye in place and provide added central magnification power for better focusing. For angle closure glaucoma, laser iridotomy lenses have offset power magnification to allow the laser emission to be directed at the peripheral iris with the eye's position in primary gaze. Even in these fairly advanced (and now routine) laser treatments for retinal disease, glaucoma and posterior opacification, the application of and control over the PI has been a skill that surgeons must hone through repetitive training.

When contact ultrasound imaging was adopted as a modality for obtaining axial length measurements, corneal tissue compression and the need to optimize the signal-to-noise ratio together introduced new PI challenges, since small deviations in the hand-held contact applanation technique required by these devices could induce large measurement errors. In response, non-applanating immersion probes were developed to index-match corneal tissue, and reduced the technical skill needed to reproducibly apply the probe to the cornea. The use of an immersion fluid bath allowed the probe to be suspended at a fixed angle and distance with respect to the corneal surface, with the added benefits of eliminating reflections from the corneal surface, improving the speed of ultrasound transmission, and maintaining the amplitude of the ultrasound wave entering and exiting the eye more so than its passage through air [5].

Evolution of Docking: From Refractive Surgery to Cataract Surgery

Our modern concept of docking for laser cataract surgery derives from corneal refractive surgery with FS lasers, so an understanding of the PIs for such devices is important. There are now at least five commercially available systems for corneal laser surgery: iFS (Abbott Medical Optics, Irvine, CA), Wavelight Ultraflap (Alcon/Wavelight, Fort Worth, TX), VisuMax (Carl Zeiss Meditec, Inc., Dublin, CA), FEMTO LDV™ Femtosecond Surgical Laser (Ziemer,

Table 6.1 Comparison on chart of requirements for FS laser LASIK vs. laser cataract surgery

	Treatment depth from corneal epithelium	Treatment plane	Treatment diameter	Imaging required	Optical system includes posterior cornea
LASIK	100–130 μm	Uniplanar 2-D	9 mm or less	No	No
Cataract	Up to 7.5 mm (7,500 μm)	Multiplanar 3D	Up to 12 mm	Yes	Yes

Port, Switzerland), and FEMTEC (Technolas Perfect Vision, Munchen, Germany).

Increased accuracy and precision requirements have driven the sophistication of coupling for corneal FS laser procedures, such as LASIK flap creation, astigmatic incisions, channels for intracorneal rings and corneal transplantation. Supine patient positioning has led to automation of portions of the docking process with controls for vacuum and system/bed motion. To improve ease of use and suction ring placement, some systems have a multipiece design with a suction ring that first attaches to the eye and then mates with an applanation cone while others use a single piece design that couples the system with the eye. To address differences in patient orbital anatomy, some manufacturers developed interfaces in multiple sizes [6].

PIs for FS corneal flap cutting applanate the cornea with a flat or curved lens to stabilize the globe, create a reference surface for treatment, and allow the laser system to focus. A reference surface is used to create a consistent flap thickness, eliminating the need for integrated imaging systems to track the eye's position in the *x*, *y* and *z* axes to guide laser energy delivery. In 2011, feasibility for applanation-free imaging and treatment of the cornea (referred to as "processing") was described in which a contact liquid layer is used with a confocal positioning system and FS laser itself rather than conventional OCT [7].

New Patient Interface Requirements for Refractive Laser Assisted Cataract Surgery (ReLACS)

New requirements have emerged for PIs intended for based on the diameter and depth of the laser treatment zone and on older patient demographics than corneal refractive surgery patients (see Table 6.1 for a comparison on chart of requirements for FS laser LASIK vs. laser cataract surgery).

Laser treatment zones for cataract surgery are different than for LASIK, and for this reason laser cataract surgery optical systems are different in several important ways from those used only for corneal surgery:

1. *Treatment is deeper inside the eye*. In ReLACS, laser pulses need to be placed as deep into the eye as the posterior portion of the crystalline lens and as peripheral as the corneal limbus. The focal depth requirements alone for ReLACS are far greater than those required for LASIK. More specifically, if one assigns a value of 0.12 mm (120 μm) for a LASIK flap compared with a distance of nearly 8 mm from the corneal surface to the posterior lens capsule of an average eye (assumes an average cornea thickness of 0.55 mm, AC depth of 3.2 mm and lens thickness of 4.05 mm [8, 9]), an FS laser must treat as much as 65 times deeper than for LASIK in order to effectively segment a cataractous lens.
2. *Treatment occurs in 3D*. Lens and corneal incisions for cataract surgery require complex three-dimensional geometries that must be image-guided and controlled. A larger treatment volume introduces the need to avoid ocular anatomical landmarks such as iris and posterior lens capsule, where FS laser pulses could cause damage or induce extra-surgical risk.
3. *Treatment diameter is wider*. Corneal incisions for cataract surgery also require a larger diameter of visible treatment area, extending out to 11–12 mm at the limbus, as compared with the central 9 mm for flaps [10, 11]. As such, a wider field of view than needed for LASIK is

required to allow for flexibility in the interface application and docking processes.

4. *Treatment times are longer*. All corneal, capsule, and lens incisions require larger treatment volumes and therefore more treatment time, as compared with the time needed to cut a flap, even if the laser repetition rate is increased substantially. As such, immobilization of the eye is of paramount importance.
5. *The cornea becomes part of the laser's optical system*. Lastly, treating through the cornea to access the capsule and cataractous lens means that the cornea becomes an integral part of the optical system. There has been a significant amount of research evaluating the optical aberrations contributed by the human anterior cornea [12] and a few papers that examine the contribution of the posterior surface to astigmatism, spherical aberration and coma [13–15]. The posterior stroma is known to easily develop folds based on its more widely spaced collagen fiber structure as compared to the tighter cohesive anterior stroma, and folds affect Descemet's membrane to become visible as striae [16]. Both anterior corneal surface irregularities and posterior corneal folds must be minimized or accounted for when focusing the laser to achieve precise incisions in the posterior cornea and lens.

The Cataract Patient Population

The laser cataract surgery patient population also has some important differences from the LASIK patient populations that are typically young and lack co-morbidities. The most apparent difference is the range of ages treated and a much older average patient age for cataract surgery. In the United States, more than 25% of people aged 65–69 have cataracts and the percentage grows to over 70% for those over 80 years [17]. Age brings with it a number of potentially complicating factors. Frail patients or those facing mobility challenges may require special considerations during head and neck positioning for both stabilization and comfort. In some populations, 25% of cataract patients have preexisting glaucoma [18]. Many will also have cardiac, peripheral vascular, or cerebrovascular disease.

There have been rare reports of acute elevations in IOP during LASIK causing optic nerve injury [19–22]. Studies examining IOP rises during various steps in the docking and laser treatment have been performed and have shown IOP greater than 90 mmHg during suction time [23–25]. Porcine and rabbit models have allowed careful analysis of IOP during suction application, suction phase, and flap cutting, showing that weak applanation with a curved interface results in less IOP rise over baseline than with strong applanation with a flat lens [26, 27]. While blood-flow responses have been shown to quickly return to normal levels in healthy eyes once suction is released, high IOP rises during ophthalmic procedures should be avoided in older patients because of the increased risk of optic nerve damage or vascular (central retinal artery or vein) occlusion [28]. Additionally, patients on anticoagulants may be more sensitive to docking and more susceptible to subconjunctival hemorrhaging [29]. While not heavily reported in the literature, a final consideration is the ocular surface, as the corneal epithelium tends to adhere less firmly in the elderly, and contact applanation devices may be more prone to cause epithelial disruption. Loose epithelium may impair laser energy transmission as well as increase discomfort and prolong visual recovery after surgery.

Important Attributes of Patient Interfaces for Laser Assisted Cataract Surgery

The functionality of the PI directly influences the safety and efficacy of laser cataract surgery. Mechanical stability of the globe and excellent optical quality are important attributes that allow the laser system to satisfy surgeon and patient expectations of efficacy and safety. Sterility and comfort are also essential. Additional important factors for the surgeon are ergonomics, reliability and economics (see Table 6.2).

Table 6.2 Important interface attributes

Optical system	Patient	Surgeon
• Optical quality • Mechanical stability	• Safety • Accuracy • Comfort • Sterility	• Ergonomics • Reliability • Economics

System Requirements: Optical Quality and Mechanical Stability

Optical Quality

The most important function of the PI is optical: the interface must ensure that the laser pulses are delivered as intended to the desired location for the desired effect. Optical systems are characterized by the location, type and size of each optic. The manufacturers of laser cataract surgical systems have spent years designing the optics of laser systems, but these devices will not function well unless coupling to the eye is performed correctly, and this last critical step is left to the surgeon to perform. When the laser system is coupled to the eye, the cornea becomes part of the optical system used to treat the capsule and lens. The patient–laser interface must allow for integration of the cornea with the optical system function in two directions: to optimize the incoming wavefront for high quality imaging of intraocular anatomy as well as subsequent outgoing uniform laser energy emanating from the laser during treatment.

Mechanical Stability

Mechanical stability of the globe is necessary to permit the optical system to account for final positioning of laser treatment and any abnormalities induced by docking the PI to the eye that might influence treatment (for example, lens tilt). The PI design must comply with anatomical variations such as corneal curvature and diameter. In addition, the PI and vacuum design must provide adequate retention force between the interface and the eye to prevent movement but also allow for safe release in the case of emergencies. Specifically, the stability of the PI should be examined during treatment for each incision as well as during image acquisition and the moment when the imaging information is used to guide the laser treatment. Eye tracking, as is used in excimer laser treatments, is not currently feasible for ReLACS because the required response times for spot placement accuracy of FS lasers are much faster than eye tracking control systems can provide. Therefore, the interface provides the function of stabilizing the eye and preventing movement.

Patient Requirements: Sterility, Safety, Comfort

Sterility

Depending on the design, the various PIs may be used with or without gel or fluid. The PI should be contained in sterile protective packaging to prevent infection or ocular surface damage and should be biocompatible to prevent toxicity on contact with the eye. It is unnecessary, however, that the actual PI application and laser treatment occur in a sterile environment. A clean environment is sufficient in FS laser flap creation because a full thickness incision into the eye is not created. Similarly, in the case of partial thickness corneal incisions in laser cataract surgery, there is no direct communication between the intraocular contents and the ocular surface until the corneal incisions are fully dissected once the patient has been sterilely draped in the OR.

Safety and Comfort

From a mechanical perspective, the PI should be designed to cause the least amount of harm as possible to the corneal epithelium and conjunctiva, so as to minimize any requisite tissue damage or cosmetic sequelae such as subconjunctival hemorrhage after surgery. Pressure sensations induced by the PI can cause patient discomfort and anxiety. As noted above, high intraocular pressure rises during suction ring placement and the duration of vacuum activation should be avoided in older patients. Additionally, the docking process may entail elevating the patient into the laser system or having the system descend towards the patient's face, which in turn can create anxiety and feelings of claustrophobia. Efforts should be taken by the surgical team to make this step as comfortable and nonthreatening to the patient as possible by explaining the procedure in advance and by using appropriate conscious sedation techniques much as one would for LASIK surgery. One potential difference is that the laser cataract surgery patient may already have IV access in place since he or she is destined for the OR.

Surgeon Requirements: Ergonomics, Reliability, Economics

Ergonomics and Reliability

Successful docking sets the stage for the remaining laser surgery and subsequent cataract removal. The PI design must provide for an easy, reproducible application method for patients with a wide range of ocular and facial-orbital anatomical variations. PI design factors for the surgical team include ambidextrous grip locations, vacuum tubing control, system controls for engaging the vacuum, and clear lines of sight for placement of the device, as good docking ergonomic design can improve both the learning curve and ease of use.

Economics

Lastly, the economics of PIs are important to surgeons, surgery centers and equipment manufacturers alike. As one of the primary drivers of variable costs in the business model, the PI cost needs to be set appropriately to create a business model that is a "win–win" for all parties involved. Multiuse PIs have strict manufacturing and optical coating requirements for reliability and optical quality, and must be sterilized in between patient uses. Sterility requirements dictate that a delay between treatment occurs while reusable devices are autoclaved, unless a sufficient quantity are purchased to accommodate the planned surgical volume for a given treatment session. Cost likely becomes an issue with this approach. Single-use disposables have lower manufacturing costs and can be provided to the center in sterile packs. For both multi- and single-use PI devices, laser cataract surgery will require inventory management as is currently done for phacoemulsification systems.

Commercially Available Patient Interfaces for Laser Cataract Surgery

There are already several commercially available PIs for FS laser cataract surgery. Each laser system has specific optical requirements for the interface and is designed around those performance variables. Single-piece PIs are comprised of one unit that attaches to both the system and the patient. Multipiece interfaces have one interface component that attaches to the patient and one or more components that secure the patient component to the system.

The PI designs also vary in the way they stabilize and attach to the globe, with flat and curved direct contact applanating interfaces and non-applanating immersion interfaces. Interface materials, optics, suction design and field of view also vary among systems. The details of design and guidelines for usage of each manufacturer's PI device are discussed at great length in the chapters on the individual laser systems elsewhere in this book: please see the table of contents for details. In this chapter, we will discuss the advantages and disadvantages of the two principal approaches to interface design: applanation designs that contact the cornea and non-applanating designs that attach to the sclera without corneal contact.

Applanation Designs

Applanation designs include both flat plates (such as the Abbott Medical Optics interface for the IFS platform) and curved lenses (such as the

Table 6.3 PIs used with laser cataract surgery systems

	OptiMedica	LensAR	LenSx/Alcon	Technolas
Applanation	Non-applanating	Non-applanating	Curved lens applanating	Curved lens applanating
# of pieces	Multipiece	Multipiece	Single piece	Multipiece

LenSx and Technolas platforms). Applanation designs are comprised of either a single- (LenSx) or two-piece (Abbott/AMO, Technolas Perfect Vision) disposable with the potential to lower costs and reduce docking steps. Applanation designs make direct contact with the cornea and may require application of a gel to reduce large changes in refraction indices at the surface boundaries. However, the radii of curvature and degree of asphericity of corneal surfaces vary widely, so it is impossible to design enough interface shapes to fit all eyes. For refractive FS laser systems, some manufacturers have offered interfaces in multiple sizes (Zeiss, Ziemer). The corneal contact interfaces have treatment zones that measure about 9 mm in diameter with respect to the central point of contact. White to white horizontal corneal diameter ranges between 10.5 and 12.75 mm [30], so a 9 mm treatment zone for the peripheral corneal incisions needed for cataract surgery will be adequate for some but not all eyes. For the smaller diameter applanating devices there may be a potential advantage when treating patients with smaller orbits, but a potential disadvantage when treating large diameter corneas, where the desired incisions may need to be placed more peripherally. If excessive pressure is applied or conformity to corneal shape is poor, the degree of applanation can cause corneal deformation, reducing the system's optical quality and increasing intraocular pressure (this issue is discussed in more detail in the following section).

Non-applanation Designs

Non-applanation designs (such as the LensAR and OptiMedica PIs) use a fluid immersion chamber and a suction ring that attaches to the sclera, thereby exposing a larger diameter of corneal tissue for imaging and laser treatment. The removal of design requirements for corneal contact and compression allows suction to be applied to the sclera, which results in less intraocular pressure rise per unit of vacuum applied to the globe, since the suction provides eye stabilization but does not deform the cornea and reduce intraocular volume. Non-applanation designs involve more disposable components, and the additional step to fill the interface with fluid makes the procedure somewhat messier. While gauze or a catchment device can be utilized to absorb any excess fluid, the sensation of fluid running down the cheek can cause unnecessary alarm, so patients should be counseled and reassured beforehand. By attaching to the sclera, these non-applanation designs may require a slightly larger orbit than some applanation devices, but also provide for a larger treatment field area. Similar to the ultrasound A scan biometry, the fluid immersion approach removes air from the optical path, improving the optical quality of the delivery system by index matching the cornea to nullify its optical power and to improve the optical coupling efficiency. By avoiding corneal and overall globe deformation, non-applanating designs minimize intraocular pressure increases and optimize the optical path into the eye to allow uniform laser energy delivery for capsule and lens incisions (see Table 6.3 for a summary of PIs used with laser cataract surgery systems and Fig. 6.1a, b for non-applanating designs and applanating designs).

Comparison of Two Patient Interface Designs: The Story of Patient Interface Product Development at OptiMedica

Through clinical experience, studies conducted by OptiMedica suggest that the design of the PI plays a pivotal role in facilitating accurate and

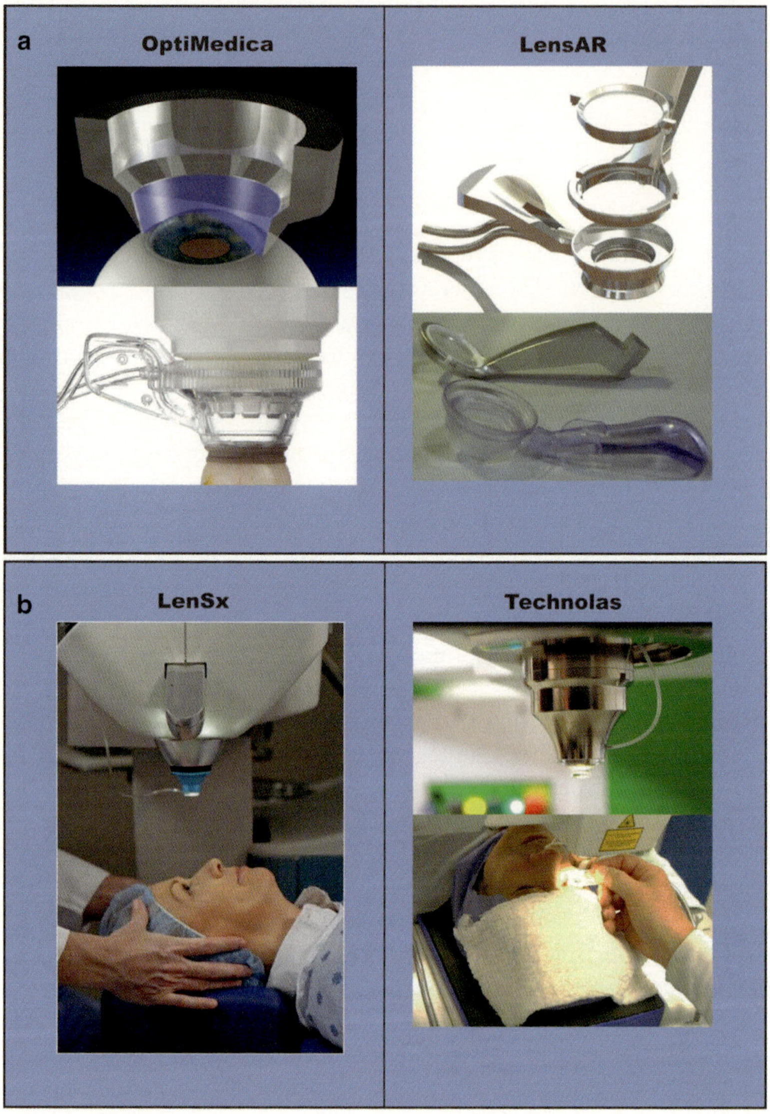

Fig. 6.1 (**a**) Non-applanating designs: OptiMedica's Liquid Optics Interface (image courtesy of OptiMedica) (on *left*) (animation image courtesy Julian Stevens FRCOphth) and LensAR's Robocone (on *right*). (**b**) Applanating designs: LenSx's PI (on *left*) and Technolas' PI (on *right*)

precise incisions in both the cornea and lens during laser cataract surgery.

OptiMedica began development and its initial clinical studies with a curved lens PI that required corneal contact applanation. With the curved lens PI, a number of barriers to precision were identified, which included deformation of the globe, poor eye stabilization, misalignment and incomplete surface identification using optical coherence tomography (OCT). Globe deformation causes IOP increases and can also cause corneal folds. Corneal folds on the posterior corneal surface can create discontinuities in the optical path of laser energy destined for the capsule and lens as it transits from the cornea into the anterior chamber, distorting the laser beam and preventing the tightly focused FS laser energy pulses needed to reach tissue photodisruption thresholds. Corneal folds were observed in the majority of patients treated with the curved applanation lens. Optical analysis of the corneal

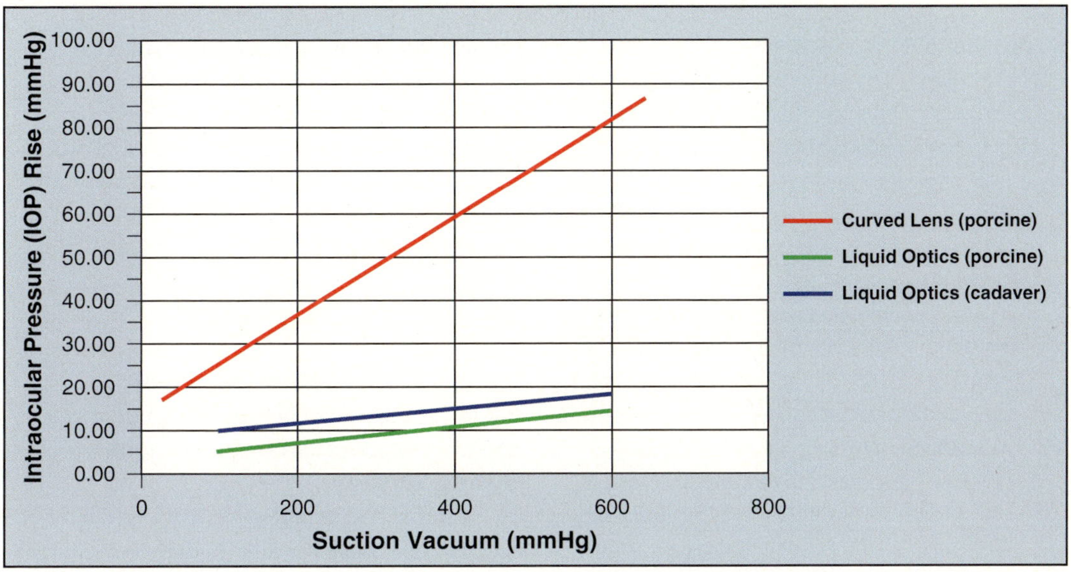

Fig. 6.2 IOP vs. suction vacuum with two OptiMedica PI designs. As applied suction reaches the 400–600 mmHg needed to adequately stabilize the globe for imaging and treatment, IOP rise with a curved applanation lens interface measured 4–6 times greater than a non-applanating immersion interface (image courtesy of OptiMedica)

folds showed beam degradation, resulting in beam defocus that led to incomplete capsulotomy. Eye movement resulting from poor eye stabilization may have also led to less precise incisions. IOP increases and subconjunctival hemorrhages were identified as barriers to safety and comfort with the curved lens design. The ease of docking for the surgeon was also an issue. The learning curve for surgeons who had no experience with docking FS laser systems was steeper, and was characterized by difficulty centering and applanating the eye using joystick- or keypad-operated remote controls. Furthermore, patients for whom head positioning was difficult to achieve and/or maintain had a tendency to become uncomfortable, as head movement placed eccentric pressure on the orbital rim, sometimes causing suction to be lost as well.

After encountering these barriers limiting precision and patient comfort in the clinical trial, OptiMedica pursued development of an alternative PI. The principal goal was to address the issues outlined above, by preventing corneal deformation to ensure that the optical path for video, OCT and laser was not compromised. The new Liquid Optics™ Interface was introduced into the clinical study [31] and the clinical results from the two PIs were compared.

Laboratory Analysis of Patient Interface Design on Suction-Induced IOP Elevation

IOP rise during suction and retention force was tested in the lab using a custom fixture for both porcine and cadaver eyes.

The graph in Fig. 6.2 shows the rise in IOP as suction vacuum is increased. At 600 mm mercury of suction vacuum, the liquid interface had five times less IOP rise than that of the curved lens direct contact interface. It is important to note that suction vacuum pressure is not the same as intraocular pressure. Please see the sidebar discussion for a more detailed explanation of the relationship between IOP and suction vacuum application with subsequent docking of the PI device.

Vacuum: IOP Vs. Suction

Although they may use the same units of measure (such as millimeters of mercury), intraocular pressure and vacuum pressure for suction-based PIs are different values.

- Pressure is defined as the force per unit area.
- In preclinical studies of intraocular pressure, eyes were pressurized to a nominal value (in the range 15–20 mmHg). Intraocular pressure was recorded as a rise above nominal.
- Vacuum pressure, sometimes referred to as suction or suction vacuum, is the pressure differential between atmospheric pressure and the vacuum created in the patient contact area. The vacuum source can be a vacuum pump under instrument control, or a manually controlled syringe. The vacuum level for the PI is much higher than the elevated intraocular pressure, on the order of hundreds of mmHg.
- Vacuum pressure plays a role in adhering the PI to the ocular tissue and stabilizing the eye.
- Preclinical studies, such as those conducted by OptiMedica, show that vacuum and IOP are related. Interface designs pull a vacuum over a surface area and deform ocular tissue, typically pulling it into a cavity in a suction ring arrangement. This deformation of ocular tissue increases the intraocular pressure. As vacuum pressure increases, more tissue is displaced and the intraocular pressure is driven up further.
- For pump-sourced vacuums, the vacuum pressure can be controlled to a level that is high enough to ensure eye stability without unnecessarily raising IOP.
- Also for pump sourced vacuums, the vacuum pressure can be controlled to a level that is low enough to be independent of altitude, since the available atmospheric pressure to generate a pressure differential decreases with altitude.
- Intraocular pressure measurements from PI studies should be referenced at a given vacuum pressure necessary for globe retention and stabilization.

Clinical Studies: Relationship of Patient Interface Design to Occurrence of Sub-conjunctival Hemorrhages During Surgery

To examine the relationship between interface designs and cosmetically bothersome subconjunctival hemorrhage, a retrospective analysis was performed using video and OCT data captured during the clinical study of laser cataract surgery using both a curved lens direct contact interface and a non-applanating liquid interface. The color threshold image analysis found a more than 50% reduction in the incidence of subconjunctival hemorrhage in the cohort treated with the liquid interface. The images presented in Fig. 6.3 clearly demonstrate the visible difference between the two PIs.

Clinical Studies: Influence of Patient Interface Design on Incidence of Corneal Folds and the Subsequent Effect of Corneal Folds on Laser Capsulotomy Treatment

Laser treatment videos as well as axial and sagittal cross sections from corneal OCT images were reviewed to identify corneal folds. Folds were apparent on video as lighter colored striae, and manifest as protrusions of the posterior corneal surface on cross-sectional OCT scans. Consistent corneal folds were found on both videos and OCT scans from subjects treated with the curved contact interface (see Fig. 6.4). Corneal folds were not detected with the liquid interface design. This qualitative improvement in the appearance of the posterior corneal surface is significant, as corneal folds

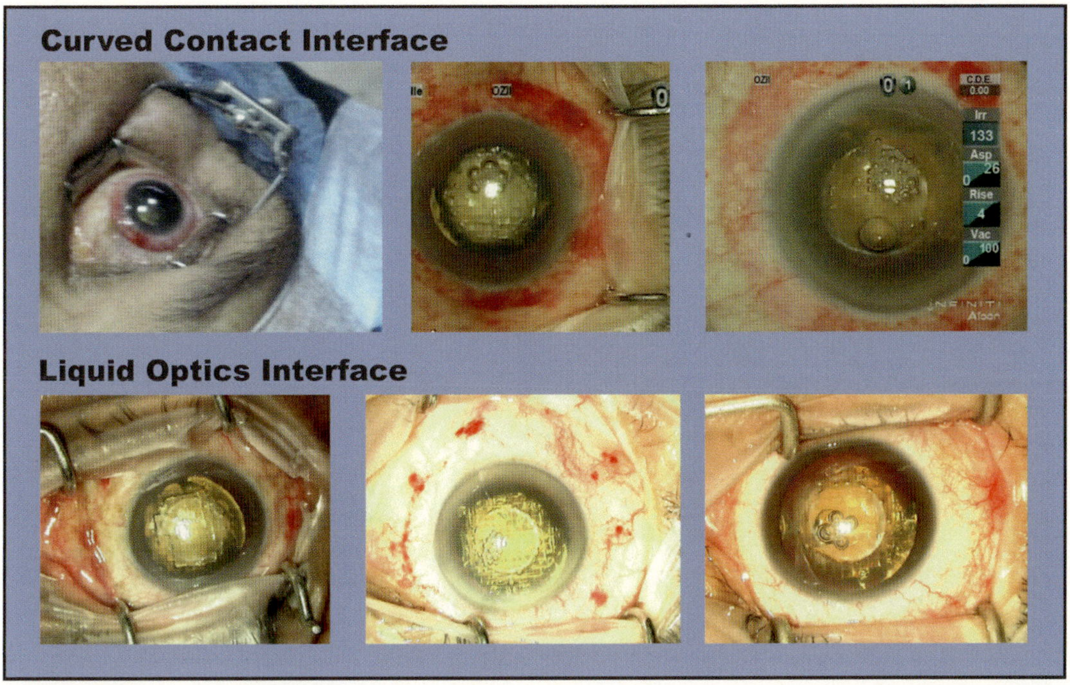

Fig. 6.3 Influence of PI design on incidence and severity of subconjunctival hemorrhage. The figure contains images from the operating room microscope immediately following laser anterior capsulotomy and lens fragmentation prior to lens removal. The *top row images* show patients treated with the curved contact interface demonstrating a *red ring* of subconjunctival hemorrhage. The *bottom row images* show patients treated with the Liquid Optics Interface demonstrating small petechiae and minimal subconjunctival hemorrhage (image courtesy of OptiMedica)

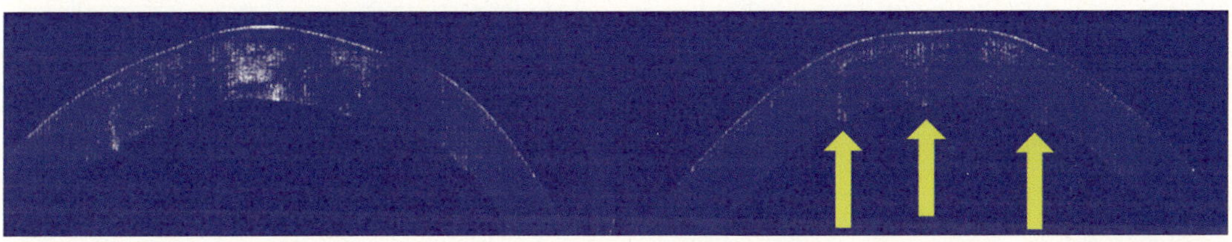

Fig. 6.4 Axial and sagittal high resolution spectral domain OCT images from a patient show numerous focal posterior corneal folds (indicated by the *arrows*) during contact applanation with a PI device just prior to FS laser treatment of the lens (image courtesy of OptiMedica)

of the degree observed in OCT images can distort the laser beam so it is unable to focus and create the threshold energy density needed for cavitation bubble formation. Optical analysis of the corneal folds showed degradation with a wavefront error of 0.94 and Strehl ratio 0.2, which are consistent with significantly aberrated optics. As points of reference, a perfect wavefront (no deviation) would have an error of 0, and the Strehl ratio for a theoretically perfect optical system is 1.0. A high quality optical system that is diffraction limited (such as a healthy human eye) will have a Strehl ratio of 0.8 or above.

Measures of optical quality. The Strehl ratio is a measure of optical quality, and is most simply defined as a metric representing the quality of the point spread function (PSF) at the image plane of an optical system (more specifically, the ratio of the intensity of the PSF at the diffraction limited Gaussian image point in the presence of aberration, divided by the intensity that would be obtained if no aberration were present). This may also be called the Strehl definition or the Strehl intensity. A Strehl ratio of 1 defines a perfect optical system [32].

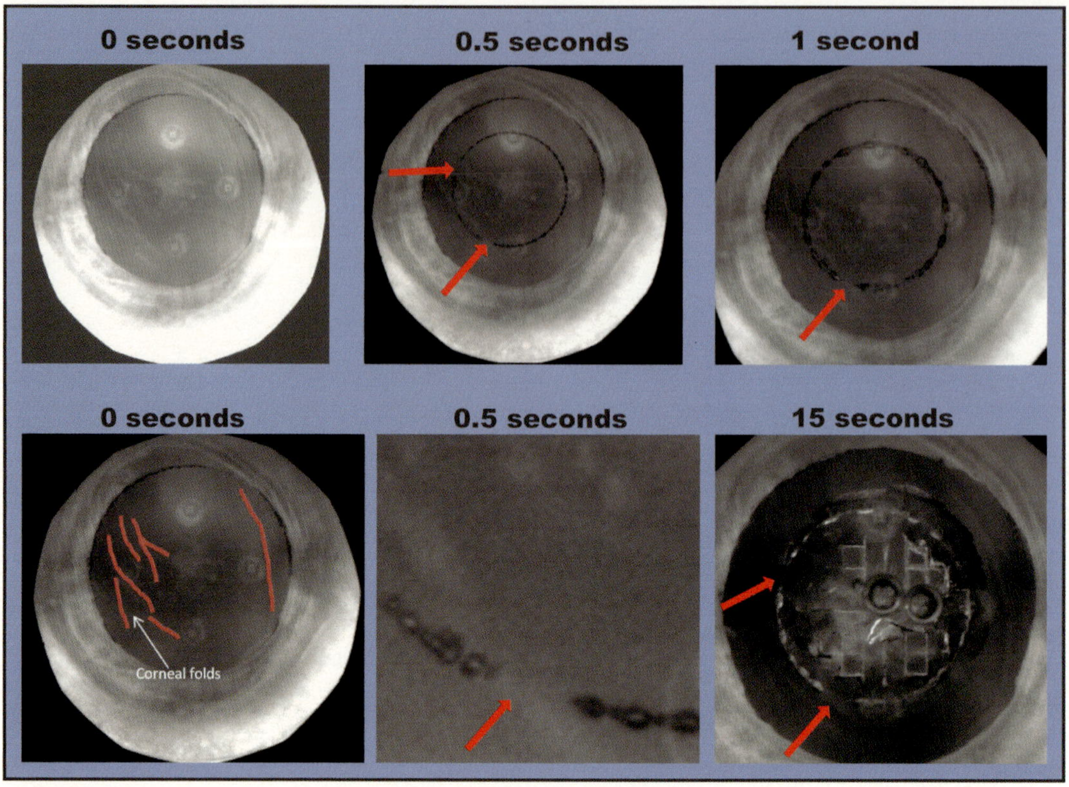

Fig. 6.5 Serial video still frames from a patient treated with a curved contact interface demonstrate corneal folds. A skip, or area of incomplete incision, is noticeable beneath the fold approximately half a second into capsulotomy formation (indicated by *arrows*). The capsule incision directly below the area of corneal fold shows the skip even after fragmentation is complete in the last still frame (image courtesy of OptiMedica)

In Fig. 6.5, a series of video still frames from the clinical study demonstrates corneal folds, highlighted in red. A "skip," or area of incomplete incision, is noticeable approximately half a second into capsulotomy formation. The capsule incision directly below the area of the corneal folds, even after fragmentation is complete, shows this skip below the folds.

The importance of achieving a complete laser capsulotomy cut cannot be understated, and will addressed in more detail in the next chapter. As any cataract surgeon knows, a focus of unexpected capsule adherence could result in an unanticipated radial anterior capsule tear if the surgeon is unaware of its existence, or if he or she does not apply the appropriate force vectors when pulling away the excised tissue. The potential result could be a radial tear that could compromise subsequent surgical steps and lead to more serious operative complications such as zonular damage, posterior capsule rupture, and vitreous loss.

Lessons Learned…

In the comparison study of applanating vs. non-applanating PI devices, the non-contact Liquid Optics Interface presented the most favorable safety and efficacy profile.

While there seem to be compelling arguments for non-applanation PI designs, the clinical experience described herein is from only one company. As laser cataract technology evolves and more experience is gained, the pros and cons of the different approaches to interface design will

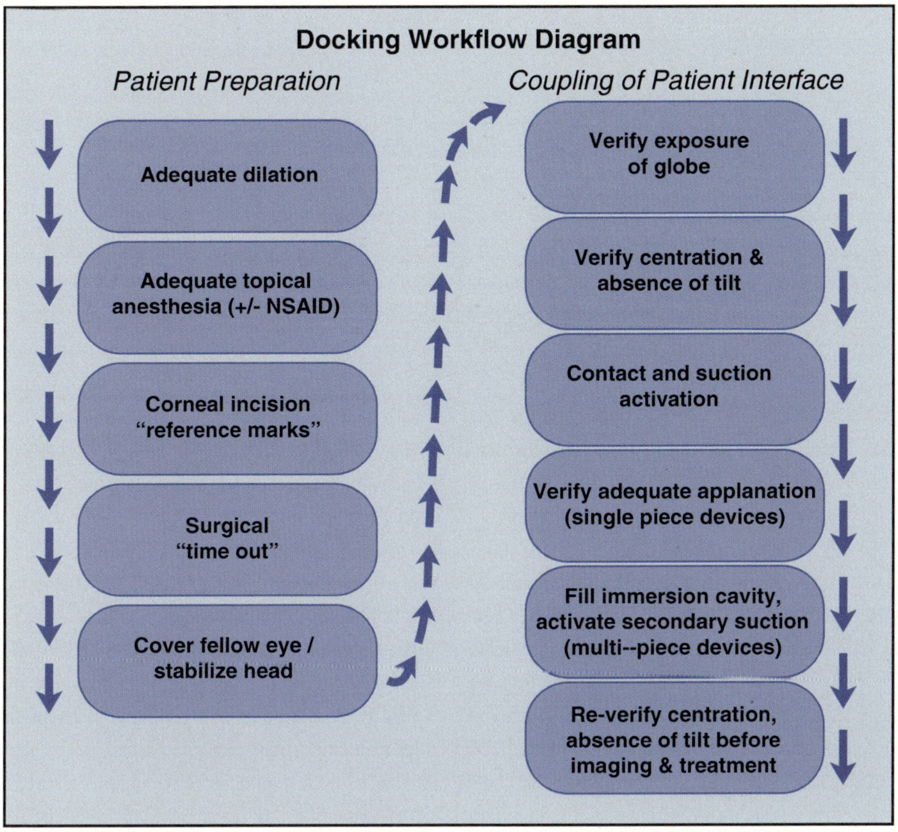

Fig. 6.6 Docking workflow diagram highlighting the important steps in the docking process starting with patient preparation through coupling of the eye, PI and laser system

become more evident, and the strategies for patient-friendly treatment will undoubtedly become more elegant and sophisticated.

Clinical Considerations for Docking During Refractive Laser Assisted Cataract Surgery

Docking Workflow

Like many clinical procedures that are performed in a high-volume setting, the docking process will benefit from a standardized workflow (see Fig. 6.6), and some elements of this process will benefit from a customized approach for each laser system. Attention paid to each step in the docking workflow can minimize the learning curve for docking and maximize procedural success. After all, docking failure prevents laser cataract surgery treatment.

The first consideration for docking is preparing the patient for surgery. The OptiMedica and Technolas platforms have dedicated patient beds. On these systems, the patient must be positioned on the bed and the bed must allow for side-to-side, head-to-toe, and floor-to-ceiling adjustments. The LensAR and LenSx systems are used with independent gurneys, do not have integrated beds and therefore require adjustment of x, y, and z axis positioning of the laser optical delivery pathway by the system itself. Before readying the patient for docking, it is necessary to carefully check to be sure that the desired degree of pupil dilation has been achieved. In addition, it is necessary to place reference marks on the globe with the patient in an upright position if astigmatic corneal incisions are planned. This is due to the fact that inadvertent misalignment from head tilt or turn may occur when the patient reclines into a supine position or as a result of globe rotation when the PI device is applied and docking proceeds. After a surgical timeout is completed to identify the correct treatment eye and the laser parameters programmed for treatment (i.e., corneal incision types size, shape, location; capsulotomy size/shape; type of lens segmentation and/or softening), the fellow eye should be covered and the head stabilized for surgery. Surgical tape across the forehead may be used to remind the patient to keep still during the procedure. Depending on the treatment plan and incision settings, the laser treatment may not require a fully sterile environment. Non-penetrating corneal incisions can be safely completed in a clean environment as demonstrated with LASIK. The surgical eye should be cleaned and anesthetic drops (typically, a few drops of 0.5% tetracaine or proparacaine) given per the recommended instructions for use. Lidocaine gel should be avoided, as viscous substances on the bulbar conjunctiva may impair adhesion following suction vacuum application. It is helpful to pretreat the patient with topical nonsteroidal anti-inflammatory medication to help with docking-related discomfort and maintain pupillary dilation.

The number of components involved in the PI has a large influence on the docking workflow. A multipiece interface requires attaching one component to the patient's eye prior to mating with the system. While this adds a step in the workflow, it may increase subsequent ease of use by decreasing the number of steps that need to happen simultaneously during docking.

Multipiece Patient Interfaces

The workflow for multipiece interfaces allow for pre-alignment prior to mating with the system. In these cases, the PI is attached to the eye and suction is applied to hold it in place. Depending on the vacuum controls and tubing constraints, the application of the PI may be completed while the patient is not yet under the system; this can provide for better access and more visibility during the attachment process. The surgeon can hold the patient's eyelids back and gently roll the PI under the inferior and then the superior lid. Patient fixation can then aid the surgeon during centering of the suction ring. A microscope can be used to ensure good alignment, which consists principally of centering the cornea within the suction ring while the corneal apex is oriented orthogonal to the laser's optical system. Alignment can be facilitated by patient fixation on a target light within the video system or microscope used to apply the suction device. Good centration of the suction device allows the laser system to perform at its fullest capability to image and treat anterior segment tissues. Moreover, both imaging and treatment of anterior segment tissues can be compromised if the PI is decentered with respect to the corneal center as defined by the limbus, or if the corneal apex (and hence the lens) is tilted with respect to the laser optics—this will be covered further in the section that follows below.

With pre-alignment using a multipiece PI, the surgeon can more easily monitor for globe rotation with suction application and final ring positioning prior to completing the full docking process, so that decentration and tilt can be avoided early in the docking process. With non-applanating immersion optic PI designs, a fluid bath must be filled after a vacuum is established between the ring and the eye in order to ensure a good seal. Multipiece PIs then require that the suction ring attached to the patient is mated with the system using additional vacuum and/or mechanical methods.

Single Piece Patient Interfaces

Single-piece PIs require that the eye mate with the laser system in one step. A speculum is sometimes helpful to hold the eyelids and lashes out of the way, to create a larger surface area to accept the interface and to free the surgeon's hands for control over the process, as unlike multipiece interfaces a suction ring is not present to hold the lids. Application of a gel (such as 1% methycellulose) may be required to fill in any gaps between the final optic-cornea plane of contact, and to assist with index matching for imaging and laser energy transmission. As noted above, great care should be taken to ensure that gel does not creep into the corneal or conjunctival suction ports. Good visualization is critical during the alignment process; final centration is achieved through video guidance and sensor feedback in some of the platforms. As the bed is raised or the system lowered to complete docking, the patient's head may need to be adjusted. The surgeon can ask the patient to move his or her chin to help align the corneal apex while keeping the iris plane parallel to the floor to avoid tilt. Some patients may need to rotate their heads laterally to avoid nose interference [6]. Once docking is completed and the patient's eye is stabilized, imaging and treatment can begin.

For both multi- and single-piece interfaces, the undocking process requires vacuum release and removal of the interface from the system and/or patient. For systems where significant applanation force on the cornea is needed to achieve adequate contact, it is helpful to encourage the patient not to look around or move the eye until treatment is complete and there is no longer any corneal contact.

Risk Factors for Docking

Depending on the docking approach and PI design, there are some challenging situations that may present relative contraindications to docking.

Uncooperative patients: A distinction must be made between anxious patients who simply require education/reassurance and uncooperative patients, who may not be good surgical candidates. General anesthesia for laser cataract surgery may be technically difficult due to the close proximity of the laser head to the airway during docking and treatment, so these individuals may best be treated without an FS laser.

Blepharospasm: Excessive blepharospasm with sustained involuntary forceful closing of the lids can prevent initial docking or cause suction loss during the treatment, even with a speculum in place (some interface designs require speculums to keep the eyelids (and eyelashes) out of the way during docking and some interfaces act as speculums). Blocking the eyelid should be considered in these cases.

Tight orbital anatomy: Docking patients with deeply set eyes can present challenges from facial feature interference and limited visibility for the surgeon. Small, narrow orbits and tight eyelids typically found in Asian populations [33] make insertion of the interface difficult, even with the assistance of a speculum. These cases should be identified in the office before surgery and noted as a potential contraindication or challenge for laser assisted cataract surgery. It can also be difficult to seat the suction ring with entrapment of conjunctiva or lashes under the ring.

Poor dilation: While not a risk factor for the docking process itself, inadequate dilation risks iris damage and necessitates a smaller capsulotomy and lens fragmentation treatment. As such, it can be an indication to abort docking.

Poor corneal epithelial adhesion: Corneal epithelial basement membrane dystrophy increases the risk of epithelial sloughing after applanation docking. This may interfere with imaging and delivery of subsequent laser treatment. In addition, visibility during surgery will be impaired, with patient comfort and visual recovery affected as well.

Conjunctivochalasis: With older patients, conjunctivochalasis can make docking more difficult due to inability to achieve sufficient suction. Additional topical vasoconstrictors may be considered preoperatively, as may conjunctivochalasis surgery using amniotic membrane (well in advance of cataract surgery) if a laser cataract approach is deemed to be very important.

Preexisting retinal or optic nerve pathology: Patients with advanced glaucoma or ocular vascular conditions such as retinal vascular occlusions or anterior ischemic optic neuropathy should be treated with a PI device that minimizes IOP rise or undergo conventional cataract surgery with great care to minimize pressurization of the globe.

Managing Docking-Related Complications

Docking for laser cataract surgery requires training and experience, and may at first be more easily mastered by those trained in docking with

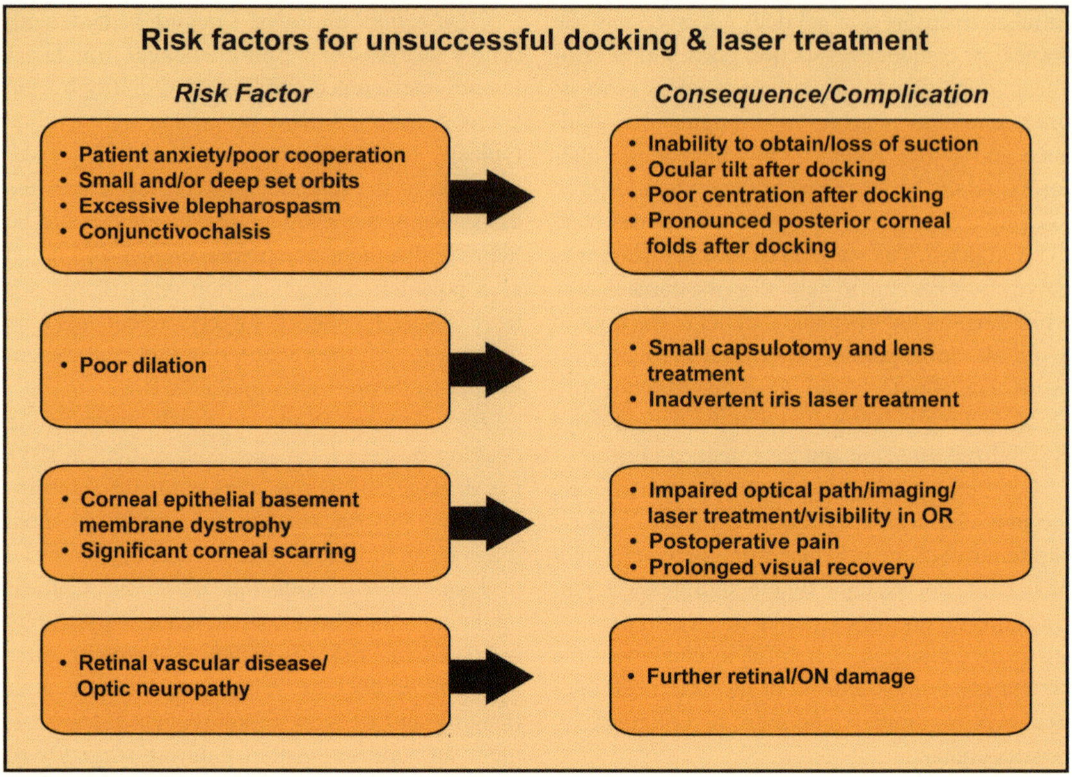

Fig. 6.7 Risk factors for unsuccessful docking and laser treatment. The figure summarizes risk factors and the associated consequence and potential complication leading to unsuccessful docking and laser treatment

refractive FS lasers. Steps that commonly require troubleshooting include the inability to dock, suction loss during treatment, inability to re-dock, and inadequate centration and/or rotational alignment [6]. There are a number of risk factors and potential complications that can result from docking that should be addressed (see Fig. 6.7).

The anxious patient: A disoriented or anxious patient may be unable to remain still for the 2–3 min necessary to dock, image and treat. It is critical to keep this in mind when selecting patients, and to take the "chair time" to educate the patient at time of the presurgical consultation. Nursing staff can also help by reminding the patient on the day of surgery what they will experience during laser treatment. While it may seem obvious, such counseling is best conducted prior to "conscious sedation."

Failure of first docking attempt: Multiple docking attempts and prolonged time under vacuum suction can increase patient anxiety and discomfort. Patient anxiety and discomfort increases the chances of inadvertent movement or suction loss, which in turn can lead to inaccurate or incomplete treatment. Excessive manipulation of interfaces may cause corneal epithelial damage, resulting in compromised imaging and laser transmission as well as postoperative discomfort. Subconjunctival hemorrhages and chemosis are not uncommon after docking, which in turn make achievement and maintenance of suction more difficult. The degree of severity and time to resolution depend on the PI and vacuum designs.

Poor corneal applanation: If a contact applanation device is used and adequate corneal contact cannot be obtained with or without lubrication due to mismatch of curvature between the PI and cornea, surgery must be aborted. If available, a non-corneal contact applanation approach may be used. All current PIs for laser cataract surgery currently have fixed diameter contact rings for suction. Future PI designs may include multiple sizes to accommodate children and smaller orbits, although variations in interface size and diameter may be limited by the design of a laser's optical system.

Corneal folds after docking (see Figs. 6.5 and 6.6): This phenomenon may be related to corneal curvature mismatch as noted above, poor centration or globe tilt (see below). Securing the PI to the eye and system completes the optical path for the laser and imaging. Imperfections in system alignment or induced corneal folds may result in incomplete incisions, especially in the anterior lens capsule.

Globe tilt or decentration after docking: Minimal eye tilt and good centration are important for laser cataract surgery treatment. The laser beam enters the eye from the fixed system, and tilted ocular structures can require increased capsulotomy height or can lead to incomplete incisions. Too much tilt or a poorly centered interface can require a surgeon to re-dock or cause inadvertent suction loss during treatment. For a contact applanation device, it is important to hold the suction ring perfectly level and to watch the contact meniscus. If the meniscus is not symmetrical, the suction ring may be tilted and the surgeon should attempt to correct the tilt to achieve a symmetrical meniscus. While some systems have the ability to account for some degree of tilt or poor centration, good docking technique can improve the speed and outcome of treatment. Additionally, if the laser system's optics are not adequately centered on the temporal corneal limbus, it may be unwise to perform the primary cataract incision with the laser. Primary incisions that are too central will impair visibility during surgery, induce astigmatism, and may result in more corneal edema after surgery.

Suction loss during laser capsulotomy: While it is fairly straightforward to re-dock and start over at any point prior to treatment, decision making becomes more complex after laser treatment is in progress. If suction loss occurs and leaves a partial laser capsulotomy, one should not attempt to recut the capsule. A recut may increase the risk of radial extension, and it is preferable to complete the capsulotomy manually at this point. Since the capsulotomy is usually the first step in treatment (lens nucleus and corneal incisions follow), it is unwise to treat the lens after re-docking if large numbers of cavitation bubbles are present within the lens. Cavitation bubbles at the level of the capsule and anterior chamber may make it more difficult to reimage the lens and posterior capsule. As more experience is gained in this area it will become clearer as to whether it is advisable to re-dock if the capsulotomy is incomplete.

Suction loss during lens fragmentation/softening: As noted above, reimaging of the lens will be necessary prior to resuming treatment. Imaging may be difficult due to media opacification and the presence of cavitation bubbles, so further lens treatment should be avoided. However, re-docking for imaging and creation of corneal incisions can proceed if the surgeon desires.

Conclusions

PIs are essential components for the success of many ophthalmic laser procedures. Prior to the introduction of FS lasers for corneal surgery, interface designs could be relatively simple as they served the singular purpose of stabilizing the eye while the surgeon manually focused and delivered treatment to structures deeper inside the eye. With FS LASIK, the requirements for PIs increased because targeting a tissue plane 100 or more microns below the corneal surface exceeded the manual focusing capabilities of a surgeon. The interface device not only had to stabilize the globe, but also provide a reference plane for precise focal point treatment preset by the laser. FS laser cataract surgery raises the demands on the PI to yet an even higher level with the requirement to provide excellent optical media to allow both imaging and treatment deep inside the eye using multiple planes of reference.

Since imaging and treatment cannot occur without successful docking of the PI to the eye, it is the most important step in laser assisted cataract surgery. As experience has demonstrated with other high volume surgical procedures, a checklist can be used to maximize accuracy and efficiency for systematic successful docking. Just as for LASIK surgery, during the procedure the clinical team is very focused on the patient and the manual docking steps being executed by the surgeon. The laser treatment then occurs very quickly so a systematic workflow approach that emphasizes not only patient comfort but also safety is critical. A surgical "time-out" should occur before docking begins, and review not only the patient's identity and eye to be treated but also all specific laser parameters that have been programmed into the laser.

As with any new, exciting and effective surgical technology, it will be tempting (and desirable) to treat as many patients as possible with laser cataract surgery. Just as different excimer lasers or IOLs may suit one patient better than another, PI designs for each FS laser cataract system may make it easier or harder to treat when confronted with certain clinical scenarios. As such, it is important to become intimately familiar with the limitations of each system, and to identify in advance situations that may compromise the ability to dock and complete treatment. If identified potential docking issues may cause harm or prevent laser treatment, proceeding directly to conventional phacoemulsification is advisable. If in doubt, a "dry run" under the laser prior to the day of surgery or counseling the patient to prepare him or her for an unsuccessful treatment attempt may be prudent.

Product launches during the time of this publication promise to reveal a period of rapid development and advancement in laser cataract surgical technology. At present, PI technology has evolved in two directions: contact corneal applanation and non-corneal applanation immersion devices. Each approach has pros and cons, and time will tell whether one strategy becomes dominant. Docking is critical to laser cataract surgery and PI designs will likely evolve dramatically over time to improve ease of use for surgeons and clinical results for patients.

Key Points

1. PI devices (PI's) are a critical component of many ophthalmic laser procedures, but are of extra importance during laser cataract surgery because they allow intraocular structures to become part of the laser's optical system for BOTH imaging and treatment.
2. Docking duration is longer than for LASIK surgery due to the need to stabilize the globe for both 3D imaging and treatment of capsule, lens and cornea. Safe and successful docking requires managing patient comfort and cooperation through education and conscious sedation.
3. Two major categories of PI's exist: corneal applanation and non-applanation designs. Each has unique advantages and disadvantages.
4. Accurate laser treatment requires adequate centration of the PI with respect to the corneal limbus to minimize tilt of intraocular structures and allow completion of peripheral corneal incisions.
5. Contraindications to docking do exist and are best recognized before surgery.
6. Suction loss can be problematic if it occurs during laser treatment, and the surgeon must know how to address this complication.
7. PI devices are not "one size fits all" and some systems may be better than others for certain clinical situations such as tight orbital anatomy, unusual corneal curvature or co-morbid conditions that require that IOP elevation during imaging and treatment be minimized.

Acknowledgements We would like to acknowledge our gratitude to Philip Gooding for his extremely valuable insights and input to our efforts while writing this chapter.

References

1. Alward WLM. A history of gonioscopy. Optom Vis Sci. 2011;88(1):29–35. doi:10.1097/OPX.0b013e3181fc3718.
2. Salzmann M. Die Ophthalmoskopie der Kammberbucht. Z Augenheilk. 1914;31:1–19.

3. Goldmann H. Zur Technik der Spaltlampenmikroskopie. Ophthalmologica. 1938;96:90–7.
4. Allen L, Braley AE, Thorpe HE. An improved gonioscopic contact prism. AMA Arch Ophthalmol. 1954;51(4):451–5.
5. Hoffer K. IOL power. Thorofare, NJ: SLACK Incorporated; 2011.
6. Faktorovich E. Femtodynamics: a guide to laser settings and procedure techniques to optimize outcomes with femtosecond lasers. Thorofare, NJ: SLACK; 2009.
7. Miclea M, Skrzypczak U, Fankhauser F, Faust S, Graener H, Seifert G. Applanation-free femtosecond laser processing of the cornea. Biomed Opt Exp. 2011;2(3):534–42. doi:10.1364/BOE.2.000534.
8. Su P-F, Lo AY, Hu C-Y, Chang S-W. Anterior chamber depth measurement in phakic and pseudophakic eyes. Optom Vis Sci. 2008;85(12):1193–200. doi:10.1097/OPX.0b013e31818e8ceb.
9. Richdale K, Bullimore MA, Zadnik K. Lens thickness with age and accommodation by optical coherence tomography. Ophthalmic Physiol Opt. 2008;28(5):441–7. doi:10.1111/j.1475-1313.2008.00594.x.
10. Binder PS. Flap dimensions created with the IntraLase FS laser. J Cataract Refract Surg. 2004;30(1):26–32. doi:10.1016/S0886-3350(03)00578-9.
11. Binder PS. One thousand consecutive IntraLase laser in situ keratomileusis flaps. J Cataract Refract Surg. 2006;32(6):962–9. doi:10.1016/j.jcrs.2006.02.043.
12. Wang L, Dai E, Koch DD, Nathoo A. Optical aberrations of the human anterior cornea. J Cataract Refract Surg. 2003;29(8):1514–21.
13. Dubbelman M, Sicam VA, van der Heijde GL. The shape of the anterior and posterior surface of the aging human cornea. Vis Res. 2006;46(6–7):993–1001. doi:10.1016/j.visres.2005.09.021.
14. Dubbelman M, Sicam VA, van der Heijde RG. The contribution of the posterior surface to the coma aberration of the human cornea. J Vis. 2007;7(7):10.1–8. doi:10.1167/7.7.10.
15. Sicam VA, Dubbelman M, van der Heijde RG. Spherical aberration of the anterior and posterior surfaces of the human cornea. J Opt Soc Am A Opt Image Sci Vis. 2006;23(3):544–9.
16. DelMonte DW, Kim T. Anatomy and physiology of the cornea. J Cataract Refract Surg. 2011;37(3):588–98. doi:10.1016/j.jcrs.2010.12.037.
17. Freeman B. 2009 Comprehensive report on the global cataract surgical equipment market. Market Scope LLC. 2009 July. www.market-scope.com
18. Chandrasekaran S, Cumming RG, Rochtchina E, Mitchell P. Associations between elevated intraocular pressure and glaucoma, use of glaucoma medications, and 5-year incident cataract: the Blue Mountains Eye Study. Ophthalmology. 2006;113(3):417–24. doi:10.1016/j.ophtha.2005.10.050.
19. Bushley DM, Parmley VC, Paglen P. Visual field defect associated with laser in situ keratomileusis. Am J Ophthalmol. 2000;129(5):668–71.
20. Weiss HS, Rubinfeld RS, Anderschat JF. Case reports and small case series: LASIK-associated visual field loss in a glaucoma suspect. Arch Ophthalmol. 2001;119(5):774–5.
21. Cameron BD, Saffra NA, Strominger MB. Laser in situ keratomileusis-induced optic neuropathy. Ophthalmology. 2001;108(4):660–5.
22. Lee AG, Kohnen T, Ebner R, Bennett JL, Miller NR, Carlow TJ, Koch DD. Optic neuropathy associated with laser in situ keratomileusis. J Cataract Refract Surg. 2000;26(11):1581–4.
23. Bradley JC, McCartney DL, Craenen GA. Continuous intraocular pressure recordings during lamellar microkeratotomy of enucleated human eyes. J Cataract Refract Surg. 2007;33(5):869–72. doi:10.1016/j.jcrs.2007.02.017.
24. Bissen-Miyajima H, Suzuki S, Ohashi Y, Minami K. Experimental observation of intraocular pressure changes during microkeratome suctioning in laser in situ keratomileusis. J Cataract Refract Surg. 2005;31(3):590–4. doi:10.1016/j.jcrs.2004.06.085.
25. Kasetsuwan N, Pangilinan RT, Moreira LL, DiMartino DS, Shah SS, Schallhorn SC, McDonnell PJ. Real time intraocular pressure and lamellar corneal flap thickness in keratomileusis. Cornea. 2001;20(1):41–4.
26. Hernández-Verdejo JL, Teus MA, Román JM, Bolívar G. Porcine model to compare real-time intraocular pressure during LASIK with a mechanical microkeratome and femtosecond laser. Invest Ophthalmol Vis Sci. 2007;48(1):68–72. doi:10.1167/iovs.06-0192.
27. Chaurasia SS, Luengo Gimeno F, Tan K, Yu S, Tan DT, Beuerman RW, Mehta JS. In vivo real-time intraocular pressure variations during LASIK flap creation. Invest Ophthalmol Vis Sci. 2010;51(9):4641–5. doi:10.1167/iovs.10-5228.
28. Conway ML, Wevill M, Benavente-Perez A, Hosking SL. Ocular blood-flow hemodynamics before and after application of a laser in situ keratomileusis ring. J Cataract Refract Surg. 2010;36(2):268–72. doi:10.1016/j.jcrs.2009.09.013.
29. Kobayashi H. Evaluation of the need to discontinue antiplatelet and anticoagulant medications before cataract surgery. J Cataract Refract Surg. 2010;36(7):1115–9. doi:10.1016/j.jcrs.2010.01.017.
30. Duke-Elder S, Wybar KC. The cornea. In system of ophthalmology. The anatomy of the visual system, vol. 2. London: Henry Kimpton; 1961. p. 92–4.
31. Friedman NJ, Palanker DV, Schuele G, et al. Femtosecond laser capsulotomy. J Cataract Refract Surg. 2011;37:1189–98.
32. Friedman NJ, Palanker DV, Schuele G, et al. Femtosecond laser capsulotomy. J Cataract Refract Surg. 2011;37:1189–98.
33. Goldberg R. Blepharoplasty: special considerations in the Asian Eyelid. In: Mauriello J, editor. Techniques in cosmetic eyelid surgery: a case study approach. Philadelphia, PA: Lippincott Williams & Wilkins; 2004. p. 217–29.

7 Laser Capsulotomy

Madeleine C. O'Meara, Jonathan H. Talamo, Neil J. Friedman, and Douglas D. Koch

Background

Capsule Anatomy

The lens capsule is the outer lining of the crystalline lens, and its elastic properties directly influence accommodation. Elasticity of the lens capsule and accommodative amplitude decrease over time, due to physiologic, age-related changes. The anterior capsule thickens by approximately 1.2% per year due to regeneration of lens epithelial cells [1]. Some believe that, as the anterior capsule thickens, it may impede the ability of the lens to become more spherical during accommodation. In addition to a reduction in elasticity, the tensile strength of the anterior capsule also decreases with time [1]. While the elastic and strength changes in the anterior capsule are independent of cataract formation, these characteristics are relevant to small incision cataract surgery, as the strength, thickness, and elasticity of the capsule opening influence the safety of the procedure as well as the refractive outcome.

M.C. O'Meara, M.S., B.A. (✉)
Department of Marketing, OptiMedica,
1310 Moffett Park Dr., Sunnyvale, CA 94089, USA
e-mail: momeara@optimedica.com

J.H. Talamo, M.D.
Harvard Medical School, Talamo Laser Eye Consultants, Ophthalmology,, Suite 184, 1601 Trapelo Rd., Waltham, MA 02451, USA

N.J. Friedman, M.D.
Ophthalmology, Stanford School of Medicine,
900 Welch Road, Palo Alto, CA 94304, USA

Cataract and Lens Surgery, Pacific Vision Institute,
San Francisco, CA, USA

D.D. Koch, M.D.
Department of Ophthalmology, Baylor College of Medicine, Cullen Eye Institute, 6565 Fannin, NC205, Houston, TX 77030, USA

The Capsule Opening in Small-Incision Cataract Surgery

In small-incision cataract surgery, the capsule opening serves as the access point for lens removal and the delivery portal for IOL implantation. It is important that this opening be resistant to tearing, as the forces exerted on the capsular bag during surgery can be substantial.

Howard Gimbel and Thomas Neuhann simultaneously and independently developed the continuous curvilinear capsulorhexis (CCC) in 1984. This technique takes advantage of the shearing properties of the anterior lens capsule—the capsule can tear with little force when the force is applied from a sharp point, but much more force is required to rupture a smooth margin [2, 3]. The CCC is created by an initial puncture of the anterior capsule with a cystotome or forceps, followed by a unidirectional arched curve tear that is progressively torn to create a full circle (see Fig. 7.1) [4]. Continuous curvilinear capsulorhexis is more resistant to tears than previous capsule opening methods, such as the can-opener.

R.R. Krueger et al. (eds.), *Textbook of Refractive Laser Assisted Cataract Surgery (ReLACS)*,
DOI 10.1007/978-1-4614-1010-2_7, © Springer Science+Business Media, LLC 2013

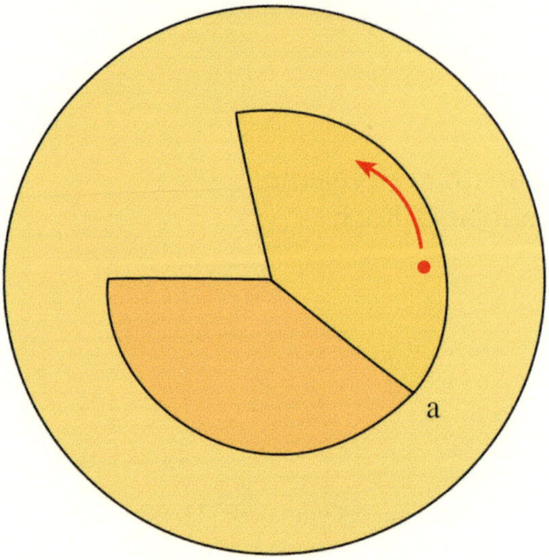

Fig. 7.1 Continuous curvilinear capsulorhexis (CCC) technique. In CCC shearing technique, flap is engaged 2–3 clock hours from the tear and is pulled counter-clockwise in curvilinear direction as indicated by *dot* and *arrow*. Reprinted with permission from SLACK Incorporated [4]

In addition to being strong, the ideal CCC is perfectly circular, predictably centered and, for most current IOL designs, slightly smaller than the diameter of the IOL optic to be implanted. Complete and consistent 360° overlap of the capsule opening with the IOL optic ensures that the IOL will sit within the capsular bag at an axial position near the zonular plane. Because the anticipated effective lens position (ELP) along the antero-posterior axis of the eye's optical path is used to determine the appropriate IOL power, the refractive outcome is directly influenced by this theoretical value and by the construction of the capsule opening [5–7]. While several technologies have incrementally improved the predictability of CCC creation—e.g., corneal rhexis marker, capsule forceps with ruler (Seibel Rhexis Ruler; MicroSurgical Technology, Redmond, WA), virtual reference rings in surgical microscope (TrueVision Systems, Santa Barbara, CA)—these instruments still require manual manipulation and are therefore subject to the variability inherent in manual techniques.

Importance of CCC: Safety

The effect of capsule opening on the safety of the procedure should be analyzed from three time points during creation of the CCC, during surgical steps following CCC, and postoperatively.

During CCC creation, the biggest safety risk is a radial extension or anterior capsule tear. For experienced surgeons, the rate of radial extension is generally between 0.8 and 2.8% [8, 9]. The incidence of anterior capsule tears by residents is almost double this value (5%) in some large studies [10]. The mechanical force required to create a CCC also puts asymmetric stress on the zonules and other lens support structures. Patients who have weak zonules due to pseudoexfoliation, an intumescent lens, trauma, or genetic conditions such as Marfan's syndrome may experience zonule damage or bag dislocation if excess unilateral pressure is applied to the anterior capsule at the site of the continuous tear.

Nearly half of all radial anterior capsule tears extend into the zonules and into posterior capsule during a subsequent surgical step [8]. A posterior capsule tear is a serious complication, with risks of vitreous loss, lens material loss into vitreous, and IOL dislocation [10]. A radial tear that does not extend to the posterior capsule remains a potential hazard, as the surgical plan will likely have to be modified with possible conversion from an in-the-bag approach to sulcus fixation.

Postoperatively, an eye with a radial tear is at increased risk for several subsequent complications:

(a) UGH syndrome

If the IOL implant or haptics are placed in the ciliary sulcus, there is increased risk of ciliary body/iris irritation that can result in uveitis–glaucoma–hyphema (UGH) syndrome from the chafing of the IOL optic or haptics against adjacent anatomical structures. Iris chafing in particular occurs if an inappropriate IOL (i.e., single piece, planar geometry) is placed in the ciliary sulcus. As its name implies, UGH syndrome can lead to chronic iritis, IOP elevation, and bleeding, as well as cystoid macular edema (CME).

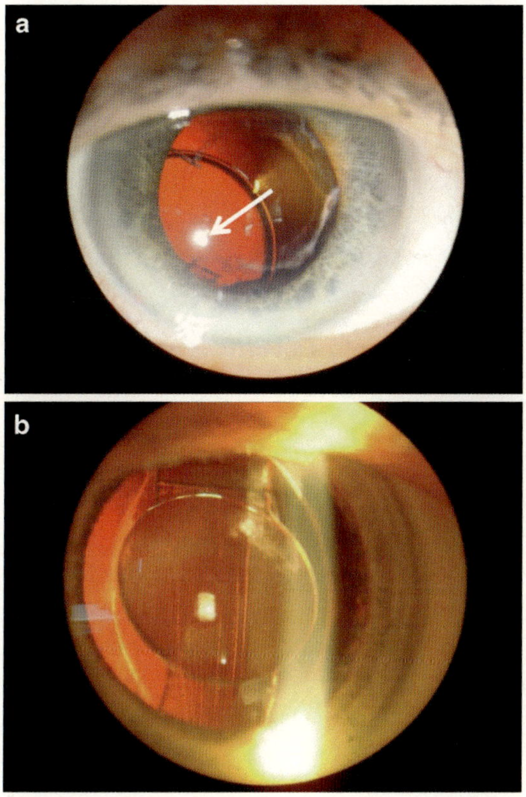

Fig. 7.2 Posterior chamber IOL dislocation. (**a**) Dislocated posterior chamber IOL. IOL dislocated in the *x*/*y* plane with direction and magnitude of shift indicated by the *arrow*. Some of this postoperative shift can be attributed to asymmetric forces of the capsular bag on the IOL. (**b**) Crystalens "Z syndrome" resulting from Crystalens® (Bausch & Lomb, Rochester, NY) implantation in the setting of an occult radial anterior capsular tear. When the Crystalens was exchanged for a three-piece monofocal IOL, the haptic footplate of the Crystalens IOL was found anterior to the capsular bag adherent to the lens zonules. Images courtesy of Jonathan Talamo

Pain, photophobia and vision loss are the symptomatic hallmarks of this condition [11–13].

(b) Occult vitreous loss

Nineteen percent of cases wherein an anterior capsule tear occurs require a vitrectomy [8]. Moreover, radial tears that extend into the zonules and vitreous may prolapse through these iatrogenic defects during or after surgery. The risk of losing lens material into the vitreous is exacerbated in this instance, as the surgeon may not yet recognize that a complication has occurred. If the IOL is implanted without recognizing vitreous loss, instability of the IOL may be noted postoperatively. When vitreous loss is not managed intraoperatively, the risks of CME and retinal detachment increase due to tractional forces from vitreous adhesions to anterior segment structures.

(c) IOL subluxation, decentration, and tilt

If large enough, an area of zonular compromise may allow migration of the IOL haptic through the defect, resulting in IOL dislocation requiring repositioning, suture fixation, or exchange (see Fig. 7.2a). Multifocal and toric IOLs perform especially poorly when decentered, and as a result should generally not be implanted in the presence of a radial capsular tear.

IOL tilt is a clinically important variant of IOL dislocation. If fixation of the IOL within the capsular bag is not symmetrical (frequently the case with radial capsule tears), the potential exists for IOL tilt even without decentration. IOL tilt induces astigmatism as well as higher order aberrations such as coma, resulting in degradation of visual acuity and contrast sensitivity uncorrectable with spectacles or contact lenses. While some degree of IOL tilt is well tolerated by monofocal IOLs, multifocal and accommodating IOLs do not function well in such circumstances (see Fig. 7.2b). Depending on the severity of tilt, IOL type, and patient to`lerance of visual aberrations, IOL reposition or exchange may be necessary.

Postoperative Complications Related to CCC Without Radial Anterior Capsule Tears

In cases without capsule tears, improper CCC sizing can play a role in the development of anterior capsular phimosis and posterior capsule opacification (PCO).

(a) Anterior capsular phimosis ("capsule contraction syndrome")

When the capsular opening is too small, there is an increased likelihood of excessive capsular phimosis [14] (see Fig. 7.3a, b). In low-level light (when pupil is more dilated), anterior capsule phimosis may compromise visual acuity and/or contrast sensitivity.

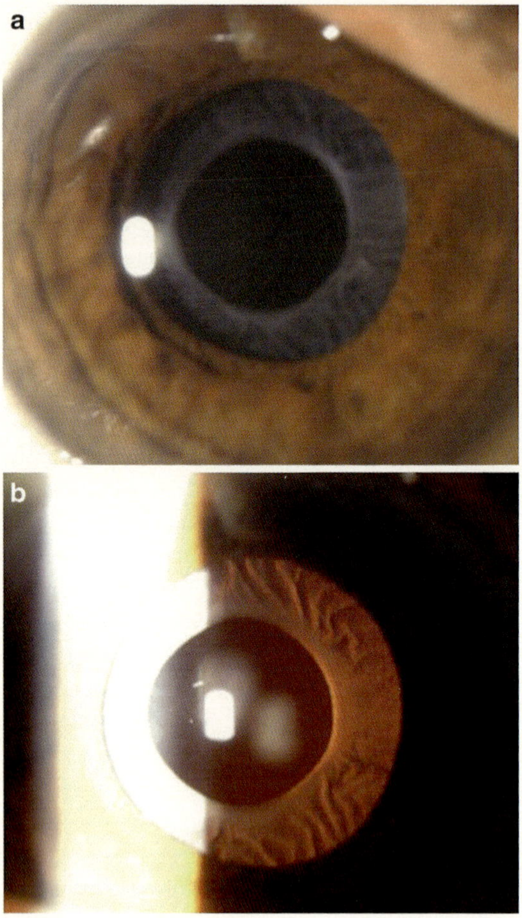

Fig. 7.3 Anterior capsule phimosis. (**a**) Direct and (**b**) retroillumination views of a manual CCC 1 year postoperatively. Significant anterior capsule phimosis is demonstrated as an opaque, wrinkled anterior capsule with a small diameter central capsule aperture. Images courtesy of Neil Friedman

Moreover, IOL decentration is higher in cases with extensive phimosis/capsule contraction syndrome [15, 16].

(b) Oversized or decentered CCC and increased rate of PCO

If the anterior capsular opening is too large, the IOL optic-capsule overlap does not provide an adequate barrier between the lens epithelial cells and the posterior capsule [17]. When these cells migrate to the posterior capsule and proliferate, posterior capsule opacification (PCO) results. PCO rates can exceed 60% when the CCC does not completely cover the IOL [18].

PCO is treated most commonly with an Nd:YAG laser. While the YAG procedure can be a quick fix, it is expensive and not without complications. Retinal detachment after Nd:YAG capsulotomy was documented in 0.4–0.81% of pseudophakic patients [19, 20]. While damage to the IOL (pitting) occurs in up to one third of cases, it is rarely of visual importance [21].

Importance of CCC: Efficacy

Capsulorhexis Size

General: Inaccurate prediction of effective lens position (ELP) has been identified as the biggest contributor to refractive error, with 35% of total refractive error attributable to deviations between intended and observed axial lens position [22]. The deviation between predicted and observed lens position is directly influenced by the amount of IOL-capsule overlap. A capsular opening that is too small results in posterior movement of the optic, which causes a hyperopic shift in the postoperative spherical equivalent refraction. In contrast, a capsular opening that is larger than the optic will result in an anterior, myopic shift [6]. Small shifts in ELP can have clinically significant effects on uncorrected visual acuity, as a 0.5 mm axial plane deviation from intended ELP results in approximately 1 D of refractive error for a 20 D lens [7]. The refractive surprise is larger than this in eyes with a short axial length and/or a higher IOL power. As such, it is not surprising that between 25 and 55% of patients have residual refractive errors of greater than 0.5 D after cataract surgery, a level that typically results in uncorrected visual acuity of 20/40 or less [23, 24].

Additional considerations for refractive cataract surgery: For premium IOL patients receiving toric, multifocal or accommodating IOLs, a principal goal is spectacle independence. In these patients, a refractive error exceeding 0.5 D can cause significant visual disturbances. Using current technology and surgical outcomes as a guide, surgeons should expect to perform refractive enhancements in 6.7–30% of these patients [25–27]. If the CCC is much smaller than intended, it can negatively influence the performance of an apodized multifocal IOL such as the AcrySof Restor® (Alcon Laboratories, Inc., Fort Worth, TX), as vision shifts from near to far when pupils dilate to 6 mm [28]. If there is significant phimosis central to 6 mm, then far vision will be compromised when the pupil dilates under mesopic conditions. A small CCC can also reduce the accommodative amplitude of an accommodative lens like the Crystalens for which most current recommendations are a 5.5- to 6.0-mm capsulorhexis. For a dual optic accommodating IOL like Synchrony (Visiogen, AMO-Abbott Santa Ana, CA), it is better to aim for a smaller CCC, as the IOL requires complete IOL-capsule overlap to prevent prolapse of the anterior optic out of the capsular bag [29, 30].

Capsulorhexis Shape and Centration

The shape and center position of the capsule opening also contribute to the postoperative refractive outcome. If the capsule opening is noncircular, the IOL can tilt or decenter as the capsule "shrink wraps" around the optic asymmetrically. Both of these phenomena can also occur in the presence of a capsule opening that is too large or contains a radial tear (see preceding section, "Safety"). The effect of CCC centration on visual outcomes has not been thoroughly studied, in part because there has been no predictable way to center using a manual CCC. Some hypothesize that centering the CCC on the center of the capsular bag is ideal, since symmetrical IOL-capsule shrink-wrap can occur. Alternative approaches include centering on the limbus, dilated or undilated pupil, or visual axis.

Preclinical Studies of Laser Capsulotomy: Focus on Safety

Laser–Tissue Interaction

A femtosecond (FS) laser creates incisions in tissue through a process called photodisruption. Photodisruption occurs as a cascade of events that is initiated when the laser spot energy exceeds a threshold fluence required for plasma formation. The plasma bubble then absorbs more energy than its surroundings, inducing a supersonic plasma expansion, shockwave, cavitation bubble and gas release. The threshold fluence for plasma formation is influenced by the pulse duration of the laser. Shorter pulse durations lower the threshold energy fluence required for plasma formation. Moreover, shorter laser pulses create smaller shockwaves, smaller cavitation bubbles, and fewer gas bubbles. FS laser pulse durations of just a few hundred femtoseconds (10^{15} pulses per second) disrupt 4×10^{-5} mm^3 of tissue [31]. The volume of tissue affected by a FS shockwave is approximately 1,000 times less than volume of tissue affected by a nanosecond shockwave [31].

The safety of FS lasers in ocular surgery has been demonstrated with FS laser corneal refractive systems [32]. FS laser energy can also be delivered posterior to the cornea. The near infrared wavelength of the FS laser can pass through translucent material (i.e., cornea) and only impact the tissue at the focus point of the laser beam [33]. Three key parameters for evaluating the safety of FS laser anterior capsulotomies involve analyzing retinal integrity, collateral tissue damage and capsule edge strength.

Retinal Safety

An in vivo study with Dutch belted rabbits ($n = 12$ eyes) was conducted using the Catalys (OptiMedica Corp., Sunnyvale, CA) Precision Laser System (Santa Clara, CA) to determine retinal safety when FS laser energy was applied in the anterior chamber. Maximum settings of laser energy (6 μJ, 100 kHz) were continuously applied for up to 60 s. No retinal damage was observed at 1 h and at 3 days [34].

Collateral Damage from Laser Capsulotomy

The laser parameters used during feasibility studies have been published for the Catalys™ Precision Laser System (OptiMedica Corp., Sunnyvale, CA) using freshly enucleated porcine eyes. A pulse duration of approximately 400 fs, wavelength of 1.03 μm, focal spot size <10 μm,

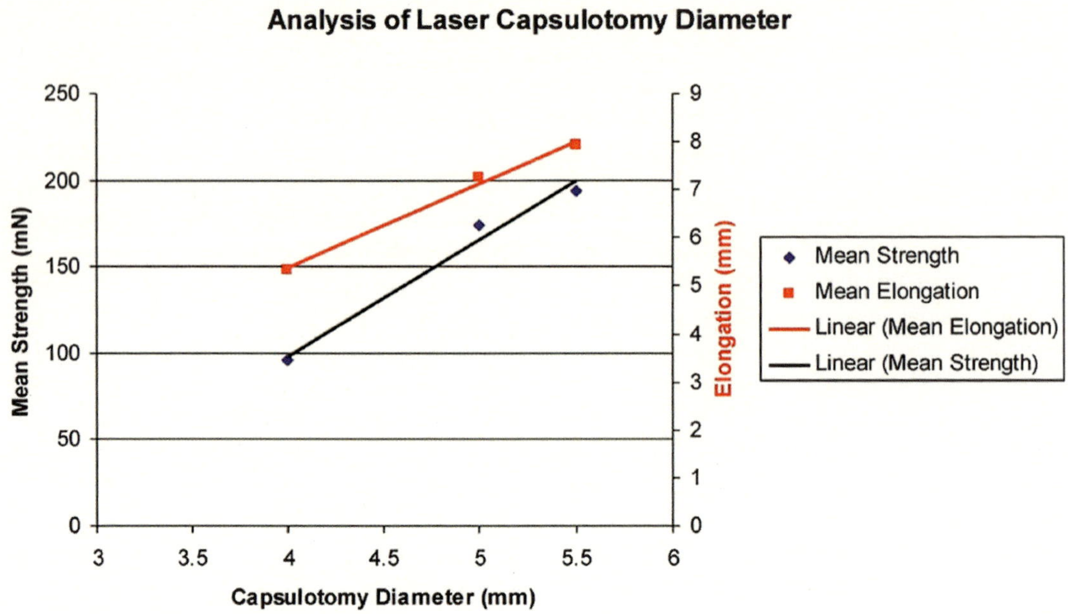

Fig. 7.4 Strength of laser capsulotomy as a function of size. LensAR laser capsulotomies of diameters 4, 5 and 5.5 mm were tested for strength and elongation at rupture. 5.5 mm laser capsulotomies had almost a two-fold increase in mean strength and elongation as compared to 4 mm diameter laser capsulotomies [36]

lateral spot spacing of 5 μm and axial (depth) spacing of 10 μm produced a continuous cut in the anterior capsule. This corresponded to a threshold pulse energy of approximately 3 μJ per laser pulse [34].

Capsular Edge Strength

Several studies have been conducted to evaluate the strength of the laser capsulotomy as it compares to manual CCC. Porcine eyes were used as a model in each study.

Nagy et al. looked at the elasticity of capsule aperture, and found that the LenSx® Laser (Alcon Laboratories, Fort Worth, TX) laser capsulotomy can stretch more before it ruptures than can a manual CCC ($p<0.001$) [35]. Frey et al. looked at the elasticity of the capsule aperture and the force registered at maximum stretch (immediately before rupture). The experimental design involved removing all nuclear and cortical tissue from within the capsular bag using ultrasound phacoemulsification. The empty capsular bag was then connected to a load cell on one side and a computer-controlled stepping motor on the other. The load (mN) and amount of displacement (mm) at the time of rupture were recorded. The manual CCC bags stretched 4.68 ± 1.01 mm with force of 125 ± 43 mN ($n=11$), while the LensAR laser capsulotomies stretched 7.45 ± 0.47 mm with a force of 177 ± 53 mN ($n=11$). Both findings were statistically significant ($p<0.05$ for force and $p<0.001$ for stretch) [36]. The study also looked at how the capsulotomy size influenced capsular elasticity and load bearing of the empty capsular bag. Larger capsulotomies ruptured at higher loads and after stretching more, as compared with smaller capsulotomies (see Fig. 7.4) [36].

In a similar study using the Catalys, Friedman et al. filled the empty capsule bag with a low viscosity liquid and then positioned the bag on an experimental stretching apparatus that simultaneously distended the capsule in equal and opposite directions (see Fig. 7.5a, b) [37]. The force was registered from both ends. The authors recorded the force at rupture for Catalys capsulotomies cut with pulse energies of 3, 6 and 10 μJ. These results were compared to the force

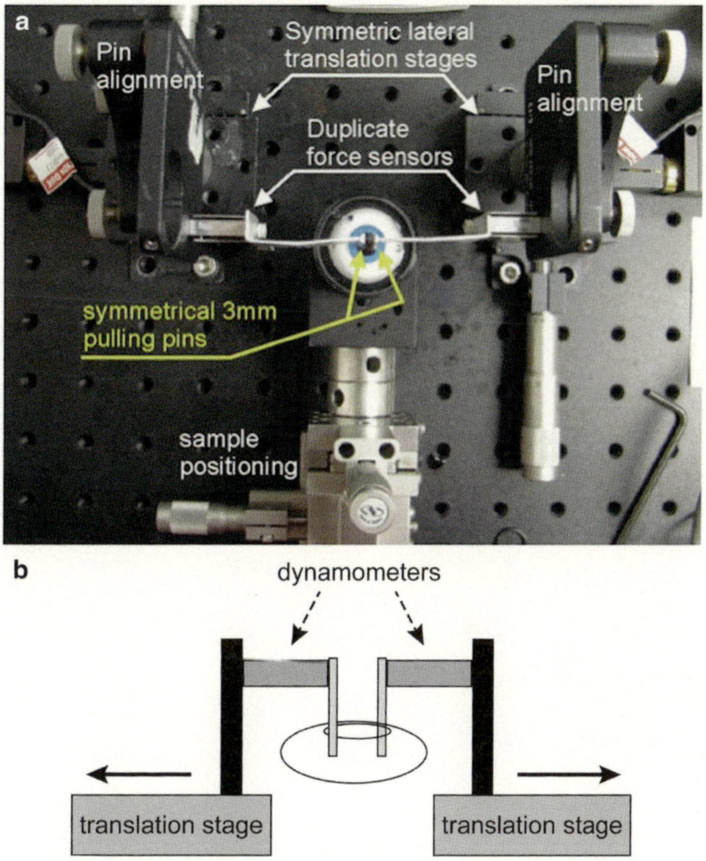

Fig. 7.5 Capsule strength testing apparatus. (**a**) Top-view photograph of capsule strength testing apparatus. (**b**) Simplified side-view illustration of same apparatus [37]. Images courtesy of Neil Friedman and OptiMedica

at rupture for manual CCC bags. For all tested pulse energies, the laser capsulotomy required more force to rupture than the manual CCC ($p<0.05$). The break force for the 3 μJ group was the highest with an average of 152 ± 21 mN, almost three times higher than the 65 ± 21 mN break force for manual CCC [37].

Capsule Edge Morphology

Capsule edge morphology was analyzed using scanning electron microscopy (SEM). When human capsules from a comparative clinical study were imaged at 2,000×, the manual CCC edge was smooth while the Catalys capsulotomy edge had microgrooves. At lower levels of magnification and in porcine eyes, the LenSx laser capsulotomies appear smooth. Further studies need to be conducted to determine if there is a direct correlation between capsule edge morphology and capsule strength (see Fig. 7.6a–d) [35].

Clinical Results: Focus on Effectiveness

As noted above, the size, shape, and centration of the CCC or capsulotomy are likely key determinants of effective lens position and can thus significantly impact refractive outcomes.

Minimizing variability from case to case (i.e., by increasing precision to achieve a lower standard deviation) is just as important as hitting the mean intended diameter value for a larger sample set (i.e., high accuracy—see sidebar "Accuracy and Precision"). For this reason, both accuracy and precision were evaluated for laser capsulotomies and manual CCCs.

Accuracy and Precision

Accuracy is an evaluation of the mean value of a sample set. If the mean value is close to the target, then accuracy is high. Precision is an evaluation of the deviation between individual samples

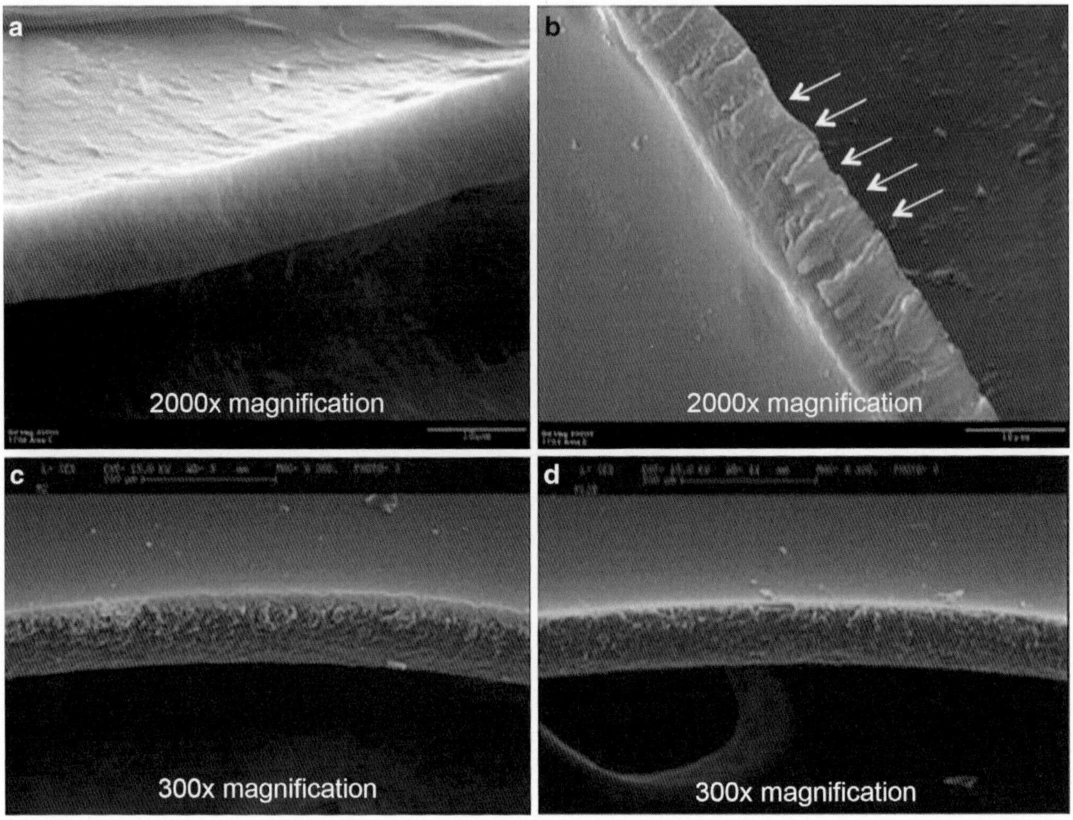

Fig. 7.6 Capsule edge morphology. (**a**) Ultrastructural appearance of manual CCC. (**b**) Ultrastructural appearance of laser capsulotomy performed with OptiMedica system. *Arrows* indicate microgrooves induced by laser cavitation on order of 5 μm. (**c**) SEM of capsule edge morphology in porcine eyes at 300× in manual CCC at 300× [35] and (**d**) laser capsulotomy with LenSx laser [35]

within the sample set. In a normally distributed sample set, precision is synonymous with standard deviation. A sample set is accurate but not precise, if the mean value of the individual samples coincides with the target value. A sample set that is precise but not accurate is populated by individual samples that are in close proximity of one another but are all off-target. High accuracy and high precision are primary goals in refractive laser-assisted cataract surgery (ReLACS) (see Fig. 7.7a–c).

Clinical Results: Laser Versus Manual Capsulotomy

Sample Study Design

In a prospective IRB-approved study, patients underwent bilateral cataract surgery with one eye randomized to laser pretreatment (capsulotomy and lens fragmentation) using the OptiMedica Catalys™ Precision Laser System, followed by cataract removal and IOL implantation [37]. The fellow eye underwent conventional cataract surgery with a manual CCC. Preceding cataract extraction, the capsule disc from each eye was excised, placed on a microscope slide and stained with Trypan Blue (see Fig. 7.8a, b). Photographs of the discs were taken using an inverted video microscope fitted with a National Institute of Standards and Technology (NIST)-traceable reticule and analyzed off-line using NIH Image software (National Institutes of Health, Bethesda, MD). The diameters along the *x*- and *y*-axis of the image and ±45° were measured and disc size recorded as the average of these four diameters. To assess the shape of the

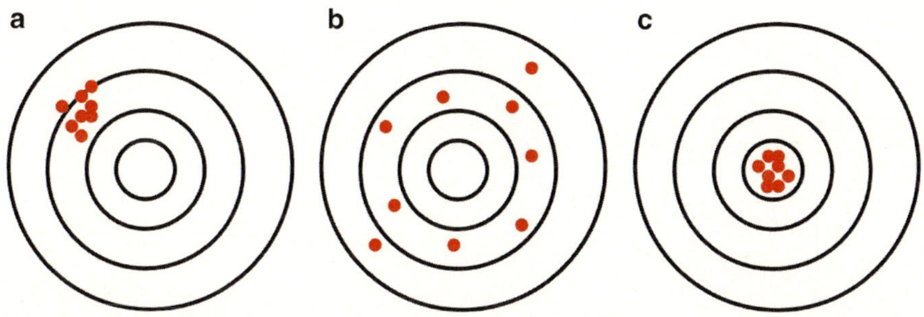

Fig. 7.7 Illustration of accuracy and precision. (**a**) Mean value of sample set is not at center of target (low accuracy) but *dots* are clustered (high precision). (**b**) Mean value of sample set is at the center of target (high accuracy) but *dots* are not clustered (low precision). (**c**) Mean value of ample set is at center of target (high accuracy) and dots are closely clustered (high precision)

excised capsule discs, the circularity equation was used ($C = 4\pi A/d^2$), where A is the area of the disc and d is the mean disc diameter. Capsulotomy centration was assessed from analyses of Catalys system video footage.

Free-floating Capsulotomies

Scientists and clinicians associated with LenSx, LensAR, and Technolas (Munich, Germany) have conducted studies targeting similar endpoints. A summary of the results recently published or presented at conferences follows.

Capsulotomy Size and Shape

Studies involving each of the four laser platforms have demonstrated significant accuracy and precision gains for size and shape of their respective laser capsulotomy as compared to manual CCC. See Tables 7.1 and 7.2 for summary of results on size and shape of laser capsulotomy versus manual CCC [34, 37–42].

Capsulotomy Centration

The average root mean square (RMS) distance from the center of capsulotomy to the intended center was 0.077 ± 0.047 mm using the Catalys [37] (see Fig. 7.9a, b). Auffarth measured the Y-axis decentration of laser capsulotomy created with the Technolas system versus manual CCC. On the Technolas system, the decentration was 0.095 ± 0.037 mm for laser capsulotomy and 0.160 ± 0.090 mm for the manual CCC ($p < 0.001$) [41].

Clinical Results of Laser Versus Manual Capsulotomy: Postoperative Effects

Capsule Aperture Size and Shape Changes Over Time

Even in cases that do not have clinically significant anterior capsule phimosis, the size and shape of the capsule aperture changes postoperatively [43, 44]. Friedman et al. investigated the amount of contraction (in diameter) for Catalys capsulotomy eyes, and compared these to manual CCC at 1 and 4 weeks postoperatively. While both the laser and manual CCC apertures contracted over time, the diameter of the laser apertures deviated just 0.1 mm with a tight standard deviation, whereas the apertures created manually deviated over 0.5 mm with a large standard deviation (see Fig. 7.10) [37]. Vukich et al. analyzed the accuracy and precision for aperture roundness ($R = 4A/\pi L^2$, where L is capsule diameter) and found that Catalys capsulotomy maintains its shape at 1 and 4 weeks [45].

Postoperative IOL Centration

Postoperative IOL centration is a function of many variables, including: capsule aperture center, size and shape at different time points, and IOL design. Nagy et al. performed a comparative prospective study that looked at IOL centration at 1 week, 1 month and 1 year after surgery for 20 lasered eyes treated with the LenSx system and 20 manual CCC eyes. Retro-illumination photographs were taken at each of these time points

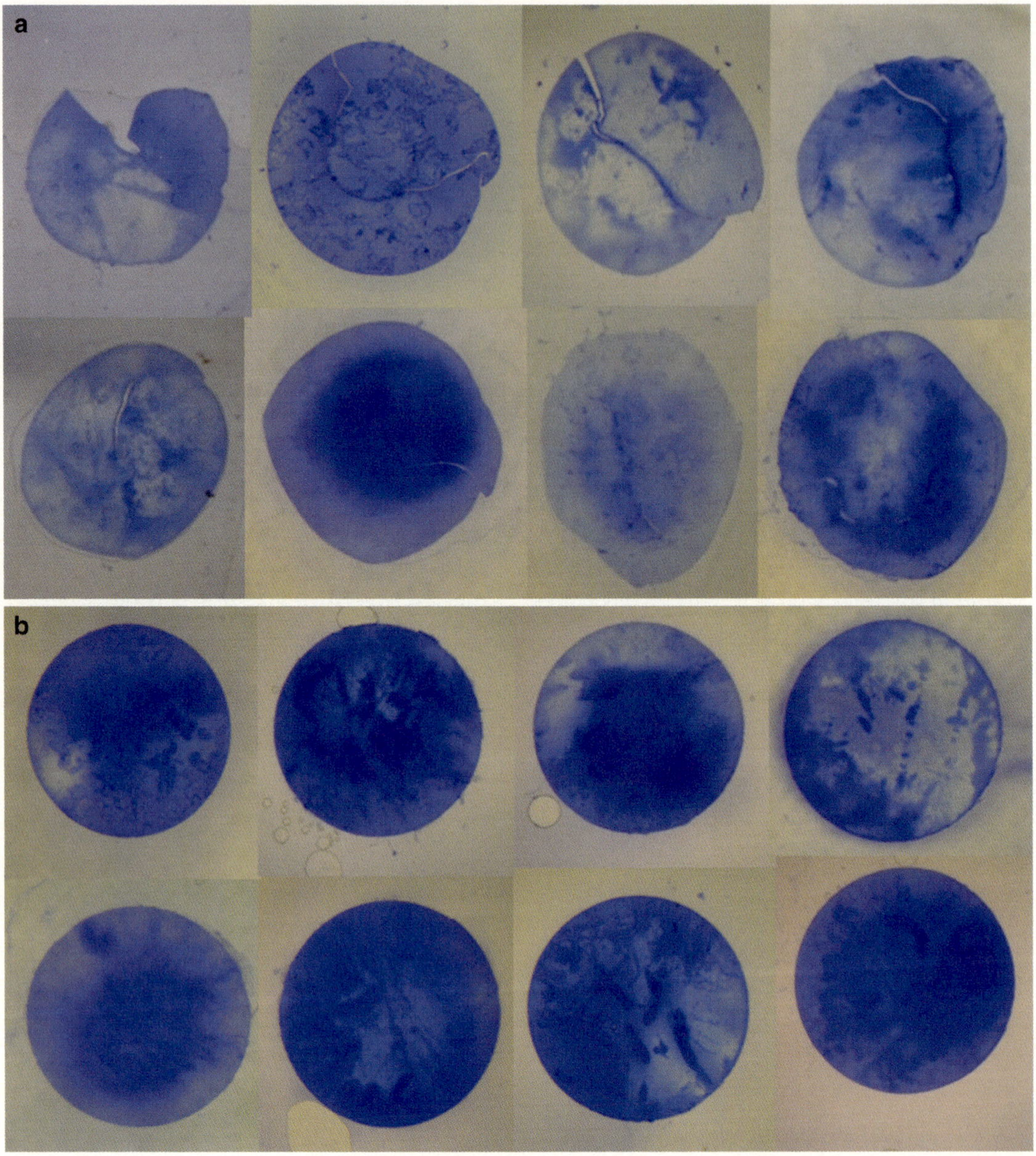

Fig. 7.8 Capsule disc morphology. (**a**) Excised CCC discs stained with Trypan Blue. (**b**) Excised Catalys capsulotomy discs stained with Trypan Blue. Images courtesy of OptiMedica

and analyzed digitally using Adobe Photoshop® (Adobe Corporation; San Jose, CA). Decentration was recorded as the distance between the center of the dilated pupil and the center of the IOL. Decentration was significantly reduced in the laser group ($p<0.01$). Moreover, multivariate analysis showed a strong correlation between the amount of IOL decentration and the irregularity of the capsule aperture shape [46, 47].

Postoperative Refraction and Effective Lens Position

Hill and Uy assessed the manifest refraction at 6 months after surgery and calculated the deviation between the manifest refraction and

Table 7.1 Capsulotomy size

Author	Laser	Measurement technique	Manual CCC	Laser capsulotomy
Yeilding et al. 2011	LensAR	Deviation from intended size	0.445 ± 0.596 mm (n = 11)	0.082 ± 0.110 mm (n = 12); (p < 0.05)
Tackman et al. 2011	LensAR	Deviation from intended size	0.42 ± 0.54 mm (n = 24)	0.16 ± 0.17 mm (n = 49); (p = 0.03)
Slade et al. 2010	LenSx (Alcom)	Deviation from intended size	10% within 0.25 mm (n = 60)	100% within 0.25 mm (n = 60)
Palanker et al. 2010	Catalys (OptiMedica)	Deviation from intended size	0.282 ± 0.305 mm (n = 30)	0.027 ± 0.025 mm (n = 29); (p < 0.001)
Friedman et al. 2011	Catalys (OptiMedica)	Deviation from intended size	0.337 ± 0.258 mm (n = 23)	0.029 ± 0.026 mm (n = 39); (p < 0.05)
Auffarth et al. 2011	Victus (Technolas)	Measure observed size (intended = 5.5 mm)	Not recorded	5.5 ± 0.12 mm (n = 31)

Summary of recent published clinical data on size of excised capsule disc for laser capsulotomy as compared to manual CCC [34, 37–41]

Table 7.2 Capsulotomy shape

Author	Laser	Measurement technique	Manual CCC	Laser capsulotomy
Yielding et al. 2011	LensAR	RMS error versus average diameter	0.346 ± 0.099 (n = 11)	0.141 ± 0.104 (n = 12); (p < 0.01)
Tachman et al. 2011	LensAR	Best fit circle—perfect circle (residuals analysis)	0.01 ± 0.03 (n = 24)	0.02 ± 0.04 (n = 49); (p = 0.09)
Nagy et al. 2010	LenSx (Alcom)	Roundness	Not reported	Significantly rounder (p = 0.028)
Palanker et al. 2010	Catalys (OptiMedica)	$4A/(\pi d^2)$ (1.00 = perfect circle)	0.77 ± 0.15 (n = 30)	0.95 ± 0.05 (n = 29); (p < 0.001)
Friedman et al. 2011	Catalys (OptiMedica)	$4A/(\pi d^2)$ (1.00 = perfect circle)	0.80 ± 0.14 (n = 18)	0.94 ± 0.04 (n = 39); (p < 0.05)
Auffarth et al. 2011	Victus Technolas	Minimum diameter/maximum diameter	0.93 ± 0.04 (n = 31)	0.97 ± 0.01 (n = 31); (p < 0.001)

Summary of recent published clinical data on laser capsulotomy shape as compared to manual CCC. The measurement technique varied by author

[a]Measurement taken for excised capsule disc unless otherwise noted [34, 37–39, 41, 42]

preoperative predicted target refraction for laser (n = 249) versus manual (n = 123) capsulotomy cases. The LensAR laser cataract surgery system was used. All cases were performed by the same surgeon (Uy). Laser-treated eyes showed a mean deviation of MRSE from target of −0.21 ± 0.39 D while the manual group value was +0.55 ± 0.41 D (p < 0.001). The absolute deviation in MRSE was less impressive (laser 0.42 ± 0.39 D; manual −0.59 ± 0.35 D) but still statistically significant, showing better predictability in the laser group. The results were more impressive when the % of cases within a certain range of the target MRSE were calculated. When a threshold of within 0.25 D of target was used, 47% of the laser group fell within this value versus 22% of the manual group. If a threshold of 0.5 D was used, 79% of the lascr group met this criterion versus 53% of manually treated eyes (p = 0.003 for both groups) [48].

Slade looked at the standard deviation in refractive error for Crystalens AO patients that underwent manual CCC versus LenSx laser capsulotomy. At 3 months, the results showed a standard deviation of 0.60 D in manual cases and 0.40 D with the LenSx laser [49].

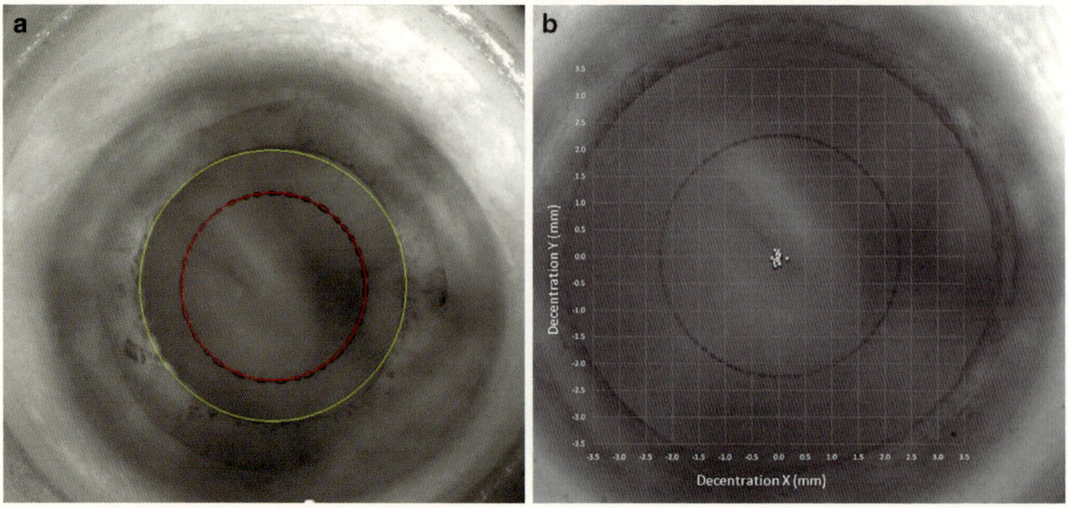

Fig. 7.9 Laser capsulotomy centration. (**a**) For human eyes, centration of the laser capsulotomy was analyzed using still frames from the Catalys video system. Centration accuracy was measured relative to the intended capsulotomy center, which was set to the center of the dilated pupil. (**b**) Each *dot* on this figure represents the observed center of the laser capsulotomy. The 0 point (*x* and *y*) represents the center of the dilated pupil. The average RMS distance between each dot and the 0 point was 0.077 ± 0.047 mm (*N* = 29) [37]. Images courtesy of Neil Friedman and OptiMedica

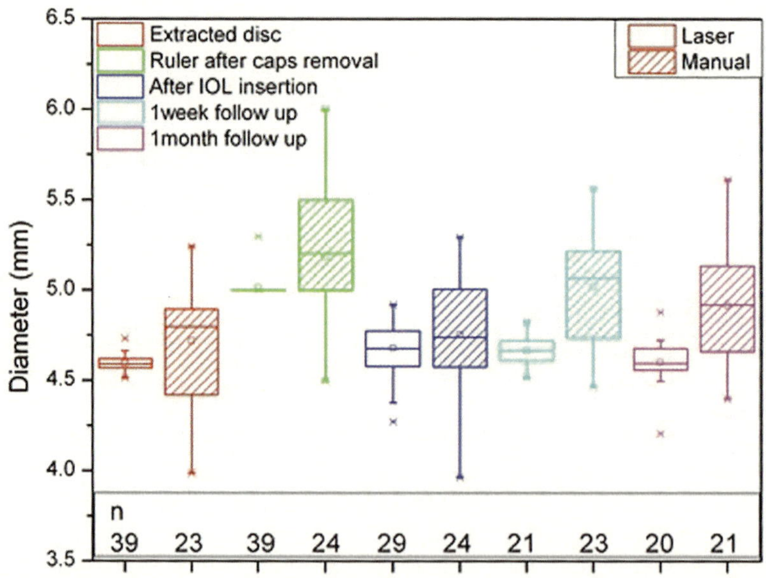

Fig. 7.10 Capsule aperture size for Catalys eyes versus manual CCC at three time points: time of surgery, 1 week postoperative and 1 month postoperative. From time of surgery through 1 month postoperative, both lasered and manual capsule apertures increased in size as a result of the tensile forces exerted on the bag. The manual CCC group experienced greater size increase and much wider size variability (as indicated by size of error bars) [37]. Image courtesy of Neil Friedman and OptiMedica

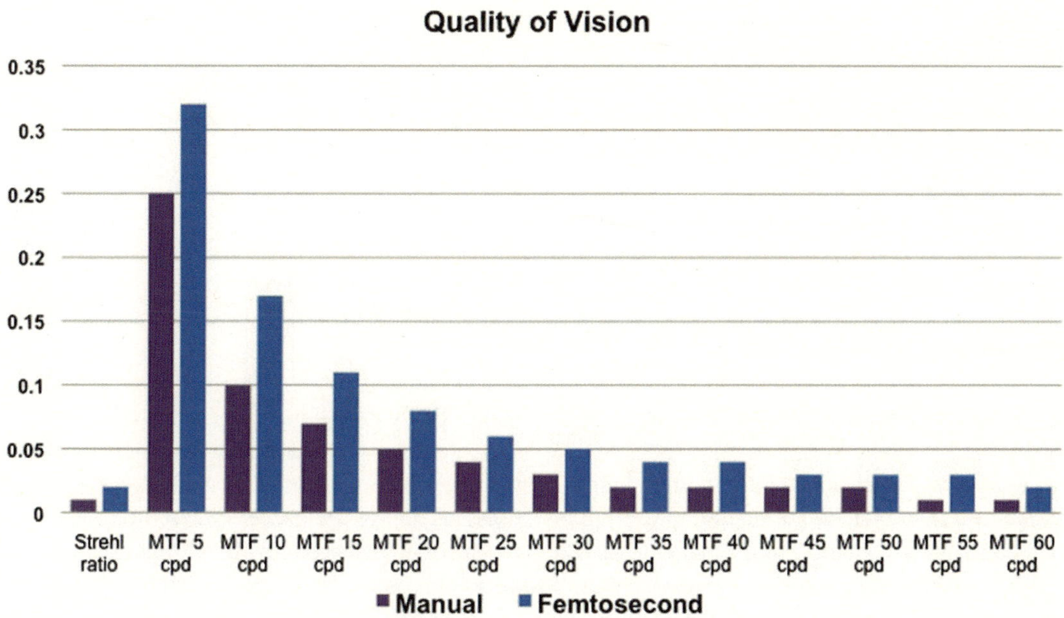

Fig. 7.11 Modulation transfer function (MTF) for LenSx laser eyes versus manual CCC. A higher MTF value is indicative of a more sharply focused image on the retina. For each spatial frequency (in cycles per degree (cpd) tested), the MTF was higher for patients who had undergone the laser cataract procedure than the manual procedure

The theoretical effective lens position (ELP) can be back calculated using variables such as postoperative refractive, keratometry readings and axial length [50]. Slade derived this theoretical ELP value at 3 months after surgery using the Crystalens patient data, and found a significantly smaller standard deviation in ELP for the LenSx laser capsulotomy than a manual control group ($p \leq 0.05$). The differential between predicted and postoperative ELP was 0.200 ± 0.074 mm for the laser eyes [49].

Visual Acuity

Preliminary studies have demonstrated the potential for laser cataract surgery to result in enhanced visual acuity. At 1 day post-op, the best corrected visual acuity for a cohort of premium IOL patients was 20/25 or better in approximately 80% of cases and 20/30 or better in all cases ($n = 50$) [40].

Higher Order Aberrations and Contrast Sensitivity

IOL position can affect higher order aberrations, such as tilt and coma, which can reduce contrast sensitivity. Preliminary studies indicate that eyes undergoing laser assisted cataract surgery had less internal vertical tilt and coma aberrations than eyes that underwent traditional cataract surgery ($p = 0.006$) [42]. In this study, Nagy also examined modulation transfer function (MTF) for laser versus manual CCC eyes and found a statistically significant difference, with laser eyes registering a higher MTF at each angular resolution level assessed (see Fig. 7.11).

Larger study sizes and additional measures of visual outcomes should be undertaken to confirm or refute many of the hypothesized beneficial effects of laser assisted cataract surgery on visual acuity and ocular higher order aberrations.

Performing Laser Capsulotomy

Performing a safe and effective laser capsulotomy involves four steps—planning, docking, image-guided customization of the plan, and treatment. The order and approach to these four steps varies by manufacturer.

Planning

For all systems, some planning can be done prior to the patient being coupled ("docked") to the laser system. For the capsulotomy, the planning parameters may include the size, shape, depth of cut, and desired center. The primary driver for the capsulotomy size and shape used in a particular case is the optic size of the IOL to be implanted. Depending on the laser system, the depth of cut may be preprogrammed or determined by the surgeon after the patient has been docked to the system.

As an example, the OptiMedica Catalys system has three automated centration methods that can be used: the pupil, the limbus, and the scanned capsule as determined by the 3D spectral domain OCT and ocular surface detection algorithms. At the time of this writing, the centration method will be based on surgeon preference as not enough clinical data is available to assess whether a certain center is optimal (capsular bag versus pupil versus limbus). Future studies should help elucidate whether or not capsular bag or limbal centration of the capsulotomy has any clinical utility.

Docking

The quality of the dock can affect the accuracy and completeness of the capsulotomy and other laser incisions. For both curved applanation and immersion lenses, if the eye is not centered in the *x*/*y* plane under the system's optical path then the centering capability and size of the capsulotomy could be compromised. If the patient interface (PI) creates corneal distortions or significant ocular tilt with respect to the laser's optics, then incomplete capsulotomies or tissue tags can occur. There is a risk of these tags extending into tears if not properly managed.

For a more detailed discussion of docking technique and other considerations, please see Chap. 6.

Image-Guided Treatment Customization

Image guidance is necessary to ensure safe treatment. Safety requirements include avoiding inadvertent laser treatment of iris and posterior capsule. Once the patient is docked, the surgeon uses an image guidance system to determine where the incisions will be placed. LenSx, Technolas, and OptiMedica use on-board three-dimensional (3D) optical coherence tomography for their imaging systems, while LensAR uses 3D confocal structured illumination (3D-CSI). In the LenSx and Technolas systems, signal processing is done manually. For the capsulotomy, this means moving the center and determining the anterior and posterior boundaries (*z*-axis) using drag-and-drop controls. OptiMedica's signal processing is done automatically using ocular surface identification algorithms, which are reviewed and modified as necessary by the surgeon. The LensAR system uses automated imaging biometry and beam placement. For a comprehensive discussion of imaging for individual laser systems, please see the specific system chapters elsewhere in this book (Chaps. 15–18).

Treatment

Order and Directionality of Incisions

Just as corneal folds can compromise laser precision in capsulotomy creation, laser induced cavitation and gas bubbles reduce the laser's ability to create cuts posterior to these bubbles. For this reason, laser energy is applied posterior to anterior for each cut. While the capsulotomy is anterior to lens fragmentation, it is usually performed first, because the precision requirements for capsulotomy exceed that of lens fragmentation, it is beneficial to provide the laser with the most accurate location of the anterior lens capsule possible when capsulotomy is performed by doing so before any other laser treatment occurs inside the lens. Capsulotomy cut time can range from 2 s to more than 15 s, depending on the system and cut parameters and the pulse energy requirements (lower pulse energy corresponds to higher allowable repetition rate or speed of cutting). The time requirements for the capsulotomy can influence cut quality, as ocular movement during capsulotomy creation can create tags or double cuts.

Moving from Laser Treatment to Lens Removal

After laser treatment, the surgeon will undock the patient and proceed with the rest of surgery. Depending on where the laser system is located within the facility, the crystalline lens removal and IOL implantation may or may not occur in the same room as the laser procedure. Before initiating lens dissection, it is critical that the surgeon confirm that there are no tags or attachment points between the capsulotomy and capsule.

Use Cases and Benefits of Laser Anterior Capsulotomy

Improved IOL Power Formula Predictability

While personal customization of A-constant or surgeon factor in IOL power formulas can reduce the average deviation from intended refraction over a large sample set, the inherent variability in manual CCC technique may result in an unexpected outcome for any particular patient. For patients opting for premium IOLs, a refractive error of just 0.5 D can be distracting or disappointing for the patient. Laser assisted cataract surgery systems give surgeons a powerful tool with which to standardize the size, shape, and positioning of the capsule aperture. As discussed above, early studies strongly suggest that FS laser capsulotomy reduces the variability in the positioning of the IOL and improves the predictability of refractive outcomes.

Complicated Cases

Manual CCC construction is especially challenging in a number of settings, such as when visibility or room to maneuver inside the eye is limited, or the integrity of the capsule and/or its zonular support is compromised.

Shallow Anterior Chamber (Short Axial Length, Small Anterior Segment, Chronic Angle Closure Glaucoma)

When working inside a small anterior chamber, it is more difficult to grasp the cut capsular edge and tear it while exerting the appropriate tangential forces to create a CCC. Furthermore, the chamber holds a smaller volume of viscoelastic than an average eye, and loss of even a small amount can destabilize the necessary posterior pressure of the viscoelastic that allows adequate control while tearing the CCC. Consequently, an unwanted radial tear/peripheral extension of the CCC can occur more easily. Clearly, the ability to create a laser capsulotomy without entering the eye and grasping capsule is a significant advantage in this setting.

Intraoperative Floppy Iris Syndrome (IFIS)

IFIS results from atrophy of the iris dilator muscle and is strongly associated with the use of selective alpha-1 blocking medications such as tamsulosin [51] and, more recently, silodosin. In this setting, the iris loses thickness and rigidity, often resulting in poor dilation. The iris may also constrict easily if touched or prolapse if an incision is made to enter the eye. The movements inside the eye associated with creating a CCC can lead to pupil constriction and/or extrusion through incisions, which makes completion of the CCC quite challenging. So again, the creation of the CCC before the eye is even entered could be tremendously helpful.

Weak or Focally Absent Zonules (Pseudoexfoliation, Trauma, Genetic defects, etc.)

The tangential, circular tearing motion needed to manually create a CCC necessitates tension on the zonules. Laser capsulotomy removes this variable, and by doing so eliminates a significant risk factor for creating further zonular damage during surgery.

Poor or Absent Red Reflex, Including Mature White Cataracts

A minimal or absent red reflex poses a technical challenge to manual CCC. The use of Trypan Blue dye is helpful, but adds an extra step to surgery. Furthermore, hypermature cataracts often contain liquefied lens material which exerts forward pressure on the anterior capsule, making it difficult to control the direction and degree of the manual CCC tear. The result can be a rapid unanticipated radial tear, which in its most severe form, creates the "Argentinean Flag Sign" as the (trypan blue-stained) capsule splits in half, sometimes resulting in a dropped nucleus. The ability to rapidly create a laser capsulotomy without entering the eye might be a major advantage for such cases.

Nonroutine Capsule Morphology

In fibrotic capsules, the capsule can be brittle and inelastic in some areas and not in others. In these cases it can be quite difficult to create a controlled CCC as the shearing force required to propagate the CCC is not circumferentially consistent. In thin, friable capsules, the capsule may fall apart or tear easily when grasped. Since laser capsulotomy creation does not rely on the shearing properties of the capsule, the laser approach may be especially advantageous for patients with fibrotic, thin, or highly elastic capsules.

Contraindications to Laser Capsulotomy

Dense Corneal Scars

Patients with significant corneal scarring should not undergo laser cataract surgery, as opacities in the cornea decrement the system's ability to image properly and deliver the laser energy precisely. When feasible, these patients should have their corneal scarring treated prior to cataract surgery, whether by manual superficial keratectomy, laser phototherapeutic keratectomy, or keratoplasty, as significant corneal scarring can skew biometry readings and also may induce irregular astigmatism. Future experience will determine how dense corneal scars can be without interfering with imaging and laser delivery.

Small Pupils

Patients that have physiologic small pupils that require intracameral extension of the pupillary boundary are also not good candidates for laser cataract surgery. Eyes exhibiting these characteristics attain suitable dilation only after the anterior chamber has been penetrated. Once the anterior chamber has been penetrated, docking the patient's eye to a laser system may be a safety risk.

Uncooperative Patients

All current laser cataract systems require that the patient be able to lie flat and remain still for several minutes while docking, imaging, and treatment occur. Disoriented or medically unstable patients who cannot remain still in a supine position are poor candidates for laser assisted cataract surgery.

Management of Potential Complications

Insufficient Pupil Dilation

Application of FS laser energy to the iris can cause miosis, hemorrhage, and pain. Therefore, the maximum size of the laser capsulotomy achievable without manual enlargement is dependent upon pupil dilation. For example, if the pupil dilates to 6.5 mm and a circumferential iris safety margin of 0.5mm is used, then the maximal capsulotomy diameter is 5.0 mm which may be smaller than the planned diameter. In these instances, the size of the capsulotomy will need to be modified after the patient is under dock. If the capsulotomy size is not reduced, then there is an increased risk for inadvertent iris treatment. The OptiMedica Catalys and LensAR systems help mitigate this risk by automatically detecting the pupil margin. Additionally, the Catalys system uses automated iris safety margins to define regions where the laser cannot fire. Systems that do not have automatic pupil detection and/or automated iris safety margins require the surgeon to manually determine the safety boundary.

Incomplete Capsulotomy

Before performing hydrodissection, the laser capsulotomy should ideally be free floating in the anterior chamber. If injection of viscoelastic does not completely separate the capsule disc from the remaining capsule, then the capsulotomy must be separated in the area of laser excision using mechanical means. In this circumstance, to minimize the chance of a radial tear, it is important for the surgeon to replicate the continuous curvilinear capsulorhexis motion that would have been used to create a manual CCC. Once the excised capsule is floating free in the anterior chamber, it can be removed using forceps or aspirated.

Suction Loss During Procedure

Suction loss is a rare event, but it can occur. Decreasing the amount of time that the patient is under dock will lessen the likelihood of suction loss. Depending on when suction loss occurs, re-docking the patient may or may not be feasible. If suction loss occurs prior to the delivery of the laser energy (i.e., during image-guided treatment customization), then re-dock could be considered by the surgeon. If suction loss occurs halfway through the capsulotomy, the surgeon has two options: (1) move to the Operating Room and complete the capsulotomy manually or (2) re-dock and create a second capsulotomy that has a diameter more peripheral than the incomplete capsulotomy.

Conclusions

Laser Capsulotomy Is More Accurate

As the data presented here show, size, shape, and centration of laser capsulotomy are more precise that manual techniques (see Fig. 7.12). While clinical experience and peer-reviewed studies are still limited, the level of precision afforded by this technology should translate into more reliable refractive outcomes after cataract surgery.

Laser Capsulotomy Is Likely Safer

Anterior capsulotomy is considered by many as the most important step in cataract surgery, as it affects the safety and accuracy of all other subsequent surgical manipulations inside the eye. While some busy cataract surgeons will argue (perhaps correctly in some instances) that they can create a manual capsulorhexis as safely as a laser, such statements will probably only hold true for routine cases that do not require precise sizing, shape, and centration of the capsular opening. However, such logic will likely break down even for the most experienced of surgeons for nonroutine, difficult cases such as small anterior chambers, mature cataracts, and eyes with compromised zonules.

If, as the laboratory experiments presented here suggest, MAY capsulotomies are actually stronger and hence more resistant to tearing than manual CCCs, MAY offer an additional safety advantage over a manual approach.

Surgical Technique will Evolve

Refractive laser-assisted cataract surgery is in its infancy. As this technology becomes more widely disseminated, new strategies for capsule manage-

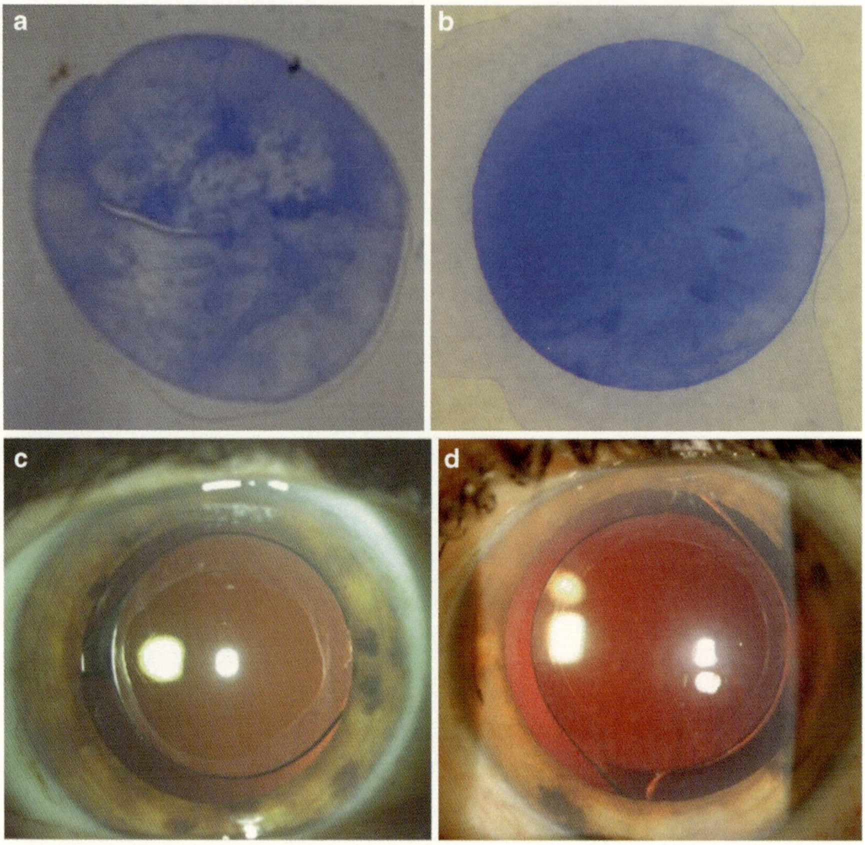

Fig. 7.12 Intraoperative-op excised capsule disc and post-op capsule aperture for manual CCC versus Catalys laser eyes. (**a**) Stained CCC disc. (**b**) Stained laser disc. (**c**) Slit lamp image of eye that underwent manual CCC. (**d**) Slit lamp image of eye that underwent Catalys laser capsulotomy. Image courtesy of OptiMedica

ment will evolve in ways that are impossible to predict at present. It may turn out that, with the ability to reliably segment and/or soften and more easily remove the cataractous lens, anterior capsulotomy openings become smaller on average.

Laser Capsulotomy will Guide the Future of IOL Design

For the past 25 years, cataract surgery has been performed by tearing a round capsulorhexis sized large enough to allow surgical manipulations to be comfortably performed inside the capsular bag but small enough to overlap an IOL optic. FS lasers give surgeons the flexibility to create capsulotomies of varied shapes and sizes that should remain more stable over time [45]. Given the highly reproducible nature of these cuts, there will be increased potential for the development of novel IOLs that must be retained (all or in part) within or by the capsular bag. Already, designs such as the Synchrony, Power Vision, and NuLens accommodating IOLs are creating greater demand for highly accurate capsulotomy dimensions. The holy grail of lens replacement surgery is the ability to achieve capsular refilling that will allow for titration of artificial lens power accompanied by maintenance of accommodation. FS lasers will allow the creation of one or more very small anterior capsular openings to achieve this end and, if the issue of posterior capsule opacification can be solved, the coming decades will witness a paradigm shift in this direction.

Key Points

1. Offers a level of accuracy, precision, and reproducibility superior to manual technique.
2. Is more resistant to rupture when compared to manual capsulorhexis (in vitro data).
3. Enhances the predictability of the effective lens position, a predominant source of error in achieving the intended refractive outcome.
4. Programmable treatment parameters include size, shape, depth, and centration coordinates. The surgical plan for these parameters should be determined in advance of the procedure to minimize dock and treatment time.
5. Proper intraoperative management of the capsulotomy disc is imperative. The surgeon should replicate the CCC technique in regions where a capsule disc may have micro-attachments to surrounding capsule tissue to mitigate the risk of a tissue bridge extending into a tear.

References

1. Krag S, Olsen T, Andreassen TT. Biomechanical characteristics of the human anterior lens capsule in relation1 to age. Invest Ophthalmol Vis Sci. 1997;38:357–63.
2. Krag S, Thim K, Corydon L. Stretching capacity of capsulorhexis: an experimental study on animal cadaver eyes. Eur J Implant Refract Surg. 1990;2:43–5.
3. Thim K, Krag S, Corydon L. Stretching capacity of capsulorhexis and nucleus delivery. J Cataract Refract Surg. 1991;17:27–31.
4. Seibel BS. Phacodynamic: mastering the tools and techniques of phacoemulsification surgery. 4th ed. Thorofare, NJ: SLACK Incorporated; 2005.
5. Hill W, Uy H. Effective lens position following laser anterior capsulotomy. In: Proceedings of the American Society of Cataract and Refractive Surgery (ASCRS) 2011 annual meeting, femtosecond laser cataract surgery session 4-E, 29 March 2011, San Diego, CA.
6. Cekiç O, Batman C. The relationship between capsulorhexis size and anterior chamber depth relation. Ophthalmic Surg Lasers. 1999;30(3):185–90.
7. Yanoff M, Duker JS, Augsburger JJ. Yanoff & Duker's ophthalmology. 3rd ed. Saint Louis, MO: Mosby; 2008.
8. Marques FF, Marques DM, Osher RH, Osher JM. Fate of anterior capsule tears during cataract surgery. J Cataract Refract Surg. 2006;32:1638–42.
9. Muhtaseb M, Kalhoro A, Ionides A. A system for preoperative stratification of cataract patients according to risk of intraoperative complications. Br J Ophthalmol. 2004;88:1242–6.
10. Unal M, Yücel I, Sarici A, et al. Phacoemulsification with topical anesthesia: resident experience. J Cataract Refract Surg. 2006;32:1361–5.
11. LeBoyer RM, Werner L, Snyder ME, et al. Acute haptic-induced ciliary sulcus irritation associated with single-piece AcrySof intraocular lenses. J Cataract Refract Surg. 2005;31:1421–7.
12. Piette S, Canlas OAQ, Tran HV, et al. Ultrasound biomicroscopy in uveitis-glaucoma-hyphema syndrome. Am J Ophthalmol. 2002;133(6):839–41.
13. Asaria RH, Salmon JF, Skinner AR, et al. Electron microscopy findings on an intraocular lens in the uveitis, glaucoma, hyphema syndrome. Eye. 1997;11:827–9.
14. Joo CK, Shin JA, Kim JH. Capsular opening contraction after continuous curvilinear capsulorhexis and intraocular lens implantation. J Cataract Refract Surg. 1996;22:585–90.
15. Werner L, Pandey SK, Apple DJ, et al. Anterior capsule opacification: correlation of pathological findings with clinical sequelae. Ophthalmology. 2001;107:1675–81.
16. Davison JA. Capsule contraction syndrome. J Cataract Refract Surg. 1993;19:582–9.
17. Ram J, Apple DJ, Peng Q, et al. Update on fixation of rigid and foldable posterior chamber intraocular lenses. Part II. Choosing the correct haptic fixation and intraocular lens design to help eradicate posterior capsule opacification. Ophthalmology. 1999;106:883–90.
18. Hollick EJ, Spalton DJ, Meacock WR. The effect of capsulorhexis size on posterior capsular opacification: one-year results of a randomized prospective trial. Am J Ophthalmol. 1999;128(3):271–9.
19. Keates RH, Steinert RF, Puliafito CA, Maxwell SK. Long-term follow-up of Nd:YAG laser posterior capsulotomy. J Am Intraocul Implant Soc. 1984;10:164–8.
20. Javitt JC, Street DA, Tielsch JM, Wang Q, et al. National outcomes of cataract extraction. Retinal detachment and endophthalmitis after outpatient cataract surgery. Ophthalmology. 1994;101:100–5.
21. Stark WJ, Worthen D, Holladay JT, Murray G. Neodymium:YAG lasers. An FDA report. Ophthalmology. 1985;92:209–12.

22. Norrby S. Sources of error in intraocular lens power calculation. J Cataract Refract Surg. 2008;34: 368–76.
23. Lim LH, Lee SY, Ang CL. Factors affecting the predictability of SRK II in patients with normal axial length undergoing phacoemulsification surgery. Singapore Med J. 2009;50(2):120–5.
24. Landers J, Goggin M. Comparison of refractive outcomes using immersion ultrasound biometry and IOLMaster biometry. Clin Exp Ophthalmol. 2009; 37(5):285–9.
25. Chow J, et al. Refractive enhancement after accommodating and apodized diffractive multifocal IOL implantation: indications, rates and outcomes. In: Proceedings of the European Society of Cataract and Refractive Surgery (ESCRS) 2010 annual meeting, aspheric IOLs/multifocal IOLs session, 07 September 2010.
26. Guttman C. Laser vision correction useful for enhancing outcomes of presbyopia-correcting IOLs. 2009. http://www.eurotimes.org/09June/LaserVision Correction. pdf. Accessed 21 May 2011.
27. Chang D. Mastering refractive IOLs: the art and science. Thorofare, NJ: SLACK Incorporated; 2008. p. 761 [Chapter 209].
28. Choi J, Schwiegerling J. Optical performance measurement and night driving simulation of ReSTOR, ReZoom, and Tecnis multifocal intraocular lenses in a model eye. J Cataract Refract Surg. 2008;24: 218–22.
29. McLeod SD, Vargas LG, Portney V, Ting A. Synchrony dual-optic accommodating intraocular lens. Part 1: Optical and biomechanical principles and design considerations. J Cataract Refract Surg. 2007;33:37–46.
30. Ossma IL, Galvis A, Vargas LG, Trager MJ, Vagefi MR, McLeod SD. Synchrony dual-optic accommodating intraocular lens. Part 2: Pilot clinical evaluation. J Cataract Refract Surg. 2007;33:47–52.
31. Juhasz T, Djotyan G, Loesel FH, et al. Applications of femtosecond lasers in corneal surgery. Laser Phys. 2000;10:495–500.
32. Stern D, Schoenlein RW, Puliafito CA, et al. Corneal ablation by nanosecond, picosecond, and femtosecond lasers at 532 and 625 nm. Arch Ophthalmol. 1989;107:587–92.
33. Niemz MH. Laser–tissue interactions: fundamentals and applications. 3rd ed. Berlin: Springer; 1996.
34. Palanker DV, Blumenkranz MS, Andersen D, Wiltberger M, Marcellino G, et al. Femtosecond laser-assisted cataract surgery with integrated optical coherence tomography. Sci Transl Med. 2010;2:58ra85.
35. Nagy Z, Takacs A, Filkom T, Sarayba M. Initial clinical evaluation of an intraocular femtosecond laser in cataract surgery. J Refract Surg. 2009;25: 1053–8.
36. Frey RW, Teuma EV, O'Suilleabhain D. Evaluation of the mechanical properties of the crystalline lens capsule following photodisruption capsulotomy and continuous curvilinear capsulorhexis. In: Poster#1141, D1103, Proceedings of the annual meeting of the Association for Research in Vision and Ophthalmology (ARVO), 3 May 2009, Fort Lauderdale, FL.
37. Friedman NJ, Palanker DV, Schuele G, et al. Femtosecond laser capsulotomy. J Cataract Refract Surg. 2011;37:1189–98.
38. Yeilding R, Villar-Kuri J, Naranjo-Tackman R, et al. Evaluation of size and shape of anterior lens capsules after photodisruption laser capsulotomy and continuous curvilinear capsulorhexis. In: Poster, D1107 #1145, Proceedings of the annual meeting of the Association for Research in Vision and Ophthalmology (ARVO), 05 May 2011, Fort Lauderdale, FL.
39. Tackman RN, Kuri JV, Nichamin LD, Edwards K. Anterior capsulotomy with an ultrashort-pulse laser. J Cataract Refract Surg. 2011;37:819–24.
40. Auffarth GU, Ruiz, LA, Reddy KP. Feasibility study of femtosecond laser cataract surgery. In: Proceedings of the American Society of Cataract and Refractive Surgery (ASCRS) 2011 annual meeting, femtosecond laser cataract surgery session 1-E, 26 March 2011, San Diego, CA.
41. Slade SG, Steinert RF, Donnenfeld ED, Doane JF. Femtosecond lasers in refractive cataract surgery. In: Proceedings of the American Academy of Ophthalmology (AAO) 2010 annual meeting. Course Number 596, October 2010.
42. Nagy Z, Mihåltz K, Kranitz K, et al. Effect of femtosecond laser vs. manual capsulotomy on IOL centration. In: Proceedings of the American Society of Cataract and Refractive Surgery (ASCRS) 2011 annual meeting, femtosecond laser cataract surgery session 1-E, 26 March 2011, San Diego, CA.
43. Park TK, Chung SK, Baek NH. Changes in the area of the anterior capsule opening after intraocular lens implantation. J Cataract Refract Surg. 2002;28: 1613–7.
44. Hayashi K, Hayashi H. Intraocular lens factors that may affect anterior capsule contraction. Ophthalmology. 2005;112:286–92.
45. Vukich JA, Culbertson WW, Batlle JF, Seibel J, et al. Characterization of femtosecond anterior capsulotomies. In: Proceedings of the American Society of Cataract and Refractive Surgery (ASCRS) 2011 annual meeting, femtosecond laser cataract surgery session 4-E, 29 March 2011, San Diego, CA.
46. Nagy ZZ, Kranitz K, Takacs AI, et al. Comparison of intraocular lens decentration parameters after femtosecond and manual capsulotomies. J Refract Surg. 2011;27:564–9.
47. Kranitz K, Takacs A, Mihaltz K, et al. Femtosecond laser capsulotomy and manual continuous curvilinear capsulorrhexis parameters and their effects on intraocular lens centration. J Refract Surg. 2011;27: 558–63.

48. Hill W, Uy H. Effective lens position following laser anterior capsulotomy. In: Proceedings of the American Academy of Ophthalmology (AAO) 2011 annual meeting, femtosecond laser cataract surgery free paper session, 23 October 2011, Orlando, FL.
49. Slade SG. Comparison of effective lens position manual vs. femtosecond laser. In: Proceedings of the American Society of Cataract and Refractive Surgery (ASCRS) 2011 annual meeting, femtosecond laser cataract surgery session 4-E, 29 March 2011, San Diego, CA.
50. Holladay JT. Refractive power calculations for intraocular lenses in the phakic eye. AJO. 1993;116:63–6.
51. Chang DF, Campbell JR. Intraoperative floppy iris syndrome associated with tamsulosin. J Cataract Refract Surg. 2005;31(4):664–73.

8 Nucleus Fragmentation and Disassembly in ReLACS

Harvey S. Uy and Ronald R. Krueger

History of Non-laser Lens Fragmentation

Nuclear disassembly lies at the heart of cataract surgery, and consists of breaking apart and removing the lens nucleus in a systematic, controlled manner. Successful disassembly involves not only complete removal of nuclear lens material, but also removal in a manner that preserves delicate surrounding ocular structures such as the capsular bag and corneal endothelium. Furthermore, in order to produce excellent refractive outcomes the procedure must take place through small, astigmatically neutral incisions.

Nuclear disassembly is the most complicated step of phacoemulsification cataract surgery, as it:

1. Requires the greatest number of intraocular surgical maneuvers.
2. Utilizes most of the expended energy during phacoemulsification.
3. Is associated with the largest number of surgical complications [1, 2].

For these reasons, nuclear disassembly engenders the most difficulty and stress for the cataract surgeon. As a testament to the intricacies of this step, a greater variety of surgical techniques and instrumentation have been developed to aid the surgeon in nuclear disassembly than for any other step in cataract surgery.

Steady technological innovation for nuclear disassembly began with the introduction of phacoemulsification by Charles Kelman and others such as Richard Kratz and James Little, who initially used one- or two-handed techniques during phacoemulsification within the anterior chamber [3–5]. This approach frequently led to corneal endothelial damage, edema and suboptimal visual outcomes. Phacoemulsification in the posterior chamber was introduced by Robert Sinskey who described a technique that involved sculpting a nuclear bowl followed by aspiration and emulsification of the rim of the bowl [6]. William Maloney popularized two-handed phacoemulsification in the iris plane [7]. The introduction of ophthalmic viscosurgical devices (OVDs) and manual capsulorrhexis further contributed to the safety and efficacy of phacoemulsification [8, 9]. In an effort to lessen the deleterious effects of excessive ultrasonic and thermal energy generated by the phacoemulsification tip, later techniques began to substitute mechanical for ultrasonic energy. Howard Gimbel and John Shepherd introduced the "divide and conquer"

H.S. Uy, M.D. (✉)
Pacific Eye and Laser Institute, Makati City, Manila, The Philippines
e-mail: harveyuy@yahoo.com

R.R. Krueger, M.D., M.S.E.
Cole Eye Institute, Department of Refractive Surgery, Cleveland Clinic Lerner College of Medicine, Cleveland, OH 44106, USA

R.R. Krueger et al. (eds.), *Textbook of Refractive Laser Assisted Cataract Surgery (ReLACS)*, DOI 10.1007/978-1-4614-1010-2_8, © Springer Science+Business Media, LLC 2013 technique, where the phacoemulsification was used to create one or more grooves in the nucleus followed by mechanical division of the nucleus into four segments that were then individually removed using further ultrasonic lens emulsification [10, 11]. Initial grooving had the advantage of creating a surgical space with which to mobilize the small segments and avoid placing stress on the capsular bag and zonules. Kinihiro Nagahara introduced mechanical chopping, which was a highly effective method for disassembling the nucleus prior to emulsification [12]. Koch wedded initial grooving followed by chopping in a technique called "stop and chop" [13]. Carrying mechanical chopping to the extreme is the technique of pre-chopping, introduced by Takayuki Akahoshi and Jorge Alio, where surgical instruments are used to stabilize and mechanically break up the lens nucleus prior to the introduction of the phacoemulsification instrument [14].

History of Laser Lens Fragmentation

The next step in the evolution of cataract surgery is the substitution of a laser in place of mechanical energy to facilitate nuclear disassembly. Laser lens fragmentation is an attractive approach because lasers accurately deliver light energy to target tissues and improve the safety and precision of the surgery. Moreover, compared to conventional phacoemulsification, laser refractive surgery can fragment lens nuclei at a fraction of the thermal energy. Cadaver studies reported a temperature rise of 7 °C after ultrasound application with continuous irrigation and 35° without irrigation, while erbium:YAG laser only produced a temperature rise of 0.5 and 2.5°, respectively [15]. Early clinical work was reported by Aron Rosa [16, 17], who utilized the short pulsed neodymium Nd:YAG lasers to create anterior and posterior capsulotomies and cut cyclitic membranes in thousands of eyes. In these seminal investigations, pigmented and non-pigmented ocular tissues were cut without significant thermal effects and without entry into the eye. The Nd:YAG laser produced ionization of the medium, plasma formation, a hydrodynamic shock wave, and was associated with insignificant temperature rise (0.002 °C).

Another precursor of femtosecond (FS) laser cataract surgery was the Dodick Photolysis system [18] which utilized a Q-switched Nd:YAG laser that delivered a laser pulse with an energy of 12 mJ to create a plasma and shock wave on the surface of a metal plate, which was utilized to fragment cataract material. The fragmented materials were then aspirated using an aspiration port integrated into the laser probe.

The transcorneal application of FS laser energy into the crystalline lens was originally proposed as a method for treating presbyopia by restoring accommodation. The Helmholtz theory of accommodation postulates age related lens sclerosis as the main cause for the development of presbyopia. As early as 1998, Raymond Myers and Ronald Krueger, postulated that photodisruption using ultrashort pulse lasers could divide the lens tissues into flexible planes that potentially restores lens flexibility, dynamic accommodation, and reversal of presbyopia [19–23]. The easy separation and fragmentation of the lens nucleus during investigations by LensAR led to its consideration for use in cataract surgery. Around the same time, several other companies including LenSx, OptiMedica, and Technolas also began independently developing their FS lasers for laser-assisted cataract surgery, including nucleus fragmentation and disassembly.

Current Limitations of Phacoemulsification for Lens Fragmentation and the FS Laser Advantage

While current phacoemulsification technology and techniques are safe and effective, there is always room for improvement, particularly for complicated cataracts.

1. *Soft Lenses*: Soft lenses will not fracture using divide and conquer strategies and are not amenable to chopping techniques, as the nucleus may be too soft to fixate using the phacoemulsification tip. Soft nuclei will often not rotate because they absorb rather than comply with the rotational forces of the instruments.

2. *Dense Nuclei*: Dense, brunescent nuclei may require large amounts of ultrasonic energy to remove, resulting in endothelial damage and incision burns. Disassembly of these hard nuclei carries with it an increased risk for capsular tears and zonular dehiscence, as forces generated from instruments during sculpting, rotation, and cracking are directly transmitted to the capsule and zonules. Brunescent cataracts often lack an epinucleus and cortex, so any cushion from nuclear fragments and the phaco tip is absent. When mobile, sharp nuclear fragments in hard cataracts may puncture the posterior capsule. Dense nuclei are often large, resulting in distended, large capsular bags. The leathery fibers within the periphery of these nuclei often prevent clean separation into mobile segments during chopping. As a result, fracturing or cracking necessitates deep sculpting close to the posterior capsule and aggressive prying apart of the segments which impart more forces to the capsular bag, increasing the chance for capsular rupture or capsular tears. Laser lens pre-fragmentation can be particularly beneficial in nuclear disassembly of dense nuclei, improving both safety and efficacy.
3. *Hypermature Cataracts*: Hypermature white cataracts also present significant challenges due to the poor visibility of the capsule because of an absent red reflex. The milky cortex can also spread out over the anterior segment and obscure the surgeon's view like smoke on a highway. In extreme cases, the liquefied cortex can create high intra-lenticular pressure which distends the capsular bag and heightens the risk of anterior capsular tears during capsulorrhexis, which, in turn, can lead to a compromised posterior capsule. A classic example of this is the "Argentinian Flag Sign," where the anterior capsule, stained with trypan blue, tears linearly to create a blue, white, blue pattern. Additionally, the white lens material and absent red flex make it difficult to judge lens thickness, increasing the risk for inadvertent puncture of the posterior capsule during sculpting [24].
4. *Poor Visualization*: Poor visualization of lens borders occurs with corneal opacities and small pupils. The inadequate view in these cases prevents correct assessment of lens width and thickness and limits sculpting excursion. Limited sculpting excursion can lead to inadequate separation of the central lens fibers making it difficult to fracture or crack the nucleus. Limited visibility increases the level of difficulty of passing a chopping instrument into the lens equator and the likelihood of accidentally damaging the anterior capsule during the chopping process.
5. *Zonular Compromise*: Zonular laxity or weakness significantly increases the level of difficulty for every type of cataract surgery. Zonular weakness may be seen in patients who are elderly, have Marfan's disease, pseudoexfoliation, retinopathy of prematurity and in eyes with prior vitrectomy, trauma, or brunescent cataracts. In these eyes, loose zonules fail to fixate the capsular bag and consequently, make it difficult to rotate and disassemble the nucleus. Sculpting and attempted rotation may break even more zonules and worsen the situation. Pronounced up and down motion ("trampolining") of the capsule may occur during phacoemulsification as well as during irrigation and aspiration. Laxity of the capsular bag may result in inadvertent aspiration and damage. When confronted with weak zonules, any maneuvers that lessen the amount of sculpting and cracking motions during nuclear disassembly, such as horizontal chopping or laser lens fragmentation, will significantly lessen the risk for complications such as vitreous loss or dropped nuclei.
6. *Posterior Polar Cataracts*: Posterior polar cataracts are associated with a thin, central posterior capsule and a higher risk for capsular rupture and vitreous loss. Care must be taken to avoid forceful hydrodissection and mechanical contact with the posterior capsule, and to prevent emptying the chamber abruptly as this will result in sudden anterior movement of the vitreous face, causing rupture of the capsule.

7. *Shallow Anterior Chambers or Compromised Corneal Endothelium*: Shallow anterior chambers, particularly in hyperopic or uveitic eyes (the latter of often manifest posterior synechiae and iris bombe), make it difficult to comfortably manipulate instruments within the anterior chamber to perform the capsulorrhexis and initiate lens removal. In these eyes, there is also a greater risk of iris prolapse, especially around the edge of the phaco probe, if the transcorneal incision is too posterior and the intraocular pressure builds up too quickly. The implementation of specially shaped laser corneal incisions and a laser capsulotomy can enhance the safety in these cases. Also, nuclear disassembly using ultrasonic energy carries a greater potential for damaging the endothelium, due to the close proximity of the phaco probe. The same situation exists for eyes with Fuch's endothelial dystrophy, where the cornea is already predisposed to decompensation from endothelial damage induced by ultrasonic energy. In both instances, laser lens fragmentation can lower the amount of expended ultrasonic energy and lessen the amount of endothelial damage.

Bimanual phacoemulsification is a strategy to reduce wound and instrument size by separating the irrigation and aspiration tubing and entering the anterior chamber through separate, smaller incisions using two handpieces. The bimanual approach provides more flexibility when manipulating nuclear segments and utilizes low inflow and aspiration rates which may be of advantage in eyes with complicated cataracts (e.g., Zonular weakness).

8. *The FS Laser Advantage*: Refractive laser assisted cataract surgery can facilitate removal of nearly all types of cataracts, and may be particularly useful in challenging cases. Several critical steps can be automatically performed with greater precision and speed, such as creation of the transcorneal surgical incisions, capsulotomy, and laser lens fragmentation. A precise, well-sealing surgical incision is important for eyes with posterior polar cataracts as this may minimize sudden emptying of the chamber, leading to capsular rupture. In the coaxial and bimanual approaches, a precise, laser created incision may prevent wound leaking and minimizes chamber instability. Laser capsulotomy is particularly useful in cases where there is poor red reflex (brunescent and white cataracts) or in eyes with smaller than optimal pupils where the surgeon wants to avoid using pupil expanding devices.

Regardless of surgeon technique, laser lens fragmentation disassembles the nucleus into smaller pieces which generally require less ultrasonic energy to emulsify, a great advantage in eyes with brunescent cataracts, shallow anterior chambers, and zonular weakness. Reduction in ultrasonic and thermal energy (40–100% depending on the cataract grade) lessens the risk for significant endothelial damage. Laser lens fragmentation creates natural fracture lines within the nucleus, which facilitate consistent, complete chopping, and is advantageous for all situations where chopping is preferred. For soft (Grades 1 and 2) lenses, laser lens fragmentation facilitates aspiration—only lens removal. Lastly, the FS laser software may be customized to create a posterior epinuclear plate or "safety zone" that protects the posterior capsule from inadvertent puncture by instruments or sharp nuclear fragments in brunescent cataracts. As more surgeons become familiar with the technology, more ways will be developed to take advantage of refractive laser assisted cataract surgery (ReLACS).

Technical Requirements for Adequate Nucleus Fragmentation Using FS Lasers

A number of companies including LensAR, LenSx, OptiMedica, and Technolas have developed FS lasers for refractive laser assisted cataract surgery. LensAR is also developing FS laser technology for accommodation restoration (AR) and hence the name LensAR.

Of all the steps in ReLACS, nucleus fragmentation is the most technically challenging because of the required depth and need for safety in laser delivery. The technical requirements are greater than those experienced in corneal surgery and can best be summarized in the following four points:

1. *Depth*: Lens fragmentation requires the greatest depth of FS laser delivery, up to a full 8 mm from the cornea. As a result, the energy parameters and depth of focus of the laser beam must be designed.
2. *Safety*: Lens fragmentation requires precise safety zones where treatment does not occur to protect delicate, adjacent intraocular tissues such as the iris and the posterior lens capsule. As such, identification of lens structures becomes the most critical for proper imaging and alignment as part of image guided FS laser surgery.
3. *Density*: The greatest variable in cataract surgery is the size and density of the lens. Lens fragmentation is most sensitive to limitations in laser energy delivery, which is highly dependent on the lens density. The ability to reliably achieve threshold energy for fragmentation, and sufficient imaging for safe localization of pulse delivery become critical differentiating factors amongst laser technology platforms. Dr. Zoltan Nagy, working with LenSx, says that in his experience, his laser can treat only up to a LOCS II grade 3.5 cataract (Personal Communication, ASCRS meeting, San Diego, CA, March 27, 2011). Dr. Juan Battle, working with OptiMedica, claims his laser can easily image and fragment LOCS II grade 4.0 cataracts, but beyond this point imaging the posterior capsule is too limiting to proceed with laser fragmentation (Personal Communication , ARVO meeting, Ft. Lauderdale, FL, May 5, 2011) [24]. In our experience with the LensAR laser, even the most advanced LOCS II and III grade cataracts can be both imaged and treated safely and effectively [25].
4. *Energy*: For lens fragmentation, the laser energy delivered to the crystalline lens must be nearly an order of magnitude greater (~10 μJ) than what is required for laser delivery to the cornea (~1 μJ). This point places a great requirement on the technical range of operation of FS lasers for cataract surgery, because both lens and corneal incisions are required.

Early Clinical Experience in ReLACS and T-LACS: Practical Considerations and Clinical Pearls

I (HSU) have worked with the LensAR system since November 2009 and as of June 2011, have performed over 400 laser-assisted cataract surgeries and over 40 FS laser photodisruptive procedures for accommodation restoration. As with any cataract surgery, preoperative evaluation and preparation are crucial to achieving optimal results. Attaining a favorable capsulorrhexis size and shape improves the ease and safety of nuclear disassembly. Careful attention should be paid to pupil dilation, size, shape, and centration. In a normally dilated pupil, a standard preprogrammed laser capsulotomy treatment algorithm may be applied. Some systems have an imaging system that detects the anterior and posterior apices of the lens and can determine lens tilt from the optical axis of the lens. This allows the surgeon to correct for errors in laser energy placement by accounting for the tilt and, if desired, to center the anterior capsulotomy over the optical axis of the crystalline lens (see Fig. 8.1).

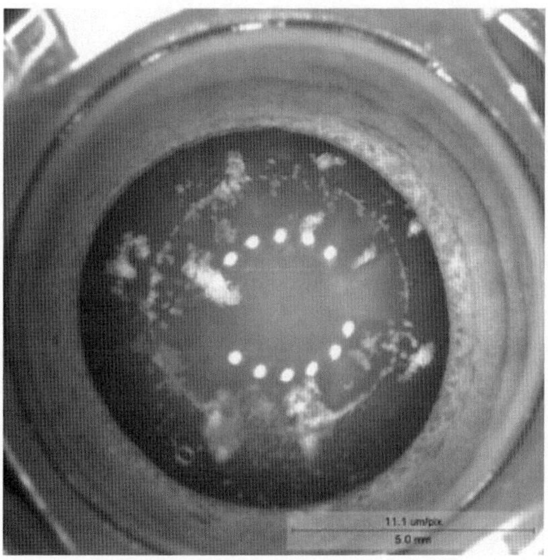

Fig. 8.1 "Down the pipe" view of laser capsulotomy using the LensAR system. Even though the laser capsulotomy is performed first, the few peripheral bubbles do not interfere with the deeper laser pulse placement for nucleus fragmentation

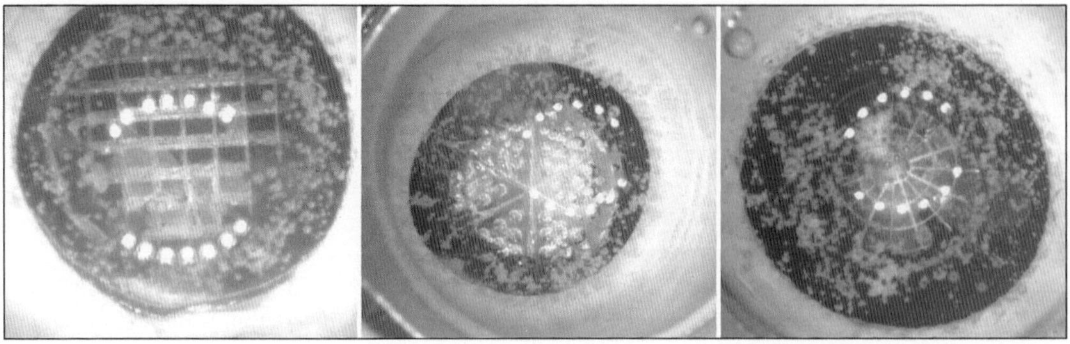

Fig. 8.2 "Down the pipe" photos of a variety of laser lens fragmentation treatment profiles (algorithms) using the LensAR system. From *left* to *right*, these are characterized as *cubes*, *spheres* and *subdivided pies*

Attaining maximal pupil dilation with mydriatics and NSAID's is ideal, as this allows the most flexibility in planning the lens fragmentation treatment zone. With small pupils, the diameter of the planned capsulotomy may be reduced to a size that still leaves a small margin of error from the pupil edge. For pupils that are off center, the treatment zone may still be centered on the presumed visual axis with reduction of the treatment zone diameter. This ability to adjust the capsulotomy parameters and center the capsulotomy as desired is especially important when premium intraocular lenses (IOLs) are used (e.g., multifocal or aspheric intraocular lenses). When IOL centration on the presumed visual axis is not considered crucial, the center of the treatment zone may be shifted in order to allow for creation of a larger capsulotomy to facilitate nuclear removal.

Depending on the laser platform, a wide variety of laser lens fragmentation treatment profiles (algorithms) may be preprogrammed and incorporated into the FS laser system's software (Fig. 8.2). The choice of treatment algorithm will depend on surgeon technique and nuclear density. The choice of treatment algorithm influences surgical efficiency and the amount of ultrasonic energy needed for nuclear disassembly. As a stop-and-chop and pre-chopping surgeon, my personal preference is the "pie" fragmentation pattern, where the nucleus is fragmented into small, pie-shaped wedges, appears to work best in reducing ultrasonic energy and facilitating nuclear disassembly. In comparison to conventionally treated eyes, the "pie" treatment algorithm, delivered by the LensAR system, reduces the cumulative dispersive energy (CDE) by 100, 64, 39, and 42% for Grades 1, 2, 3, and 4 cataracts, respectively (LensAR company data on file). The "pie" pattern divides the nucleus into 20 pie slices with each wedge further subdivided into inner, middle, and outer segments (Fig. 8.3). As a point of differentiation, surgeons using the LenSx laser and OptiMedica Catalys FS laser have preferred and achieved somewhat similar results using a laser pattern that fragments the lens into four quadrants (see Chaps. 15 and 17).

After maximal dilation, the patient is placed on a treatment bed which is positioned adjacent to the FS laser. Topical anesthesia provides sufficient comfort for the application of the suction ring. Some eyes with small palpebral fissures or abnormally strong blink reflexes may require periocular lidocaine injections to relax the periorbital muscles and facilitate placement of the suction ring. In some machines, the laser head is on a motorized extending arm that is used to dock a movable interface device to the suction ring. In other systems, the patient is on a motorized bed which is used to attach the suction ring to a fixed interface device attached to the laser head. In the LensAR system, the laser head is under servo control and maintains a predetermined force on the eye at all times. The docking process is monitored via the surgeon's screen and controlled using a joystick device.

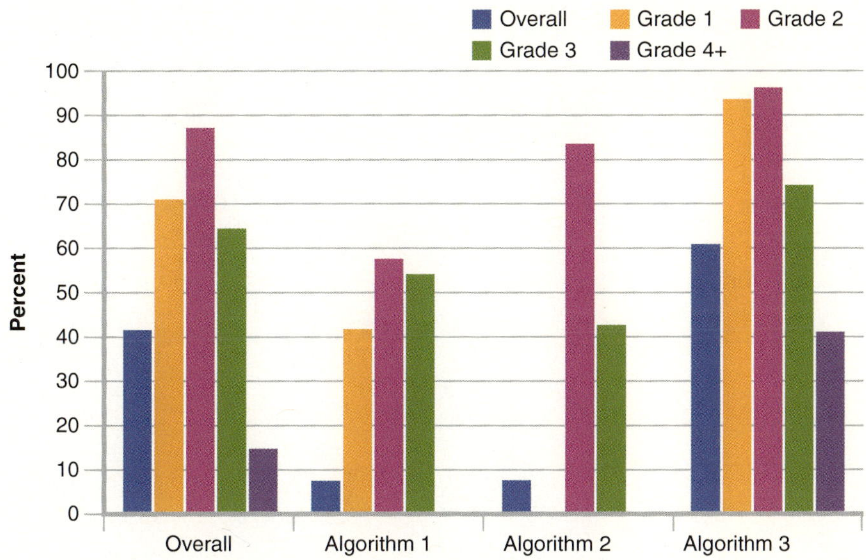

Fig. 8.3 Reduction of cumulative dispersive energy according to lens nucleus grade and treatment profile (algorithm) (1 = cubes; 2 = spheres; 3 = subdivided pies). Data presented at the American Academy of Ophthalmology Annual Meeting, 2010

After docking, an imaging system is used to image and measure the dimensions of the anterior chamber and lens. The LensAR system uses a confocal scanning laser device (SLD), incorporating the Scheimpflug principle, while the LenSx, OptiMedica, and Technolas systems utilize optical coherence tomography (OCT) (see Fig. 8.4). The acquired images are then used to create a 3D reconstruction of the key ocular structures (Fig. 8.5).

After 3D reconstruction, the software creates patient-specific parameters for surgical incisions, capsulotomy and lens fragmentation. The treatment algorithm is customized to surgeon preferences that take into account preferred incision site, IOL to be implanted and, depending on laser hardware and software options, may account for nuclear density and preferred fragmentation patterns. Some systems take into account lens tilt and provide a predefined capsular clearance to maintain a safety margin from the capsule. The crucial parameters can be visualized and adjusted if necessary using the graphic user interface on the operator screen. Once the surgeon is satisfied with the planned treatment parameters, the FS laser is then activated.

The FS laser treatment process is monitored in real time using the surgical screen, and can be halted at any moment. As the FS laser energy is applied, gas bubbles may be observed (Fig. 8.1). Most of the time, the capsulotomy is performed first (few, peripheral bubbles) followed by laser lens fragmentation in a posterior to anterior direction with the corneal incisions last. The surgical duration from initiation of docking to end of treatment ranges from 3 to 4 min, but occasionally will be a little longer in eyes that need repeat docking or imaging. Although it may seem intuitive to apply the FS laser for the lens fragmentation (from posterior to anterior) before the capsulotomy, bubble interference and distortion of the lens anatomy is actually greater if it is done this way, since there is no release of the expanding bubbles from within the lens. The few bubbles generated within the lens and anterior chamber during the laser capsulotomy procedure are sufficiently peripheral and of small size and number so as not to interfere with the lens nucleus fragmentation done afterwards.

Fig. 8.4 LensAR software screen, demonstrating the side angle (Scheimpflug) image highlighting the key anterior segment structures within the dilated pupil (posterior cornea, anterior lens capsule and posterior lens capsule) used for FS laser cataract surgery planning and image-guided surgery

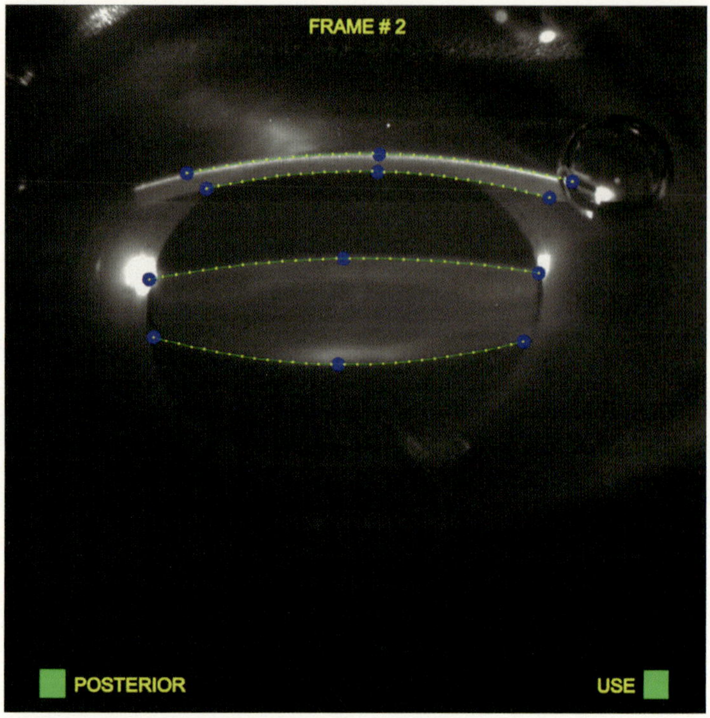

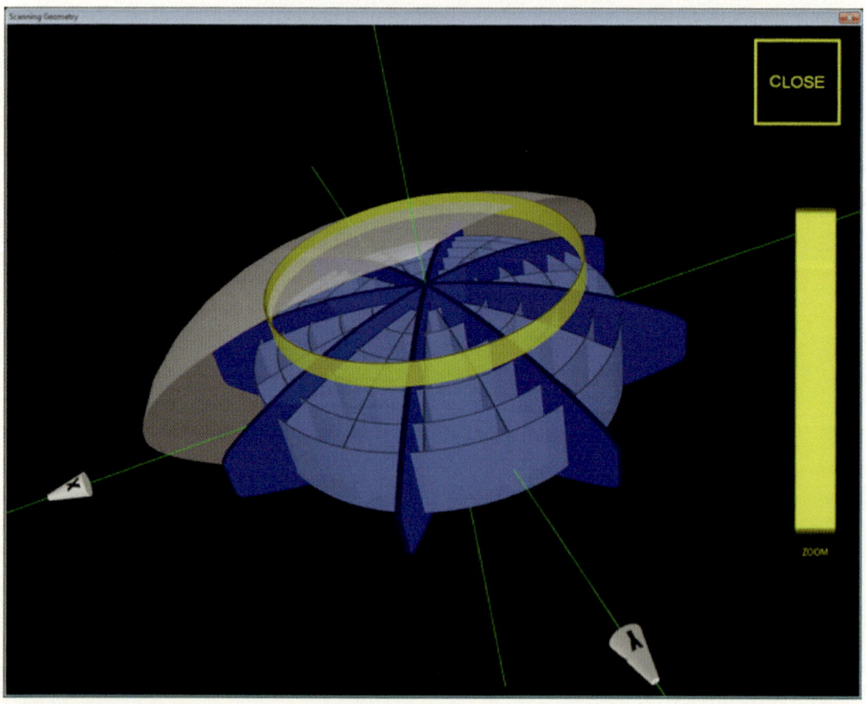

Fig. 8.5 LensAR screen image demonstrating the software generated treatment profile (algorithm) for capsulotomy (*lighter shade top circle*) and laser lens fragmentation (*darker shade central pattern with multiple rings*). The capsular bag is represented in *gray*

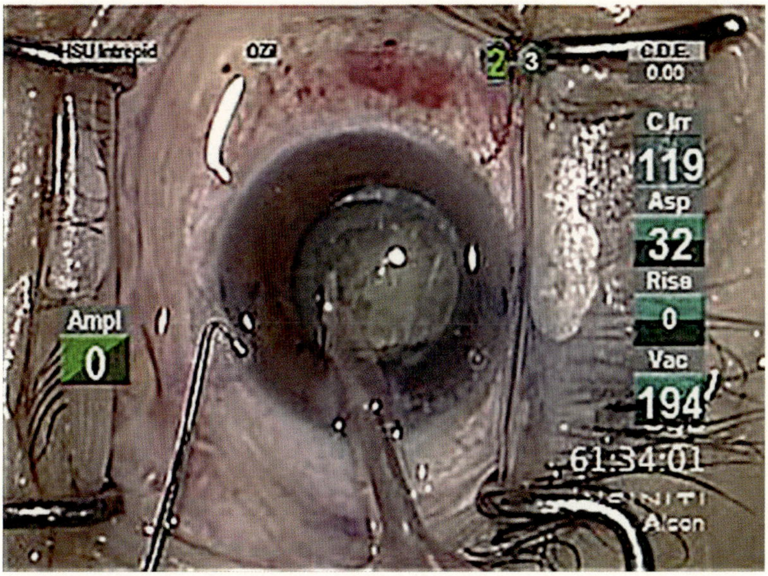

Fig. 8.6 Surgical microscope image, demonstrating phacoemulsification of a laser fragmented nucleus. Note zero cumulative dissipated energy indicating aspiration only lens removal

After FS laser treatment, the patient may be transferred into another room (the operating suite) for phacoemulsification. Alternatively, the FS laser may be positioned inside the operating suite and moved out of the way, if mobile, so the phacoemulsification machine and operating microscope can be positioned for cataract surgery. Efforts should be made to minimize any delay from FS laser treatment to phacoemulsification (<30 min) because the intraocular pressure may, on rare occasion, increase if sufficient lens proteins leak from the "opened" capsule and clog the trabecular meshwork.

As most incisions are partial thickness or require dissection for full thickness opening, the usual steps of asepsis and nonsterile draping are carried out during the laser pretreatment process. Additional anesthetic drops as well as a lid speculum may be applied. During the extraction procedure in the surgical suite, the usual sterile draping and preparation is required. After opening the surgical incisions and injecting an ophthalmic viscoelastic device (OVD), the capsulotomy button is then removed using forceps. In occasional instances, some adhesions to the capsulotomy edge may be present but these are usually severed with gentle pushing of or pulling on the capsulotomy button. This is followed by hydrodissection and hydrodelineation in the usual manner. The nucleus can be rotated to assure adequate separation from the cortex, even though the laser fragmentation step facilitates easy disassembly. Gas bubbles may be released during this step and additional OVD may be placed to push out the gas bubbles from the anterior chamber.

Nuclear disassembly can then proceed according to surgeon preference. Laser lens fragmentation facilitates nuclear disassembly regardless of preferred technique. For divide and conquer surgeons, the fragmented nucleus will require less ultrasonic power during sculpting and segment removal as the smaller fragments are already broken down extensively and easily aspirated by the instrument tip (Fig. 8.6). For surgeons who utilize chopping maneuvers, the pretreated cleavage planes created during laser lens fragmentation facilitate easy fracturing or division of the nucleus during the emulsification process. For pre-choppers, laser lens fragmentation creates pretreated cleavage planes that allow for more complete and controlled division of even very dense nuclei into several segments (Fig. 8.7).

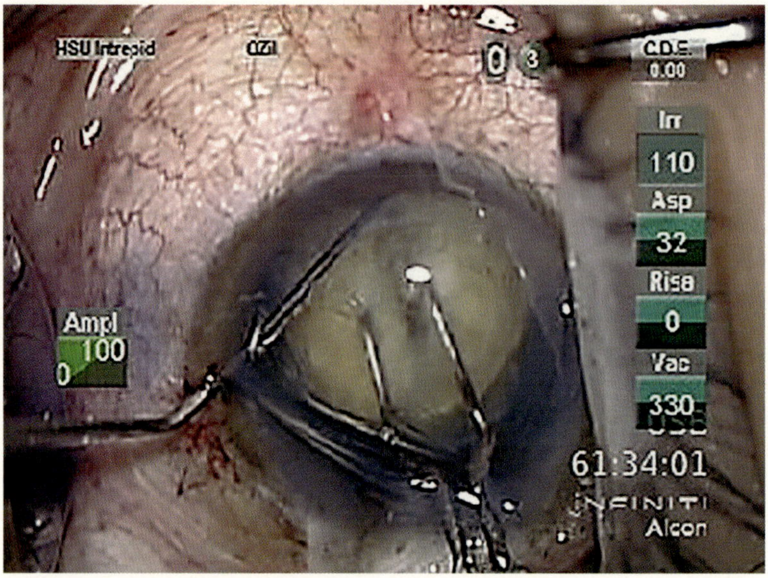

Fig. 8.7 Surgical microscope image, demonstrating prechopping of a laser fragmented dense nucleus. Note clean and complete bisection of the brunescent nucleus following laser lens fragmentation

For soft nuclei, fragmentation may be accomplished by just passing the hydrodissection cannula or phaco tip through the nuclear segments. For harder nuclei, a relatively small mechanical force is required, when using chopping or prechopping instruments, to completely separate the precut segments. With treatment algorithms that further subdivide the segments beyond that of four quadrants, the removal of nuclear fragments will require less ultrasound energy.

One major safety advantage of FS laser lens fragmentation is the ability of the machine software to create a protective posterior epinuclear plate or safety zone between the nucleus and the posterior capsule. When desired by the surgeon, this layer serves as an armor plate that lessens the risk of posterior capsular rupture or puncture by surgical instrumentation or hard/sharp lens material. This epinuclear plate is easily removed using aspiration or gentle phacoemulsification after the primary bulk of nuclear material is removed. The cortex is then removed using conventional irrigation and aspiration.

Surgical Complications

The only foolproof way to avoid surgical complications is to avoid doing any surgery at all. Even with all the safety advantages offered by laser-assisted cataract surgery, complications may still occur so patients have to be counseled of the risks of surgery. While the combination of computer-directed laser application coupled with surgeon monitoring and control has provided refractive laser assisted cataract surgery with a great safety profile, phacoemulsification still has to be performed and complications may still result.

Laser Related Complications

IOP Rise

In over 400 laser assisted cataract surgeries, the only laser-related complication I (Harvey Uy) have encountered is the occasional transient intraocular pressure rise after application of the

FS laser. IOP rise may occasionally ensue from the creation of gas bubbles or from blockage of the trabecular meshwork by lens proteins released after the capsulotomy is opened for an extended period (>20 or 30 min). This was observed in our initial studies when we checked the IOP before and immediately after surgery with the FS laser in both cataract and accommodation restoration (AR) procedures. Very mild IOP rise was observed, due to the creation of bubbles, in both procedures, which quickly dissipated in the AR procedures due to the intact lens capsule. In the cataract procedures, however, a marked IOP spike was observed in some eyes after 30 min, presumably due to the liberation of lens proteins or ensuing inflammation. Completion of the surgery and removal of all lens proteins lowered the pressure and minimized any adverse sequela from this complication. Consequently, we recommend avoiding the possible risk of a blown pupil or optic nerve damage from IOP rise by performing phacoemulsification without delay.

Capsular Block and Rupture

Although we have not experienced this with the LensAR laser, several reports of posterior capsular rupture during hydrodissection were reported in Australia with the LenSx laser (Chap. 14). This was presumably due to the expanded volume of the lens after laser pretreatment, leading to an anterior capsular block, with posterior trapping of the rapidly injected fluid during hydrodissection and subsequent capsular rupture.

Suction Loss

Another phenomenon we have not yet experienced with the LensAR laser, but has been reported with the LenSx laser (Chap. 15) is the loss of suction during laser pretreatment. One should carefully observe the execution of the laser pretreatment throughout the procedure to make sure there is no shifting of the laser pattern and potential risk to the adjacent lens structures due to suction loss.

Enhanced Management of Unrelated Complications

Beyond the scope of the laser pretreatment, the anterior and posterior capsules may still be torn during nuclear disassembly by inadvertent contact with an active phacoemulsification tip or sharp/hard nuclear fragment. An inherently compromised posterior capsule may still rupture from minimal manipulation of nuclear segments. Loose and weakened zonules may still break, causing an undesirable posterior displacement of the capsular bag, and increase in the difficulty of nucleus removal with a likelihood for damage to the capsular bag.

Posterior Capsular Rupture and Vitreous Loss

The management of posterior capsular rupture and vitreous loss in refractive laser assisted cataract surgery follows the same principles as management of vitreous loss in conventional phacoe-mulsification: remove remaining lens material (nucleus, epinucleus and cortex), perform an anterior vitrectomy, preserve capsular support and implant the IOL. The laser cataract surgeon should be prepared at all times to meet these situations. From personal experience, there seems to be no additional difficulties in the management of these challenging complications when performing ReLACS. If anything, the circular, well-centered laser capsulotomy provides more than adequate support for sulcus implantation of the IOL.

Fragile Zonules

Fragile zonules cause difficulties for capsulorrhexis and nuclear disassembly. Laser capsulotomy facilitates creation of a smaller, optimally sized capsulorrhexis and allows the surgeon to avoid the risk of capsular tears associated with a noncompliant peripheral capsule. Horizontal chopping is recommended for cataracts with weak zonules as this reduces the stress placed on the zonules during sculpting and rotation and minimizes lens tilt and displacement. Laser lens fragmentation creates cleavage planes within the nucleus and greatly facilitates horizontal chopping and nuclear removal. Flaccid posterior capsules are associated with weak zonules and the epinuclear plate or safety zone created by laser lens fragmentation reduces the trampolining effect of these flaccid posterior capsules. At the end of nuclear disassembly, the epinuclear plate can be easily prolapsed into the anterior chamber away from the loose posterior capsule, and removed. In the supra-capsular flip technique described by David Brown, a large capsulorrhexis is required to allow anterior displacement of the nucleus into the anterior chamber for phacoemulsification. In these cases, laser capsulotomy greatly facilitates creation of a large capsulorrhexis to facilitate this technique. In extremely loose zonules, it may be necessary to support the capsular bag using capsule retractors. The edges of the laser capsulotomy appear robust enough to withstand the stresses produced by capsule retractors as well as implantation of capsular tension rings.

Learning Curve

Apart from training to operate the FS laser user interface and docking the patient interface (PI) device to the eye, the learning curve for laser assisted cataract surgery is very short. Upon entering the eye after laser pretreatment, one needs only adjust to the presence of gas bubbles, which are easily removed by aspiration or injecting more OVD. For the most part, surgeons can utilize the same techniques and instrumentation they normally use for conventional phacoemulsification. Transitioning surgeons will discover that phaco chop and pre-chop will be greatly facilitated by FS laser lens fragmentation. As more experience is gained, the surgeon may adjust machine settings to reduce phaco power and increase vacuum and flow in order to fully take advantage of the laser fragmented lens particles.

The surgeon should be mindful of the presence of an epinuclear plate which should be removed only after the nuclear disassembly in order to maximize posterior capsular protection. Careful attention to capsulorrhexis size and centration should help the surgeon obtain the best visual outcomes from premium IOL implantation. In my overall experience (HSU), I have found the use of the FS laser for lens fragmentation and disassembly to be a comfortable, easily manageable and enjoyable process. I encourage you to have fun and enjoy it too.

Conclusion

The FS is a precise cutting tool that can effectively and safely be applied to the human lens for laser lens fragmentation. Laser-assisted cataract surgery results in more efficient nuclear disassembly with significant reduction in utilized ultrasonic energy.

Key Points

1. FS laser lens fragmentation significantly simplifies lens removal for most densities of lens nuclei (exception is a white cataract) and can offer significant safety advantages in complicated cases.
2. It is advantageous to utilize different fragmentation and/or softening patterns depending on nuclear density.
3. It is advantageous to utilize different fragmentation and/or softening patterns depending on surgical technique.
4. The ability to image and fragment hard lens nuclei may vary among laser systems.
5. The interval between laser treatment and surgical lens removal should be minimized to prevent IOP spikes between laser treatment and entry into the eye.

References

1. Dooley IJ, O'Brien PD. Subjective difficulty of each stage of phacoemulsification cataract surgery performed by basic surgical trainees. J Cataract Refract Surg. 2006;32:605–8.
2. Bhagat N, Nissirios N, Potdevin L, Chung P, et al. Complications in resident-performed phacoemulsifi-

cation cataract surgery at New Jersey Medical School. Br J Ophthalmol. 2007;91:1315–7.
3. Kelman CD. Symposium: phacoemulsification. History of emulsification and aspiration of senile cataracts. Trans Am Acad Ophthalmol Otolaryngol. 1974; 78:OP5–13.
4. Kratz RP. Symposium: Phacoemulsification. Difficulties, complications, and management. Trans Am Acad Ophthalmol Otolaryngol. 1974;78:OP18–21.
5. Wilkinson CP, Anderson LS, Little JH. Retinal detachment following phacoemulsification. Ophthalmology. 1978;85:151–6.
6. Chang DF. Phaco Chop: mastering techniques, optimizing technology and avoiding complications. Thorofare, NJ: Slack Incorporated; 2004.
7. Maloney WF, Dillman DM, Nichamin LD. Supracapsular phacoemulsification: a capsule-free posterior chamber approach. J Cataract Refract Surg. 1997;23(3):323–8.
8. Pedersen OO. Comparison of the protective effects of methylcellulose and sodium hyaluronate on corneal swelling following phacoemulsification of senile cataracts. J Cataract Refract Surg. 1990;16(5):594–6.
9. Koch DD, Liu JF, Glasser DB, Merin LM, Haft E. A comparison of corneal endothelial changes after use of Healon or Viscoat during phacoemulsification. Am J Ophthalmol. 1993;115(2):188–201.
10. Gimbel HV. Divide and conquer nucleofractis phacoemulsification: development and variations. J Cataract Refract Surg. 1991;17(3):281–91.
11. Shepherd JR. In situ fracture. J Cataract Refract Surg. 1990;16(4):436–40.
12. Can I, Takmaz T, Cakici F, Ozgül M. Comparison of Nagahara phaco-chop and stop-and-chop phacoemulsification nucleotomy techniques. J Cataract Refract Surg. 2004;30(3):663–8.
13. Koch PS, Katzen LE. Stop and chop phacoemulsification. J Cataract Refract Surg. 1994;20(5):566–70.
14. Henriques JS, Alió JL, Akahoshi T, Escaf L, et al. Prechopping surgical techniques. Tech Ophthalmol. 2009;7:139–45.
15. Berger JW, Talamo JH, LaMarche KJ, Kim SH, Snyder RW, D'Amico DJ, Marcellino G. Temperature measurements during phacoemulsification and erbium:YAG laser phacoablation in model systems. J Cataract Refract Surg. 1996;22:372–8.
16. Aron-Rosa D, Aron JJ, Griesemann M, Thyzel R. Use of the neodymium-YAG laser to open the posterior capsule after lens implant surgery: a preliminary report. J Am Intraocul Implant Soc. 1980;6:352–4.
17. Aron-Rosa DS, Aron JJ, Cohn HC. Use of a pulsed picosecond Nd: YAG laser in 6,664 cases. J Am Intraocul Implant Soc. 1984;10(1):35–9.
18. Dodick JM, Lally JM, Sperber LT. Lasers in cataract surgery. Curr Opin Ophthalmol. 1993;4(1):107–9.
19. Myers RI, Krueger RR. Novel approaches to correction of presbyopia with laser modification of the crystalline lens. J Refract Surg. 1998;14:136–9.
20. Heys KR, Cram SL, Truscott RJ. Massive increase in the stiffness of the human lens nucleus with age: the basis for presbyopia? Mol Vis. 2004;10:956–63.
21. Krueger RR, Kuszak J, Lubatschowski H, Myers RI, Ripken T, Heisterkamp A. First safety study of femtosecond laser photodisruption in animal lenses: tissue morphology and cataractogenesis. J Cataract Refract Surg. 2005;31:2386–94.
22. Gerten G, Ripken T, Breitenfeld P, Krueger RR, Kermani O, Lubatschowski H, Oberheide U. In vitro and in vivo investigations on the treatment of presbyopia using femtosecond lasers. Ophthalmologe. 2007; 104:40–6.
23. Lubatschowski H, Schumacher S, Fromm M, Wegener A, Hoffmann H, Oberheide U, Gerten G. Femtosecond lentotomy: generating gliding planes inside the crystalline lens to regain accommodation ability. J Biophotonics. 2010;3:265–8.
24. Batlle JF, Feliz R, Culbertson WW. OCT-guided femtosecond laser cataract surgery: precision and efficacy. Association for Research in Vision and Ophthalmology Annual Meeting. Poster #D633, 5 May 2011, Fort Lauderdale, FL.
25. Uy HS. Laser lens fragmentation of higher grade cataracts. American Society of Cataract and Refractive Surgery Annual Meeting. Poster #984231, March 2011, San Diego, CA.

Primary Transcorneal Laser Incisions

9

Roger F. Steinert and James C. Loden

Principles of Cataract Wound Incisional Architecture

The cataract incision has a major impact on several key aspects of cataract surgery. Instruments must be passed through the incision without excessive manipulation and, during surgery, the instruments must be able to maneuver adequately within the eye to accomplish their goal. The intraocular lens (IOL) must be able to be inserted through the incision. After surgery, the incision may have an impact on astigmatism, generally in the direction of causing flattening of that meridian. Finally, any leakage from the incision has two major associated risks. The first is damage to the corneal endothelium from shallowing or emptying of the anterior chamber, particularly if implanted devices such as an IOL come in contact with the endothelium. The second and worst of the potential complications is the ingress of organisms, resulting in endophthalmitis. All of these factors determine the ultimate selection of incision size and configuration.

R.F. Steinert, M.D. (✉)
Department of Ophthalmology, Gavin Herbert Eye Institute, University of California, Irvine, CA 92697, USA
e-mail: steinert@uci.edu

J.C. Loden, M.D.
Loden Vision Centers, 907 Rivergate Parkway, Suite C2020, Goodlettsville, TN 37072, USA

Instrument Insertion

For ease of instrument insertion, the incision size must be matched to the instruments being employed. Typically, the largest instrument is the ultrasonic phacoemulsification tip and sleeve. Because the ultrasound tip is round, in order to give as much volume as possible for aspiration of ultrasonic material, the mechanical requirement is for a slit incision that has width but no height to nevertheless admit a round object that inherently deforms the incision in order to be inserted. That deformation not only presents a mechanical challenge during the insertion, but also carries the potential for stretching of the incision. In order to facilitate insertion but keep the overall incision width as small as possible, a common strategy is create a "funnel" shape to the incision so that the external opening is larger than the internal opening, making the initial introduction of the ultrasound tip easier.

The Intraocular Lens

The IOL and the incision have had a long history of influencing each other. The development of IOLs that pass through a smaller incision has stimulated the development of smaller gauge ultrasound tips for lens removal, but conversely, the improvement in ultrasonic technology has, in turn, stimulated IOL manu-

R.R. Krueger et al. (eds.), *Textbook of Refractive Laser Assisted Cataract Surgery (ReLACS)*,
DOI 10.1007/978-1-4614-1010-2_9, © Springer Science+Business Media, LLC 2013

facturers to develop new lenses and new lens insertion systems to reduce the requirement for the incision size.

Incision Width Versus Height

In general, the width of the incision is the largest factor in the slippage of the wound that results in flattening of the corneal dome in the meridian of the incision. The relationship of incision width to astigmatism is not linear, however. While there is yet to be agreement about a minimum incision size, below which there is no further benefit of reduction of astigmatism, the curve of the improvement is with one that approaches an asymptote in the vicinity of 2 mm. In addition to incision width, the distance of the incision from the optical zone also reduces the impact of the incision. Because the cornea is not circular, but rather somewhat elliptical in the temporal direction, a temporal incision at the limbus has less potential for inducing an astigmatic shift than an equal-sized incision elsewhere, such as superiorly or nasally.

Postoperative Incision Behavior

Postoperatively, an incision must be sealed and resistant to reopening due to normal day-to-day activity. At the time of surgery, it is common for incisions, particularly clear corneal incisions, to ooze when the anterior chamber is pressurized. Stromal hydration is often used to counteract this. Critics of stromal hydration state that it is a temporary effect and that, while the incision is secure and not leaking at the end of the case once hydration has been performed, the subsequent dehydration of the stroma will allow leakage to resume. Advocates of stromal hydration, however, invoke the theory that stromal hydration forces the collagen within the stroma edges of the incision into contact. When the endothelium pumps the water of the cornea, the apposed tissue planes remain in contact with each other and, therefore, the incision remains secure. It has long been accepted that the endothelial pump function creates a negative pressure, functioning as a vacuum, at a level of about 50 mmHg.

Postoperatively, the incision is subject to forces both internal and external. Internally, high pressure in the early postoperative period is common, especially attributed to retained viscoelastic material, as well as in patients with increased inflammation or retained lens material. Conversely, the pressure may be low, in which case a sealed incision could gape open. Externally, patients may rub their eyes, put pressure on the eye while administering eye drops, transmit pressure onto the globe while asleep, and have fluctuation in pressure from the simple act of blinking.

Structural Principles

For all of these reasons, a structurally secure incision is a key property of an acceptable incision [1]. During the evolution of clear corneal incisions, Dr. Paul Ernest demonstrated that the most secure configuration of a clear corneal incision is a truly square incision. In other words, if the incision is 3 mm wide, the length of the tunnel into the cornea should also be 3 mm. The difficulty with a truly square incision is that a long tunnel length presents other challenges to the surgeon. The surgeon typically finds that a long tunnel makes manipulation of instruments more difficult, and, in particular, may make visualization of the anterior chamber more challenging when instruments are tilted posteriorly, because the cornea will be deformed with a degradation of the corneal optics. The narrower the width of the incision, the less this is a problem, of course. A 2 mm wide incision can be square with only a 2 mm tunnel length, which represents a 33% reduction in the restriction on instrument movement and the potential for corneal optical degradation.

In addition to the basic concept of the ratio of width to tunnel length, much attention has been paid to different configurations of manual blade incisions. Some surgeons advocate two or three plane incisions, believing that creating a more complex geometry is more likely to result in a self-sealing incision. Dr. David Langerman strongly advocated a very deep vertical groove at the limbus as the first plane in a multi-plane incision. He argued that this configuration would create more flexibility in the inner portion of the incision "flap," acting like a hinge that would make it more likely that the inner aspect of the incision would be easily apposed to the anterior aspect of the incision. This principle became known as the "Langerman Hinge" [1]. Other surgeons were concerned that this type of deep initial groove would act like a small limbal relaxing incision, increasing any tendency for astigmatic shift beyond the shift that would occur due to the width of the incision alone. Another approach, pursued especially by Dr. I. Howard Fine, modified the shape of the keratome blade in an effort to gain better structural configuration of the entry through Descemet's membrane, attempting to take into account the three-dimensional structure of the corneal dome and its impact on the actual configuration of the penetration of the blade into the incision [1].

All of these modifications were designed to reduce the potential for endophthalmitis, hypotony, and iris prolapse.

Other Issues

In addition to the structural issues, the integrity of the incision is degraded if there is thermal injury to the incision during ultrasonic phacoemulsification. Generation of heat will cause shrinkage of collagen. Extreme wound burns are easily detected but very hard to seal and can cause permanent high levels of astigmatism. More subtle thermal injury is more easily overlooked, however, but will markedly reduce incision integrity and, if persistent leakage is detected at the time of surgery, necessitate the placement of one or more sutures.

The final aspect of creating the ideal incision is to avoid tearing and subsequent detachment of Descemet's membrane. In addition to the initial incision itself, the passage of instruments in and out of the incision has the potential to catch the edge of Descemet's membrane, leading to detachment. A detachment of Descemet's membrane is challenging to treat and may never be adequately repaired, necessitating subsequent corneal transplantation.

Scleral Tunnels

The alternative to a clear corneal incision is, of course, a more traditional scleral tunnel. The advantage of a scleral tunnel is that a conjunctival flap must be created. In addition to the tunnel itself being more peripheral than a clear corneal incision, the conjunctival flap can be placed over the scleral incision, providing an additional seal to protect against ingress of organisms. The disadvantages to this approach, however, include prolonged surgical time due to the extra manipulation, the requirement for higher levels of anesthetic due to the discomfort of the conjunctival dissection and the use of cautery, and the postoperative appearance of the eye which will typically include visible subconjunctival hemorrhage. An intermediate approach is to start the incision through the very thin, transitional conjunctiva at the limbus, which therefore does not require dissecting a conjunctival flap. This area, being more vascularized, has the potential for more accelerated healing than a purely clear cornea incision. However, small amounts of bleeding may be problematic, and there is the potential for introducing epithelium into the anterior chamber, resulting in the severe complication of epithelial ingrowth. This, fortunately, is quite rare. The more common difficulty with entry at the limbus is ballooning of the conjunctiva as the irrigating fluid becomes entrapped within the conjunctiva. Profound chemosis can occur intraoperatively. Although this will resolve rapidly postoperatively, with no permanent sequelae, the expansion of the conjunctiva can result in a "donut" of conjunctiva around the cornea for 360°, which may trap the irrigating fluid and make visibility during surgery a major challenge.

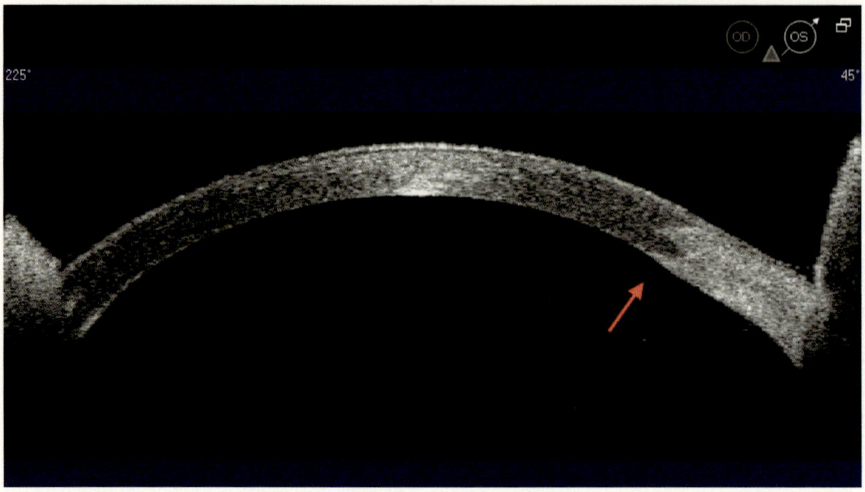

Fig. 9.1 OCT of a zigzag shaped penetrating keratoplasty incision created by the FS laser on the donor and the host (*arrow*)

Femtosecond Laser Corneal Incisions

The femtosecond (FS) laser has unique properties in the creation of corneal incisions, opening a new set of incision parameters that may improve incision performance and reduce or eliminate incision-related complications associated with blade incisions.

Incision Planes

A laser may be programmed to create an infinite variety of patterns, many of which cannot be created with a manual blade. This capability has been explored in penetrating and deep anterior lamellar keratoplasties [2–6]. In that application, the most common incision configurations have been called "top hat," "mushroom," and "zigzag," based on their cross sectional profile appearance. An optical coherence tomography (OCT) image of a zigzag incision is shown in Fig. 9.1. The FS laser incision yields less astigmatism and has better wound-sealing properties, avoiding excess suture tension and faster recovery of vision compared to manual incisions [3, 5, 6].

Lessons relevant to cataract incisions can be learned from the keratoplasty studies. First, the precise inter-locking incision patterns can create an inherently effective "hermetic" seal. Second, the precise replication of the incision pattern will likely yield more predictable results for all incision-related outcomes. Third, the lamellar and flexible structure of the cornea places some limitation on the practical configuration of clinically acceptable patterns. Patterns that can be drawn on paper and programmed into the laser will not necessarily behave well when opening incisions and passing instruments.

Incision Width

The width of a laser incision is precisely repeatable, readily modified for different aspiration instrumentation and IOL implant injection devices, and not restricted to the same width at all depths. In other words, the surgeon would have the option of creating width variations such as an external "funnel" to facilitate the initial instrument entry, an internal funnel to reduce restriction in instrument manipulation, or perhaps an "hourglass" shape that would provide both an internal and external funnel configuration.

Incision Location

In programming the laser, the location of the main and the side-port incisions is precisely programmed into the laser computer. As part of

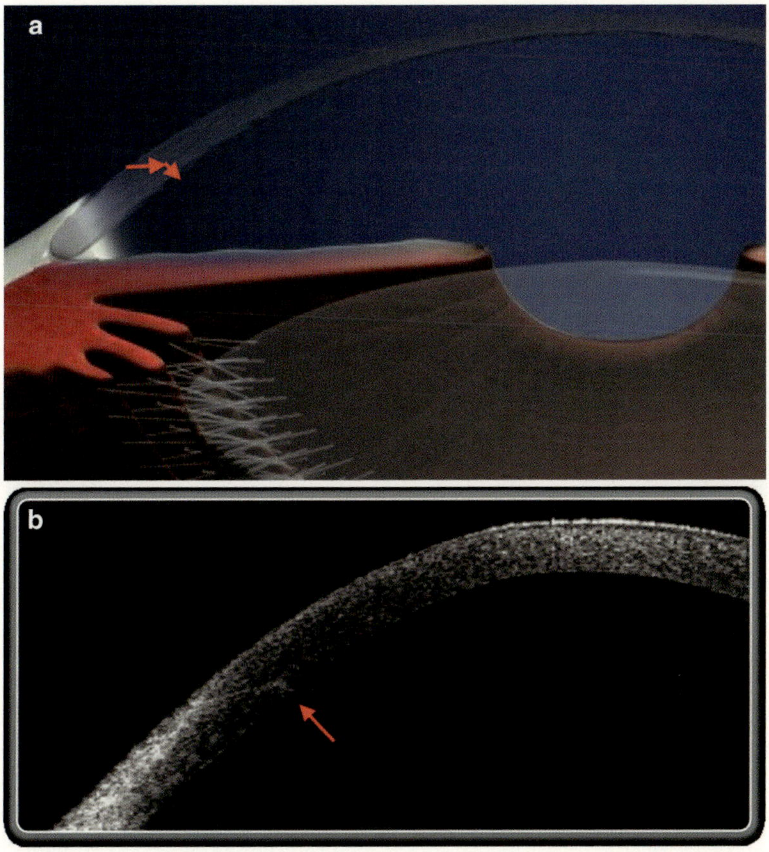

Fig. 9.2 (**a**) Drawing of concept of a two plane corneal incision. (**b**) OCT of a FS laser two plane corneal incision 2 weeks postoperatively (figures courtesy of Zoltan Z. Nagy)

astigmatism management, the surgeon has the option of readily placing the incision at any desired position over 360°.

Initial Incision Integrity

Unless the incision is created in the operating room under fully sterile conditions, initial incision integrity is essential to prevent leakage with fluid ingress or egress. FS laser incisions in the cornea leave small uncut tissue bridges between the two layers. These fine collagen strands are readily broken by instrumentation at the time of the intraocular surgery, but provide added integrity to the incision, in addition to the incision shape, when the laser is located outside the operating room.

Early Results of Femtosecond Laser Cataract Incisions

In 2009, Zoltan Nagy, M.D., and I studied the sealing properties of FS laser incisions (initially presented at the American Academy of Ophthalmology Annual Meeting, San Francisco, CA, Oct 23–27, 2009). We compared the outcomes of 18 eyes with a Langerman-style manual blade incision (three planes), 15 eyes with a "dimple down" manual blade incision (two planes), and 42 eyes with a FS laser incision approximating the two plane configuration of the manual "dimple down" incision (Fig. 9.2). The incision width was 2.75 mm in all cases. The endpoint was a dry, external incision edge when the anterior chamber was pressurized. No eyes required sutures.

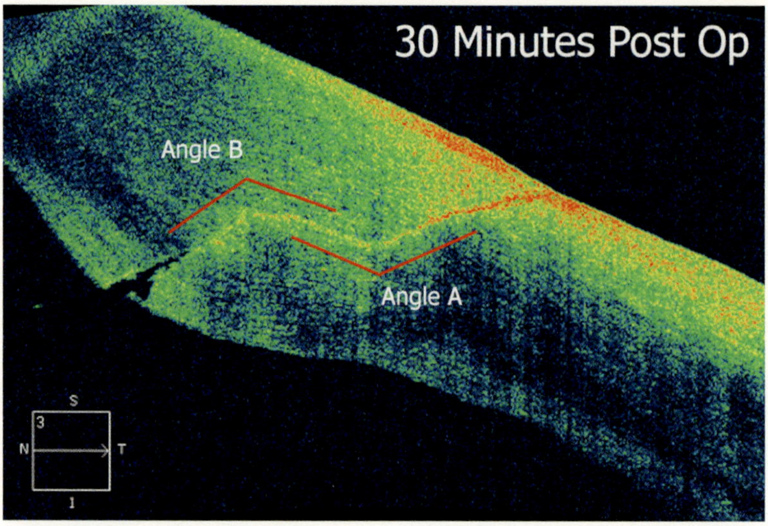

Fig. 9.3 Thirty minutes post-op in the three-plane FS incision OCT analysis. Note the tight wound apposition at angle "A" (image courtesy of James C. Loden)

Seventeen (94%) of the eyes with the manual Langerman-style three plane incision and 13 (87%) of the manual "dimple down" two plane incision required stromal hydration to fully seal, whereas none of the FS laser incision eyes required stromal hydration. Postoperatively, none of the eyes had complications such as iris prolapse or endophthalmitis.

This marked and highly significant difference may reflect better apposition of tissue planes in the FS laser incisions because of the incision creation, the reduced instrumentation and surgical time after FS laser capsulotomy and nuclear softening, or a combination.

Masket and coworkers, using a cadaver eye and an IntraLase, demonstrated high resistance to wound leakage with FS laser incisions of 3 mm width and 2 mm length [7].

In 2011, James Loden, MD conducted studies comparing OCT images of three-plane FS clear cornea incisions created with the IntraLase™ platform to two-plane clear corneal incisions made with a steel 2.5 mm keratome. The three-plane FS incision OCT analysis of 30 eyes in 30 patients showed consistent uniform outcomes with a complete seal noted in all 30 eyes at 30 min post-op (Fig. 9.3), 1 day post-op (Fig. 9.4), and 1 week post-op (Fig. 9.5). Analysis suggest that the tight wound apposition noted at angle "A" may provide a clear cornea incision that will result in a significantly lower incidence of postoperative ingress or egress of aqueous. In addition, no epithelial or external wound gape was documented.

Internal wound gape was noted in all 30 eyes that resolved over the course of 1 week. This gape prompted Loden to study OCT images of ten eyes with two-plane keratome "dimple down" clear corneal incisions. All ten eyes were noted to have internal wound gape that sealed over the course of 1 week (Figs. 9.6, 9.7, and 9.8). The wound architecture by OCT was noted to be uniplanar in all ten eyes despite the attempt to create a "dimple down" two-plane incision. In two of the ten eyes significant external wound gape was visualized even after stromal hydration being performed in all eyes [8].

Further trials of different incision patterns and different surgeons are underway.

Conclusions

Corneal cataract incisions performed by the FS laser are feasible. Laser incisions are highly reproducible in size. The laser can create patterns

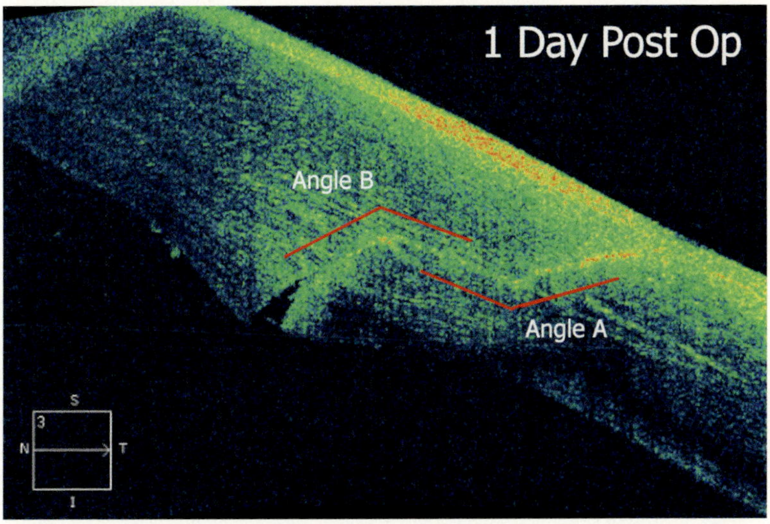

Fig. 9.4 One day post-op in the three-plane FS incision OCT analysis. Note the tight wound apposition at angle "A" (image courtesy of James C. Loden)

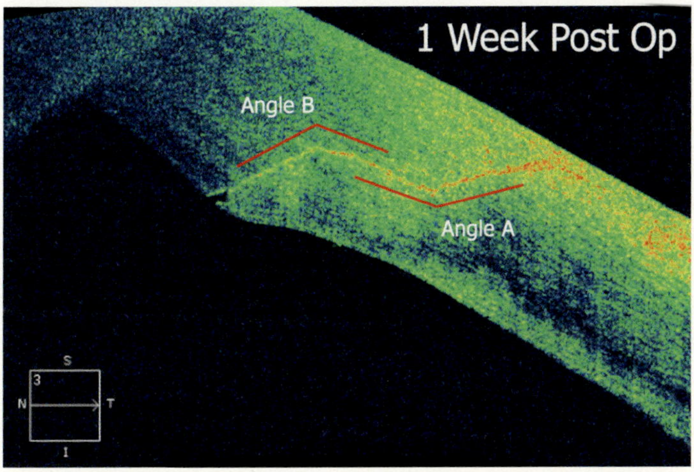

Fig. 9.5 One week post-op in the three-plane FS incision OCT analysis. Note the tight wound apposition at angle "A" (image courtesy of James C. Loden)

that are difficult or impossible to create with manual techniques. Preliminary experience suggests that a laser incision may seal more readily than a manual incision, with the potential for reduction in postoperative complications, especially endophthalmitis.

Key Points

1. Incisions must be large enough to allow both insertion and manipulation of instruments as well as the IOL.
2. The astigmatic effect of incisions is minimized when placed as peripherally in the temporal

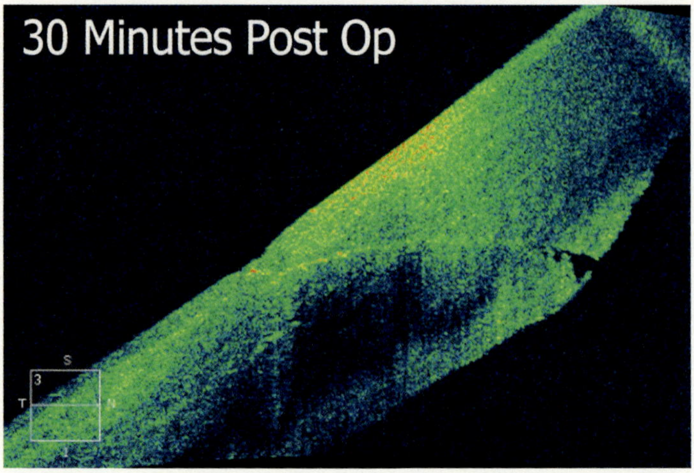

Fig. 9.6 Thirty minutes post-op in study with two plane keratome "dimple down" clear corneal incisions (image courtesy of James C. Loden)

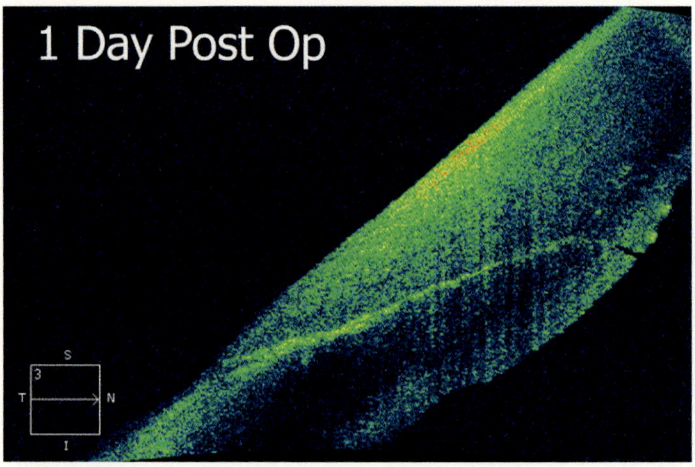

Fig. 9.7 One day post-op in study with two plane keratome "dimple down" clear corneal incisions (image courtesy of James C. Loden)

cornea and width (chord length) rather than height is as short as possible.

3. Scleral tunnel incisions cause the least astigmatism, but are more difficult to create, insert and manipulate instruments through and require more anesthesia.
4. Wound leakage is a serious complication of clear corneal incisions, particularly due to the increased risk of infectious endophthalmitis.
5. Stromal hydration is generally necessary to seal clear corneal cataract incisions created by manual techniques using a blade, while early studies of FS laser incisions show they do not.

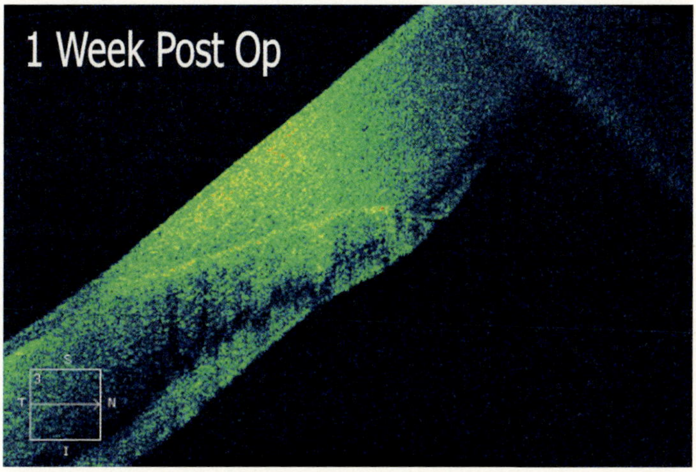

Fig. 9.8 One week post-op in study with two plane keratome "dimple down" clear corneal incisions (image courtesy of James C. Loden)

References

1. Fine IH. Incision construction. In: Steinert RF, editor. Cataract surgery. 3rd ed. London: Saunders Elsevier; 2010. p. 141–62.
2. Steinert RF, Ignacio TS, Sarayba MS. Top hat-shaped penetrating keratoplasty using the femtosecond laser. Am J Ophthalmol. 2007;143:689–91.
3. Farid M, Kim M, Steinert RF. Results of penetrating keratoplasty performed with femtosecond laser zig-zag incision initial report. Ophthalmology. 2007;114:2208–12.
4. Farid M, Steinert RF. Deep anterior lamellar keratoplasty performed with the femtosecond laser zigzag incision for the treatment of stromal corneal pathology and ecstatic disease. J Cataract Refract Surg. 2009; 35(5):809–13.
5. Farid M, Steinert RF, Gaster RM, Chamberlain W, Lin A. Comparison of penetrating keratoplasty performed with a femtosecond laser zig-zag incision versus conventional blade trephination. Ophthalmology. 2009;116(9):1638–43 [Epub 2009 Jul 31. PMID: 19646760].
6. Farid M, Steinert RF. Femtosecond laser-assisted corneal surgery. Curr Opin Ophthalmol. 2010;21(4):288–92.
7. Masket S, Sarayba M, Ignacio T, Fram N. Femtosecond laser-assisted cataract incisions: architectural stability and reproducibility. J Cataract Refract Surg. 2010;36: 1048–9.
8. Loden J. "Laser Cataract Surgery with Femtosecond Technology" Presented at the Annual Meeting of the American Society of Cataract and Refractive Surgery, session 1E, March 26, 2011, San Diego CA.

Relaxing Incisions for Astigmatism Correction in ReLACS

Section A: Peripheral Corneal Laser Relaxing Incisions

Section B: Conic Intrastromal Relaxing Incisions (CIRI) Roberto Zaldivar and Roger Zaldivar

10

Ana P. Canto, Sonia H. Yoo, and Roger Zaldivar

Abbreviations

AK	Astigmatic keratotomy
BCVA	Best-corrected visual acuity
D	Diopter
IOL	Intraocular lens
LRI	Limbal relaxing incision
PCRI	Peripheral corneal relaxing incision
UCVA	Uncorrected visual acuity

Section A: Peripheral Corneal Laser Relaxing Incisions

Introduction

Cataract surgery in the last decade has undergone significant changes, with the primary focus shifting from reducing complications to improving refractive outcomes. Refractive cataract surgery refers to the uncomplicated removal of a cataract with a major objective of minimizing postoperative spectacle dependence. The reduction of refractive astigmatism is an important component of minimizing postoperative spectacle dependence and is facilitated by the availability of femtosecond (FS) laser technology.

According to a recent study, the degree and prevalence of corneal astigmatism before cataract surgery is greater than 1.00 D in 36% of the patients, and greater than 1.50 D in 17–22% of patients [1]. Since the presence of 0.5 D or more of astigmatism materially affects unaided visual acuity, a significant number of patients undergoing refractive cataract surgery could benefit from concomitant reduction of their astigmatism in order to maximize their refractive outcomes.

History of Astigmatic and Limbal Relaxing Incisions for Cataract Surgery

The first description of the use of corneal incisions to modify corneal curvature dates back to the nineteenth century. In 1869, Snellen suggested that anterior corneal incisions could flatten the steep corneal meridian [2].

In 1885, Hjalmar August Shiøtz was the first surgeon to report the treatment of astigmatism using keratotomy. In a case report, Shiøtz described how a 3.5 mm incision at the patient's upper limbus using a Graefe's knife decreased the patient's with-the-rule astigmatism of 19.5 D,

A.P. Canto, M.D. • S.H. Yoo, M.D. (✉)
Department of Ophthalmology, Bascom Palmer Eye Institute, University of Miami Miller School of Medicine, 900 NW 17 St., Miami, FL 33136, USA
e-mail: syoo@med.miami.edu

R. Zaldivar (✉) • R. Zaldivar , M.D.
Department of Cataract & Refractive Surgery, Instituto Zaldivar, 685 Emilio Civit St., Mendoza, 5500 Argentina
e-mail: zaldivarroberto@gmail.com

R.R. Krueger et al. (eds.), *Textbook of Refractive Laser Assisted Cataract Surgery (ReLACS)*, DOI 10.1007/978-1-4614-1010-2_10, © Springer Science+Business Media, LLC 2013 induced by cataract surgery, to just 7.00 D of cylinder [3].

In 1894, William H. Bates from New York suggested an operation to correct astigmatism based on observing six patients who had peripheral surgical or traumatic corneal scars and developed flattening of the cornea in the same meridian that intersected the scar, with no effect on the meridian 90° away. He concluded from his study that incisions on the cornea should be made at right angles to the most convex meridian, and the number, depth and location of these incisions could regulate the amount of correction [4].

In 1895, Faber reported reduction of naturally occurring astigmatism from 1.50 to 0.75 D in a 19-year-old, using perforating corneal incisions [5], and in 1896, Lucciola reported ten cases of reduction of astigmatism with non-perforating corneal incisions [6].

In 1898, Leendert Jan Lans published experiments in rabbits describing corneal section, resection, and cauterization to reduce astigmatism. He assumed that change in the tension of the tissue near the limbus would alter the cornea curvature [7].

In 1943, after a long period of either a mysterious abandonment of or lack of reporting on this topic, Japanese physician Tsutomu Sato and his staff reported results of experimental studies on radial and tangential incisions in rabbits to correct astigmatism [8]. Then, in 1950, Sato suggested posterior corneal incisions to treat regular astigmatism of more than 2 D and described it as the only remedy to treat a strong astigmatism of an oblique axis that could not be corrected by spectacles [9].

This was followed by the work of Fyodorov and his colleagues in the Soviet Union in the 1970s, who developed numerous patterns of incisions to correct astigmatism [10].

The correction of preexisting congenital or acquired astigmatic errors at the time of cataract surgery was first described by Troutman in 1973, who performed corneal incisions on the flatter meridian, in addition to excising a wedge from the wound edges [11].

In 1989, Osher published a study initiated in 1983, which determined if simultaneous peripheral corneal relaxing incisions in the steep meridians could reduce moderate preexisting cylinder as well as preventing eyes with low astigmatism from gaining induced cylinder after cataract surgery [12].

Later on, in the 1990s and early 2000s, several other surgeons contributed to the investigation of astigmatic keratotomy techniques, including Nordan [13], Lindstrom [14], Thornton [15], and Nichamin [16].

Nordan proposed three keratotomy patterns to be performed in combination with cataract surgery to reduce preexisting astigmatism [13]. Lindstrom developed a technique, as well as a nomogram for straight and arcuate astigmatic keratotomy that included an age factor [14].

Thornton's technique involved making paired straight or arcuate T incisions at different optical zone sizes. Multiple pairs of incisions were included on his nomogram [15].

Nichamin developed an extensive nomogram for limbal relaxing incision at the time of cataract surgery [16].

With the advent of refractive laser-assisted cataract surgery (ReLACS), it is possible to perform corneal incisions, capsulorrhexis, lens softening, and for neutralizing astigmatism, either astigmatic keratotomy or limbal relaxing incisions all in one single procedure.

Clinical Results for Astigmatic Relaxing Incisions with Phacoemulsification

Clinical Results of Relaxing Incisions Combined with Phacoemulsification

Studies have shown that astigmatic keratotomy (AK), limbal relaxing incisions (LRI) and peripheral corneal relaxing incisions (PCRI) performed concurrently with cataract surgery can safely and effectively reduce preexisting corneal astigmatism [17–27].

The astigmatic keratotomy incision is usually placed at the 5–7 mm optical zone on the steepest astigmatism axis, whereas a peripheral corneal relaxing incision is an incision placed outside the 7 mm optical zone, but greater than 1 mm anterior to the limbus. The effect of a relaxing astigmatic incision also depends on the optical zone: the closer the incision to the corneal center, the greater relaxing effect [27]. A limbal relaxing incision is an incision placed adjacent to the limbus, just anterior to the vascular arcade.

Wang et al. [24] analyzed the effectiveness of peripheral corneal relaxing incision (PCRI) in 115 eyes that had the procedure combined with phacoemulsification. They also proposed an improved nomogram in which the length and number of PCRIs are determined based on age and preoperative keratometric corneal astigmatism.

In 2007, Carvalho et al. [28] reported the refractive outcomes of limbal relaxing incisions in 26 eyes, using the Nichamin nomogram, which takes into consideration the degree and axis of the astigmatism and the patient's age. In this study, a significant reduction in the topographic astigmatism with a stable postoperative refraction was observed, but also reflected a trend towards under-correction.

Kulkarni et al. [29] reported long-term refractive stability following combined astigmatic keratotomy and phacoemulsification in 2009. They used the Buzard nomogram that recommends paired arcuate incisions, 600 μm deep in the cornea, varying the arc length based on the age and magnitude of astigmatism to be corrected, with results showing a postoperative reduction of the astigmatism with no complications during or after surgery.

In 2010, Ouchi et al. [30] achieved an accurate correction of preexisting astigmatism, leading to good uncorrected visual acuity by performing limbal relaxing incisions combined with microincisional cataract surgery in 96 eyes. They used the Fukuyama's nomogram for limbal relaxing incisions, which determines the degrees of the incision arcs based on the amount of astigmatism and the steepest axis (against-the-rule, oblique and with-the-rule astigmatism) and incision depth based on the patient's age.

Current nomograms for combined phacoemulsification and astigmatic relaxing incisions. Over time, numerous nomograms were developed and enhanced to improve accuracy and outcomes in the performance of astigmatic incisions combined with cataract surgery. Currently, the length and number of the astigmatic incisions are determined based on the preoperative corneal astigmatism and patient's age.

Pioneers and developers of their own nomograms for LRI at the time of cataract surgery include Louis D. "Skip" Nichamin [31], James Gills [32], Douglas Koch [24], Kevin Miller [33], and Eric Donnenfeld [34].

It is noteworthy that the literature emphasizes that every nomogram requires customization for each surgeon's personal technique, instrumentation, and outcomes [35].

The Nichamin-NAPA nomogram [35] is effective between 0.75 and 3 D of cylinder. The maximum suggested length for a LRI is 90° (3 clock hours). This nomogram is unique because it is the only one in which the cataract incision can overlap the relaxing incision.

The Donnenfeld-DONO nomogram [34] is effective between 0.5 and 3 D of astigmatism. The maximum suggested length for an LRI is also 90°. Each 90° LRI provides approximately 1.5 D of correction. The incisions are placed 0.5 mm from the limbus at a depth of 600 μm.

Complications and Limitations of Blade AK/LRI

Manually performed astigmatic relaxing incisions are usually successful in correcting corneal astigmatism. Nevertheless, this procedure has well-acknowledged limitations and complications. The poor predictability of this procedure is its foremost limitation, as a seemingly identical operation in two different patients can produce completely different results [36].

The final effect of a corneal astigmatic incision depends upon multiple incision variables, including length, depth, optical zone size, number, correct placement on the steepest axis and configuration. Other factors that contribute to the final outcomes are the surgeon's experience, corneal healing process, patient's age, cause of the astigmatism (naturally occurring or surgically induced), and blade calibration [37].

Table 10.1 Limitations and complications of corneal relaxing incisions performed by a blade

• Surgeon's personal technique and experience may vary the results
• Imprecision of the blade used may interfere with the results
• Lack of precision in obtaining a regular, smooth, uniform and perfect incision
• Difficulty in achieving and maintaining the exactly incision depth
• Difficulty in performing the exactly planned arc incision extension
• Difficulty in maintaining the incision curvature
• Difficulty in maintaining the incisions symmetry
• Only allows incisions perpendicular to the cornea
• Perforation
• Infection
• Decreased corneal sensation
• Misalignment
• Shift of the astigmatism axis
• Distortion of the cornea
• Wound gape
• Wrong axis incision
• Induced irregular astigmatism
• Over- and undercorrection
• Corneal abrasion

Performing an astigmatic incision with the precise intended length, at a uniform depth along the entire incision, keeping the entire length of the incision at the calculated optical zone, is a challenge when performing it manually. It is very difficult to produce a precise and perfectly reproducible incision.

Possible complications of corneal relaxing incisions performed by a blade include perforations, over- or undercorrection, shift of the astigmatism axis, distortion of the cornea, irregular astigmatism, infection, wound gape and corneal abrasion [21, 38, 39]. See Table 10.1 for complications and limitations (see Fig. 10.1).

Rationale for Image Guided Laser Relaxing Incisions

The lasers that perform ReLACS are equipped with image-guidance systems to make the incisions more precisely and reproducibly. This technology provides real-time determination of the corneal thickness, which is critical for making consistent incisions at a uniform depth in the planned position of the arcuate incisions.

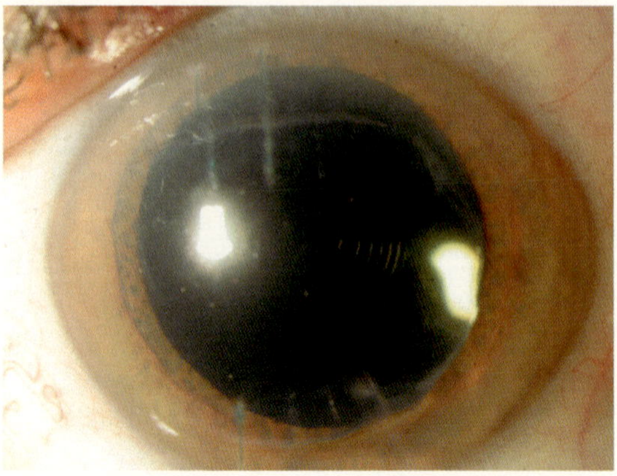

Fig. 10.1 Manually performed astigmatic keratotomy to correct astigmatism after a multifocal IOL. Overcorrection after the procedure was noticed and sutures had to be placed at the astigmatic incisions to compensate

Astigmatic Incisions with the Femtosecond Laser

Why Adopt Femtosecond Laser Technology?

FS laser incisions eliminate the mechanical variability related to manually performed astigmatic keratotomy. The laser allows greater precision in incision orientation, depth, and length, and eliminates the surgeon's personal technique and experience. While greater precision will not completely negate the variability conferred by corneal healing, incisional wounds with consistent architectural characteristics will likely produce superior results, increase patient satisfaction and reduce the chance of complications.

While results of laser LRI's for post-cataract astigmatism are just beginning to emerge in mid 2011, several studies have shown that FS assisted astigmatic keratotomy is a safe, effective and a promising treatment option for both naturally occurring and post-keratoplasty astigmatism [22, 40–43] (see Fig. 10.2).

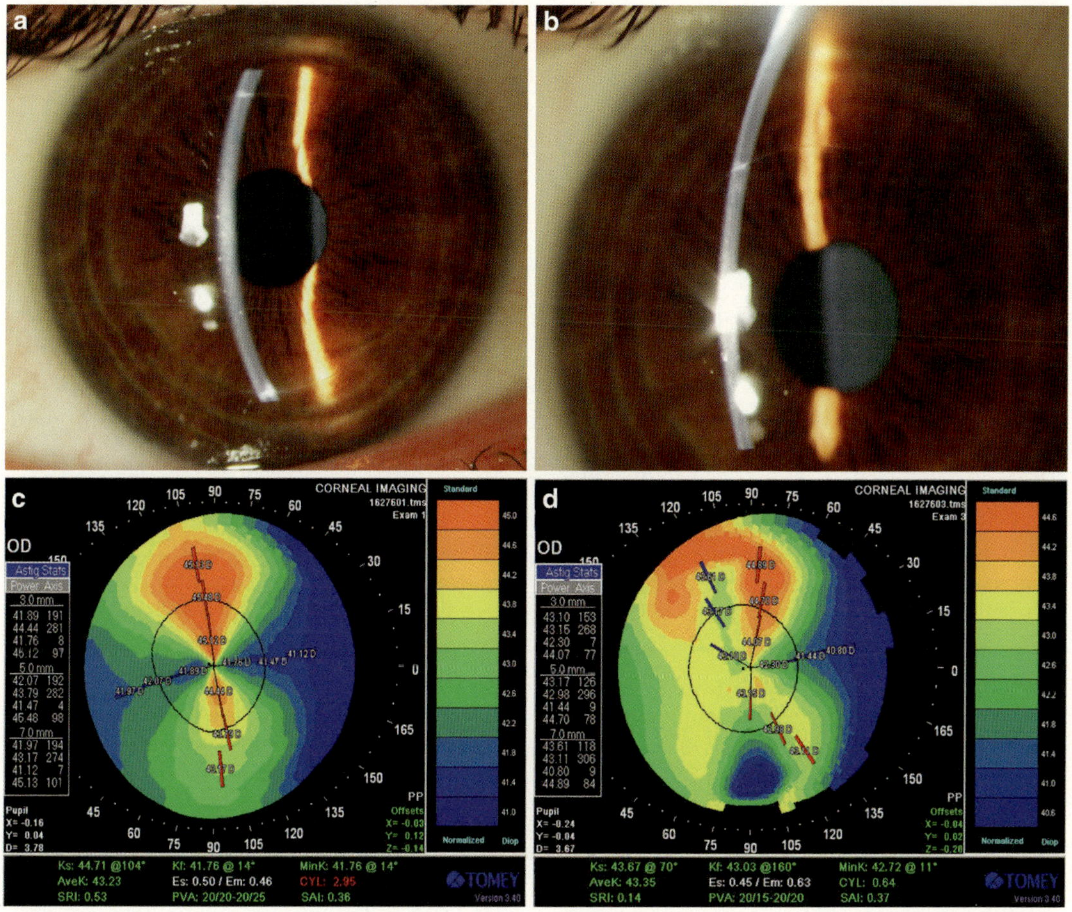

Fig. 10.2 FS-assisted astigmatic keratotomy for naturally occurring astigmatism. (**a**) incisions, (**b**) higher magnification of superior incision, (**c**) preoperative topography, (**d**) postoperative topography

Straight Vs. Arcuate Incisions

Transverse keratotomy incisions can be straight or arcuate, and placed as AK, PCRI or LRI's. However, the limbal vasculature limits the length of straight incisions placed as LRI's. Incisions can be single or multiple, symmetric or asymmetric. Asymmetric incisions are useful to treat asymmetric astigmatism.

A straight transverse incision is made tangential to the optical zone circle mark and is measured in millimeters. The arcuate transverse incision is made along the optical zone circle mark and is measured in degrees. Straight (equidistant from the center) lines on a spherical surface are curved to follow the circumference, while straight transverse incisions are actually inverse arcs and are semiradial.

Arcuate incisions in theory have the potential for greater effect than straight incisions with the same chord length. Although the chord length is the same, the actual length is about 10% longer on the curve, and the entire length of the incision is equidistant from the center of the cornea [44]. Arcuate incisions are said to be more difficult to perform manually, since it is difficult for most surgeons to make a precise concentric arc incision. Despite this fact, arcuate incisions are most commonly used, and the evolving FS laser nomograms and software all utilize arcuate incisions.

Limbal Vs. Peripheral Corneal Incisions

The preference for utilizing an LRI instead of an AK with a smaller optical zone in combination with phacoemulsification is based on the coupling ratio effect. The coupling ratio for corneal astigmatic incisions was described by Thornton [15] as the relationship between a transverse incision that flattens the meridian it incises and the compensatory steepening that occurs in the uncut meridian 90° away. Coupling is proportional to the length and proximity of the incisions to the corneal center.

It is important to consider the coupling ratio when planning AK, PCRI or LRI incisions during cataract surgery since its value can affect the resulting spherical equivalent refraction. If the coupling ratio is 1, the flattening of the incised meridian will equal the steepening of the opposite meridian, and the spherical equivalent will not change after astigmatic keratotomy. If the incision ends up with a coupling ratio >1 (flattening of the incised meridian was greater than the steepening of the opposite meridian) the spherical equivalent will shift toward hyperopia. If a coupling ratio is <1 (the flattening of the incised meridian was less than the steepening of the opposite meridian), the spherical equivalent will shift toward myopia [45].

Limbal relaxing incisions have a coupling ratio of 1:1. No change in the IOL power is needed, because the cornea's spherical equivalent does not change.

When planning the correction of astigmatism during manual or FS refractive cataract surgery only the keratometric cylinder should be considered to calculate the astigmatic correction since lenticular astigmatism is eliminated with the cataract removal and intraocular lens implantation.

Surface Vs. Intrastromal Incisions

FS laser assisted astigmatic keratotomy allows the surgeon to create new incisional techniques and change the architecture or shape of the incision (see Fig. 10.3).

With the FS laser, instead of creating an incision from the corneal surface through the desired corneal depth and opening the epithelium with a Sinskey hook or other fine-tipped instrument, it is possible to create an intrastromal incision. Intrastromal incisions are placed entirely within the corneal stroma, leaving the epithelium and Bowman's layer intact. Investigators studying this approach feel it may yield greater precision and postoperative comfort while reducing the chance of infection. However, experience to date is limited and nomograms are likely to be very different from those currently available as these wounds may heal differently.

Nichamin and coworkers [46] have developed a model of the human cornea created with finite element analysis that predicts tissue response to corneal incisions. This model is being used to study LRIs and helps to develop optimal nomograms for astigmatic incisions using FS laser technology. Their initial results showed that the model's results were consistent with existing LRI nomograms. The group has been also studying the sub-Bowman's incisions with promising outcomes.

Abbott Medical Optics (AMO) has been conducting a prospective single center study to evaluate the feasibility of intrastromal arcuate keratotomy performed with the IntraLase iFS™ FS Laser System. Dr. Gunther Grabner and colleagues in Austria are evaluating this treatment for natural occurring astigmatism as well as residual astigmatism after cataract surgery of 0.75–7.00 D [47]. Preliminary results have not been released by AMO at the time of this publication (July 2011). Dr. Roberto Zaldivar and colleagues in Argentina are also working with AMO as part of an investigator initiated study, and have also developed a nomogram for sub-Bowman's corneal relaxing incisions. Please see "Section B" for Dr. Zaldivar's data and discussion of this topic.

Perpendicular Vs. Angled Incisions

In 2010, during the American Academy Ophthalmology Meeting, Dr. David Huang presented his experience with beveled astigmatic keratotomy performed with the FS laser in post-keratotomy eyes. He performed 135° beveled astigmatic keratotomy incisions (inverse 45° from perpendicular) instead of perpendicular incisions in six eyes post-keratoplasty using the IntraLase™ FS laser (AMO, Irvine, CA). He reported an average gain of 5.1 lines in the uncorrected visual acuity (UCVA), 1.4 line gain in the best-corrected

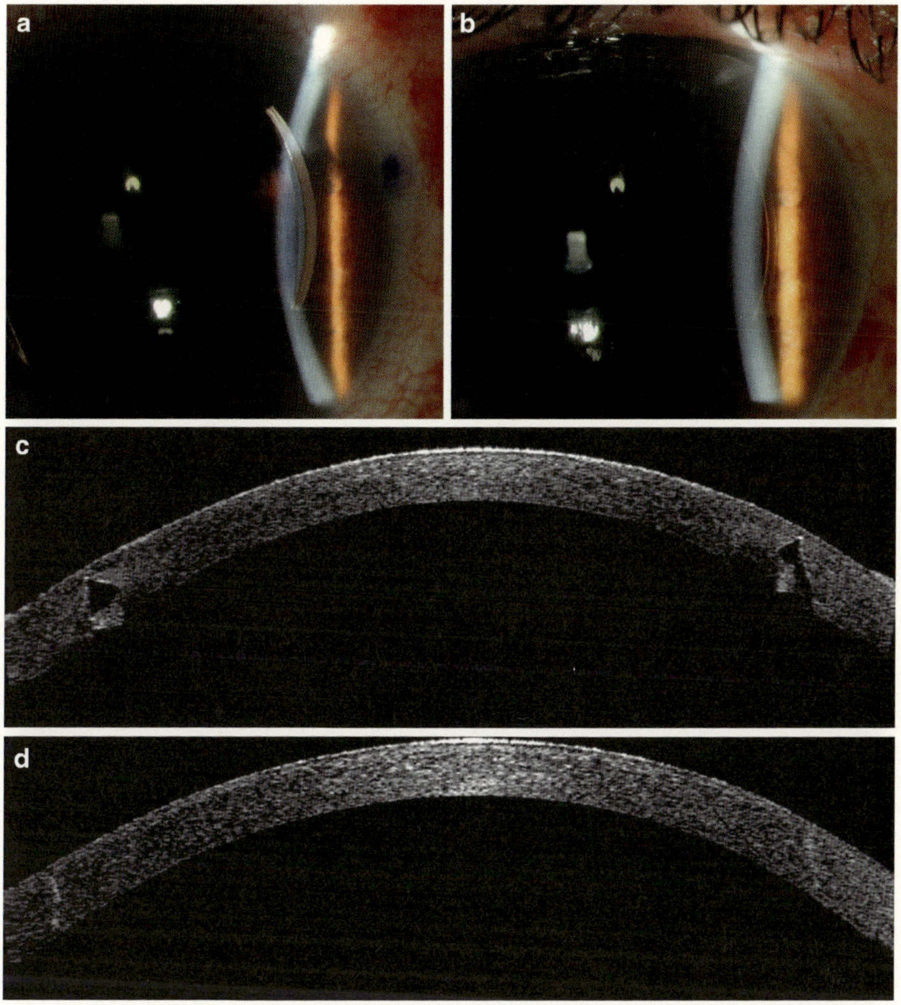

Fig. 10.3 FS-assisted intrastromal beveled arcuate incisions for treatment of residual corneal cylinder after multifocal IOL cataract surgery. (**a**) Incisions immediately post-op showing the intrastromal beveled incisions created by the photodisruption, (**b**) the same incisions on first post-op day (note that only a intrastromal corneal line is noticed), (**c**) anterior segment optical coherence tomography immediately post-op showing the space created intrastromally, (**d**) anterior segment optical coherence tomography on first post-op day (image Courtesy of Dr. William W. Culbertson)

visual acuity (BCVA) and a 72% reduction on the magnitude of the keratometric cylinder. The astigmatic outcome was stable by 1 month postoperatively in five of his six patients. In one patient, there was significant regression between the first and third months after surgery.

Dr. Huang postulates that the advantage of using a beveled incision is that the incision wound does not gape, minimizing dellen formation, epithelial defects and chronic discomfort for the patient. Another advantage is that no epithelial plug is formed on the epithelium surface of the incision, which is common following perpendicular incisions and contributes to the variability of results [48]. While the data reported were from eyes that had undergone penetrating keratoplasty, it is reasonable to infer that these same advantages should apply to LRI, PCRI and AK in other situations. If wound behavior were to become more predictable due to beveled architecture,

Table 10.2 FS laser-assisted arcuate keratotomy nomogram for naturally occurring astigmatism

Astigmatism (D)	Zone diameter (mm)	Incision depth (%)[a]	Angular length (°)
1.5–2.5	7.25	90	60
2.6–3.6	7	90	70
3.7–4.8	7	90	80
4.9–5.9	6.75	90	80
6.0–7.0	6.75	90	90
7.1–8.0	6.5	90	90

Add 0.5 D per year for each year under 30 years of age. Subtract 0.05 D per year for each year over 30 years of age. Subtract an additional 0.02 D per year for each year after 50 years of age

[a]The depth of the incision is calculated from the lowest pachymetry reading along the intended arcuate incision

Table 10.3 FS laser-assisted arcuate keratotomy nomogram for post-keratoplasty astigmatism

Astigmatism (D)	Zone diameter (mm)	Incision depth (%)[a]	Angular length(°)
1.5–2.5	7.25	75	60
2.6–3.6	7	75	70
3.7–4.8	7	75	80
4.9–5.9	6.75	75	80
6.0–7.0	6.75	75	90
7.1–8.0	6.5	75	90

Add 0.5 D per year for each year under 30 years of age. Subtract 0.05 D per year for each year over 30 years of age. Subtract an additional 0.02 D per year for each year after 50 years of age

[a]The depth of the incision is calculated from the lowest pachymetry reading along the intended arcuate incision

routine use of more central incisions (PCRI or, less likely, AK) at cataract surgery may be possible, expanding the potential range of astigmatic effect and reducing the likelihood that healing effects related to the proximity of limbal vasculature could influence outcomes.

Nomograms for Femtosecond Astigmatic Keratotomy (AK)

Abbey et al. [49] have proposed a FS laser-assisted arcuate keratotomy nomogram based on a modified Lindstrom nomogram (Table 10.2). Subsequently, Hurmeric and Yoo [50] proposed a modified version of the previous naturally occurring nomogram to be used on post-keratoplasty astigmatic incisions (Table 10.3). For naturally occurring astigmatism the depth of the incision should be 90% of the lowest pachymetric reading along the intended arcuate incision, whereas for post-keratoplasty astigmatism, the incision depth should be 75% of the lowest pachymetry reading.

Nomograms for FS Laser LRI's

At this time, there are no published peer-reviewed data comparing naturally occurring astigmatism treated with any variation manual or FS laser assisted astigmatic keratotomy (LRI, PCRI, or AK). However, early experience (personally communicated at ASCRS Summer Town Hall Meeting 2011) with the LenSx laser (LenSx Lasers, Aliso Viejo, CA) system by Drs. Stephen Slade, Eric Donnenfeld. and others recommends that the LRI's should be performed at 80% of the corneal thickness measured with the anterior segment optical coherence tomography. If the AMO LRI calculator (Donnenfeld nomogram—www.lricalculator.com) is used, they recommend subtracting 33% from the recommended treatment.

Table 10.4 Contraindications for astigmatic keratotomy

• Corneal ectatic disorders
• Highly irregular astigmatism
• Limbal peripheral corneal pathology
• Extreme dry eye
• Ocular surface disease

When planning the astigmatic keratotomy incisions during the cataract surgery the surgeon needs to take into consideration the induced astigmatism caused by the location and size of the primary corneal phacoemulsification incision.

Performing FS Laser AK and LRI

Planning the Procedure

1. Indications: Naturally occurring astigmatism, astigmatism after cataract surgery, astigmatism after penetrating keratoplasty. See contraindications (Table 10.4).
2. Measure the astigmatism power and axis. That can be done performing a corneal topography using Placido disk imaging, Scheimpflug camera, or a combination of both.
3. Get the best refraction. If the procedure will be performed at the time of the cataract surgery, only the keratometric astigmatism should be treated since the lenticular component will be corrected by surgical removal of the lens. However, if the procedure will be performed in eyes not undergoing concomitant lens surgery, treat the astigmatism detected by refraction. This should correspond with the keratometric astigmatism. Discrepancy in the refractive and keratometric astigmatism is a relative contraindication to treatment.
4. Choose the surgical plan based on a nomogram. Nomograms take into consideration the age of the patient, the axis of the astigmatism, and the magnitude of the astigmatism. Based on the nomogram, an optical zone diameter (mm), the depth (%) and the angular length (°) of the incisions will be determined.
5. Identify the accurate thinnest pachymetry along the intended site of the incisions. This can be measured using an ultrasound pachymeter, anterior segment optical coherence tomography, or the real-time corneal image provided by the FS cataract laser devices (Fig. 10.4).
6. Calculate the depth of the incision based on the nomogram and pachymetry.
7. Enter the surgical plan on the FS laser screen: posterior depth of the incision (μm), anterior side-cut diameter (mm) that refers to the optical zone diameter determined by the nomogram, anterior side-cut energy (mJ), the cut position of the first incision (°), cut angle of the first incision (arc length), the cut position of the second incision (°) that might be 180 degrees away from the first incision, cut angle of the second incision (arc length), side cut angle (°), side cut spot separation, side cut layer separation, depth in contact glass (selected according to manufacturer recommendations). Usually it is 50 μm for the Intralase™ (AMO, Irvine, CA) but a minus value can be used to stop the incision before reaching the glass for Sub-Bowman's incisions.

The Procedure

1. At the slit-lamp, under topical anesthesia and using a surgical marking pen, mark the 0°, 90°, 180° and 270° corneal axes.
2. Under the laser surgical microscope, mark the center of the pupil with a marking pen. Use an axis marker to mark the planned locations of the incisions.
3. Use an optical zone marker centered on the pupil to mark the optical zone diameter.
4. Align the corneal marks with the reticle lines from the FS device.
5. Engage the FS suction ring, followed by the cone applanation centering on the pupil (Fig. 10.5).
6. The treatment screen shows the location of the incisions and the suction ring can be used to rotate the eye to ensure proper axis alignment. The centration of the optical zone can be modified on the screen, if necessary.
7. After the laser treatment, the incisions are opened with a Sinskey hook.
8. Antibiotic and steroid eyedrops are prescribed four times daily for 1 week.

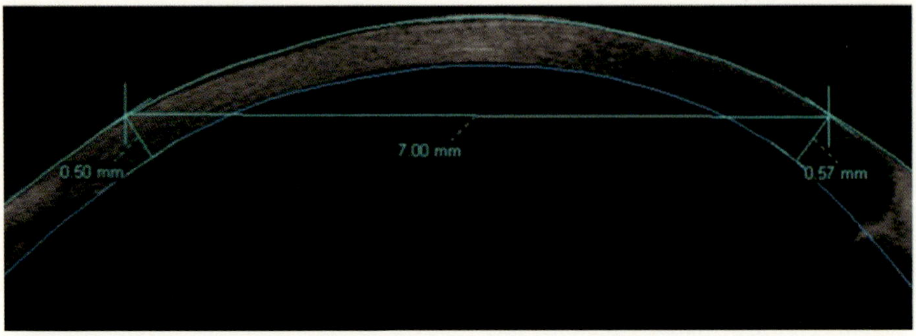

Fig. 10.4 Anterior segment optical coherence tomography used to measure the corneal thickness at the planned astigmatic keratotomy optical zone

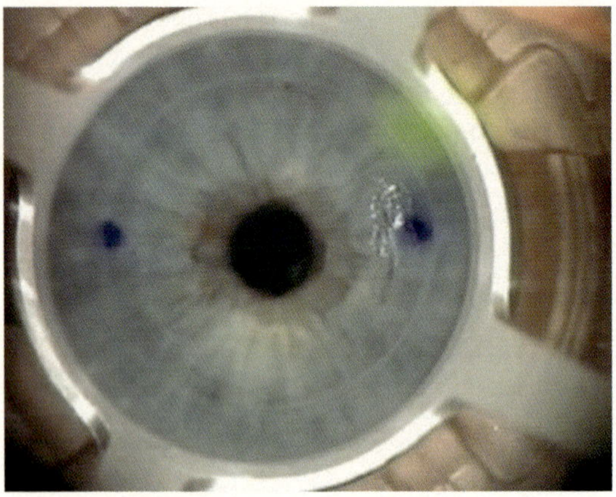

Fig. 10.5 Astigmatic keratotomy being performed. Note the 0° and 180° corneal marks and the first incision being performed

9. The patient is instructed to avoid rubbing the eye and to use artificial tears frequently.

Comparison of Techniques to Treat Astigmatism During Cataract Surgery

Manual AK Vs. Femtosecond AK

Bahar et al. [43] compared the outcomes of FS astigmatic keratotomy to manual astigmatic keratotomy after penetrating keratoplasty in a retrospective study. Dr. Bahar described results of 20 eyes that underwent manual astigmatic keratotomy with a diamond blade and 20 eyes that underwent Intralase™ FS astigmatic keratotomy. The FS group showed improved UCVA and BCVA compared to the manual AK group, had more reduction in the absolute cylinder and greater improvement in the defocus equivalent, however, they were not statistically significant.

Both procedures reduced the amount of astigmatism, but, while manual AK induced a large shift in axis from with the rule to against the rule, the FS AK brought the mean astigmatism vector closer to neutral. FS laser astigmatic keratotomy was shown to be a safe and effective procedure in this setting.

Hoffart et al. [51] in a prospective, randomized study compared the effectiveness of arcuate keratotomy performed with a FS laser or Hanna keratome (Moria, Anthony, France) for correction of post-keratoplasty astigmatism. They found a significantly ($P=0.011$) higher reduction of preoperative refractive cylinder in the laser AK group than in the mechanical AK group. No complications occurred with the FS group while in the mechanical AK group they had one case of microperforation and one case where the incisions were off-center.

Abbey et al. [49] reported their results in a 30 year-old patient with a naturally occurring astigmatism of 5.25 D in both eyes. The treatment plan was based on a modified Lindstrom nomogram, which they have designated the FS astigmatic keratotomy nomogram. An improvement in the UCVA and BCVA was seen in both eyes 1 year after procedure. The corneal topography showed a significant improvement in the astigmatism, with no significant change in the axis.

For guidance on the performance of FS laser LRI's, please see the above section "Astigmatic Incisions with the FS Laser".

Toric Intraocular Lens Vs. Limbal Relaxing Incisions

Poll et al. [52] compared toric intraocular lens (IOL) implantation to peripheral corneal relaxing incisions to study if the two methods were equally efficacious in astigmatism correction at the time of cataract surgery. They did a 2-year retrospective analysis, the group receiving peripheral corneal relaxing incision (115 eyes) had a single-piece aspheric, acrylic IOL (Acrysoft IQ SN60WF, Alcon Laboratories Inc.) implanted and the group receiving the toric intraocular lens (77 eyes) received a single-piece, non-aspheric, toric, acrylic IOL (Acrysof SN60T3, SN60T4, or SN60T5, Alcon Labs, Fort Worth, Texas). The amount of astigmatism was assessed by three different methods, with Humphrey Atlas videokeratography (Carl Zeiss Meditec Inc., Dublin, California), IOLMaster (Carls Zeiss Meditec), and manual keratometry. Both groups had comparable keratometric astigmatism values. For the relaxing incisions they used a previous nomogram published by Wang et al. [24]. Their results support the use of both toric IOL and peripheral corneal relaxing incisions as effective in reducing mild-to-moderate preoperative corneal astigmatism at the time of surgery. However, for greater amounts of astigmatism (>2.25 D), the data supported the use of a toric IOL.

Conclusions

FS laser technology allows surgeons to effectively treat corneal astigmatism during cataract surgery, potentially obviating the need for subsequent refractive enhancement procedures. The intraoperative reduction in astigmatism will lead to improved refractive outcomes after cataract surgery. Nomograms are currently under refinement for conventional incisions which cut through Bowman's layer and epithelium, while those using beveled and/or sub-Bowman's astigmatic corneal incisions are in the initial stages of development.

Key Points

- Femtosecond-assisted corneal relaxing incisions (FS-CRIs) have less possible complications than manually performed incisions.
- FS-CRIs can be programmed to the exact desired length, depth, and location.
- Corneal relaxing incisions are an excellent option to correct the corneal astigmatism during cataract surgery.
- FS-CRIs are customizable.

Section B: Conic Intrastromal Relaxing Incisions (CIRI): A New Surgical Technique

Summary

We describe a new technique to correct astigmatism using femtosecond (FS) laser technology, which consists of creating an inverted bevel intrastromal cut in the steepest axis. This procedure offers clear advantages for the treatment of astigmatism in difficult cases such as residual astigmatism after premium intraocular lens (IOL) surgery, patients with extreme dry eye syndrome, post-penetrating keratoplasty (PK), and other combined intraocular surgeries where one wishes to address existing astigmatism in the presence of ocular surface disease.

Introduction

In the year 2006, the need to obtain long-term biomechanical stability of laser in situ keratomileusis (LASIK) flaps led us to propose to Abbott Medical Optics (AMO, Santa Ana, CA, USA) a change in their FS laser's profile from the conventional 90° side cut to a 120° oblique incision profile in order to ensure a more stable

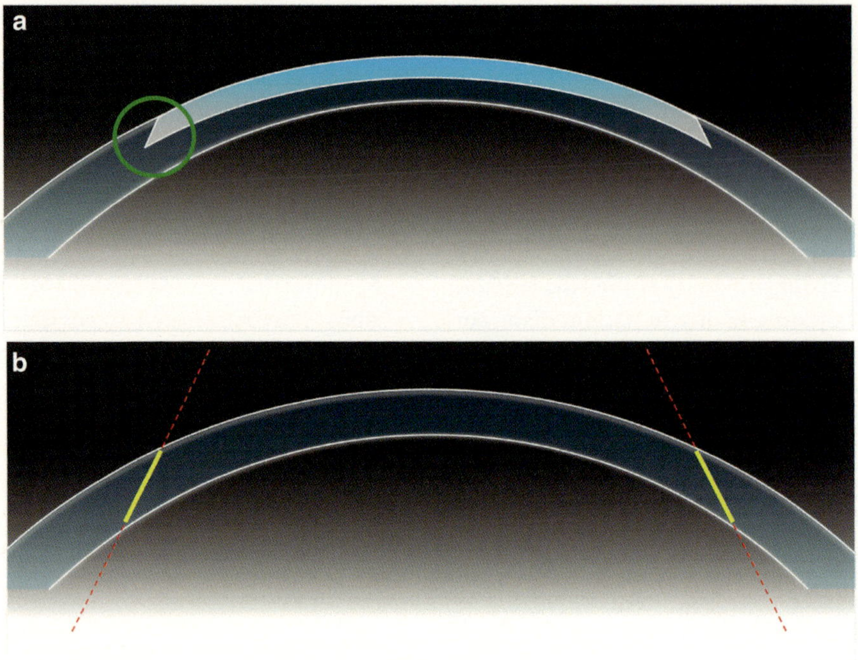

Fig. 10.6 (**a**) Illustration showing an inverted bevel-in side cut in a LASIK flap (IFS, AMO). (**b**) Illustration of a 150° side cut CIRI

positioning of the corneal flaps (Fig. 10.6a). In 2008, the Cadaver Cornea Data Study led by Prof. John Marshall revealed that bevel-in (inverted) side cuts produced less strain when compared to vertical side cuts enhancing the biomechanical stability of flaps [53, 54] in LASIK procedures.

Based on the biomechanical stability achieved with LASIK flaps using the inverted bevel cuts, we developed an intrastromal pattern for correcting astigmatism with the INTRALASE laser (AMO, Santa Ana, CA) which we named CIRI, or "Conic Intrastromal Relaxing Incision," based on the incision's profile (Fig. 10.6b). Since CIRI's do not penetrate the corneal epithelium or Bowman's layer, they are designed to minimize drawbacks associate with disruption of the corneal surface. With few exceptions (see results on "Group C" below) these incisions are completely intrastromal, sparing the epithelium, Bowman's layer and Descemet's membrane/endothelium.

Surgical Technique

The initial part of the procedure takes place at the slit lamp mark, where 0° and 180° reference axes are marked to account for the ocular cyclotorsion [55–61] which can occur when assuming the supine position necessary for the FS laser intervention. All cases are performed under topical anesthesia. Proper centering of the laser suction ring on the cornea is mandatory; therefore, marking the cornea intercept of the center of the entrance pupil is performed first using a gentian violet marker. Once good suction is achieved and the ring is centered appropriately, the 180° mark from the suction ring is aligned with the 180° axis previously marked at the slit lamp (Fig. 10.7) in order to avoid cyclotorsion. The value of the steepest axis is entered into the FS laser software. Other variables are also entered and may vary depending on the amount of astigmatism we are aiming to correct. These variables include the following: optical zone diameter, incision length,

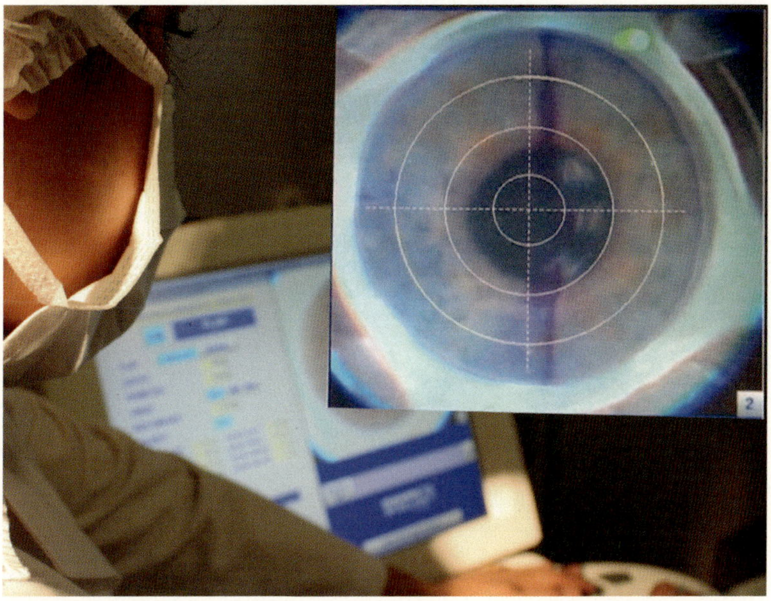

Fig. 10.7 Image showing how the 180° mark from the suction ring is aligned with the 180° axis previously marked at the slit lamp in order to avoid cyclotorsion

intrastromal depth, energy level, incidence angle, and the desired number of incisions. Once the incisions have been performed, the laser suction ring is removed and postoperative medication is instilled.

Retrospective Analyses

Group A

The purpose of this subgroup analysis was to demonstrate the use of the CIRI procedure in patients with previous ocular surgeries such as the following: BIOPTICS, cataract extractions, LASIK, pterygium excision, penetrating keratoplasty (PK), as well as in patients with mixed astigmatism (see Table 10.5). The objectives of the study were to determine:

1. If the incisions have any effect under different eye characteristics.
2. To determine the coupling ratio of the procedure.
3. To evaluate any potential drawbacks of the technique.

In this first study, 25 eyes were treated with the CIRI procedure. The patient's age ranged from 22 to 70 years (mean: 50 years old). With the aid of the INTRALASE™ FS 60 (AMO, Santa Ana, CA, USA) laser the procedure was performed with an optical zone set at 6-mm and incision arc length at 90°. The incision depth (100%) was set to extend anteriorly from a point at 60 μm from the endothelium and finish 100 μm from the surface (epithelium) with the pulse energy of 1.5 μJ. The profile's design included two-paired incisions with an incidence angle of 150° (see Table 10.6).

Table 10.5 Different eye characteristics combined in group A

Optical zone	6 mm
Incision length	90°
Depth	100%—60 μm
Energy	1.5 μJ
Angle of incidence	150°
Number of incisions	2

Table 10.6 CIRI profile design for group A

Optical zone	5.50, 6.00, 6.50, 7.00, 7.50, 8.00 mm
Incision length	90°
Depth	100%—60 μm
Energy	1.5 μJ
Angle of incidence	150°
Number of incisions	2

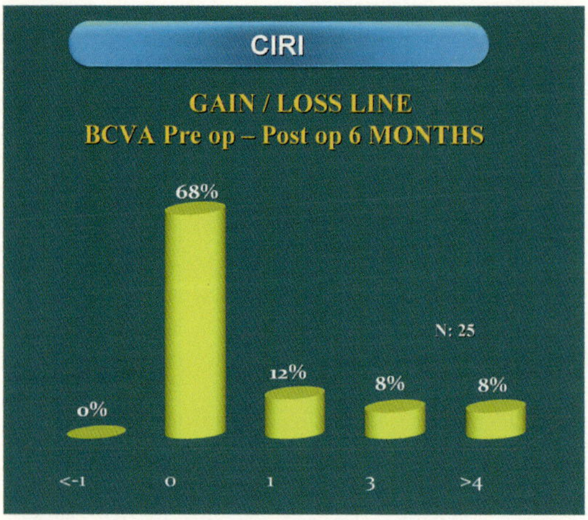

Fig. 10.8 Graph showing gain/loss lines of BCVA 6 months after the CIRI surgery

The results shown in Fig. 10.8 revealed that none of the eyes treated lost best corrected visual acuity (BCVA). Seventeen eyes (68%) exhibited no improvement while three eyes (12%) improved one line, two eyes (8%) improved three lines, and two eyes (8%) improved four lines in their BDVA. The coupling ratio was 1.02 and no complications were encountered in any of the procedures.

The astigmatic effects of the CIRI technique varied depending on the type of surgery with which it was associated. Fifteen of the 25 treated eyes (63%) had CIRI performed the day prior to the intraocular surgery (phaco or ICL) and in these eyes the entry wound (tunnel) was located at the steepest axis. The other seven eyes (31.8%) received CIRI as the only treatment option in either a virgin or postsurgical cornea. Among these, the patient who experienced the least astigmatic correction was one of the mixed astigmatism virgin corneas where neither topographic nor refractive changes were demonstrated after 6 months. The patient who experienced the largest astigmatic correction was one of the previous LASIK eyes with a very thin stromal bed (380 μm). In this case, CIRI corrected 4.50 D of refractive astigmatism when last measured at 6 months after surgery. It is our impression that eyes with thin corneas, especially those with previous refractive surgery, experience more astigmatic correction when compared to untreated virgin eyes with thicker corneas. Overall, eyes with thick corneas seem to have less effect with the CIRI procedure.

The patient that experienced the highest intended cylinder correction had a previous PK, where CIRI was performed with a 5.5-mm optical zone and was combined with paired-incisions at 6.5-mm (150° side cut). Additionally, Descemet's membrane was incised in order to induce more cylinder correction (see Fig. 10.9). As a result, 8.8 D of topographic astigmatism correction was achieved after 9 months ("D" of Fig. 10.9) and 12 D after 18 months, which remained stable out to 33 months ("E" of Fig. 10.9). In two other eyes with prior PKs, we changed the optical zone to 6.5-mm, combined with only one pair of incisions (150° side cut), and we preserved Descemet's membrane (see Fig. 10.10a, b). As a result, we induced less cylinder correction but increased the stability and predictability of the result.

Group B

The purpose of this analysis was to demonstrate the differing effects of the CIRI procedure in relation to the optical zone size in patients undergoing a BIOPTICS procedure with a posterior chamber phakic IOL (STAAR Visian ICL, STAAR SURGICAL AG, Nidau, Switzerland). A total of 40 eyes with corneal astigmatism received an ICL with CIRI with both the entry incision (3 mm) and CIRI along the steepest axis predefined optical zones of 5.50, 6.00, 6.50, 7.00, 7.50, and 8.00 mm axis. The incision length was 90° and the depth was set at 60 μm anterior to the endothelium and 100 μm below the epithelium. The energy level used was 1.5 μJ. The CIRI's profile design included one paired incisions with an incidence angle of 150° (Table 10.7).

The results of this group are shown in Table 10.8. As expected, the highest degree of correction was achieved using the smallest optical zone (5.5 mm). All treated optical zones demonstrated refractive stability between 1 and 6 months post-op. The amount of correction observed with the conic intrastromal incisions between the 5.5 and 8.0 mm optical zones appeared to be less significant when compared to traditional corneal surface incision procedures (AK and LRI).

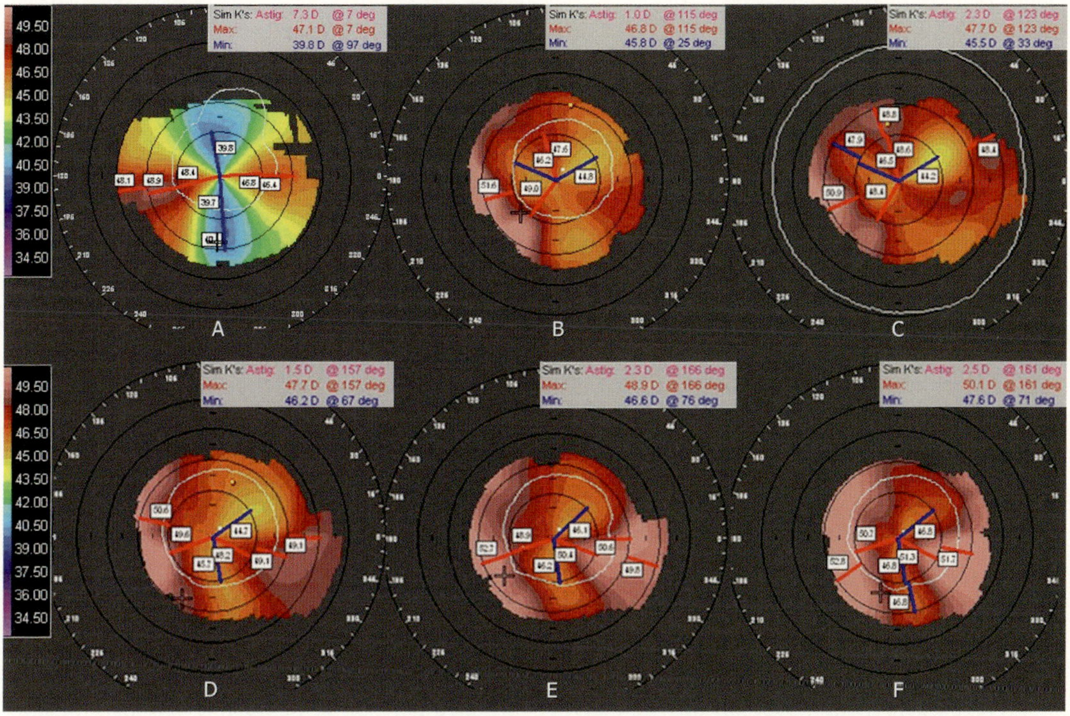

Fig. 10.9 Topographic images obtained with an Orbscan II from a patient with previous PK. (**a**) Pre-op patient. (**b**) 1 Month post-op. (**c**) 6 Months post-op. (**d**) 9 Months post-op. (**e**) 18 Months post-op. (**f**) 2 Years and 9 months

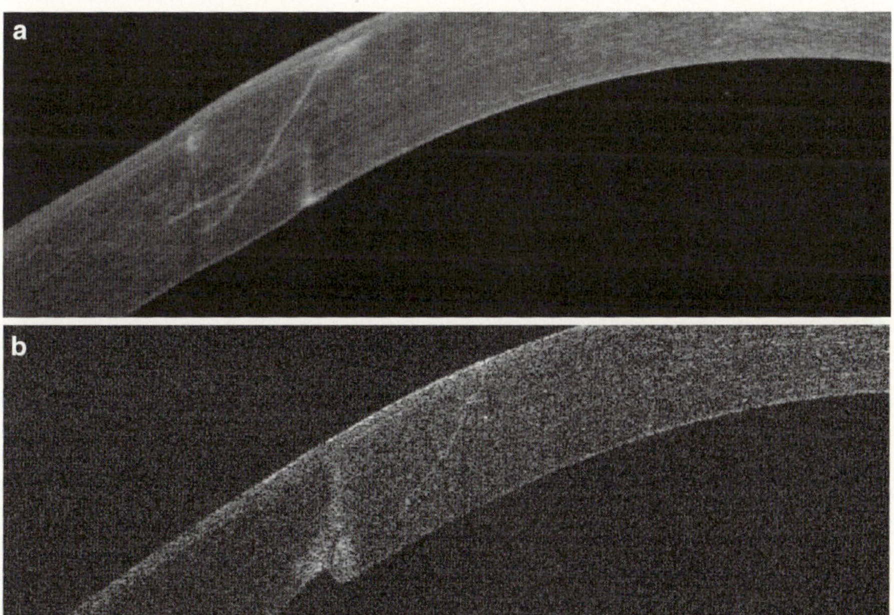

Fig. 10.10 (**a**) OCT image (Optovue) of a mushroom type PK performed with the AMO-Intralase laser with a 150° side cut CIRI for residual astigmatism. (**b**) OCT image (Optovue) of a PK performed with trephine after addition of a 150° side cut CIRI

Table 10.7 CIRI profile design for group B

Optical zone	5.50, 6.00, 6.50, 7.00, 7.50, 8.00 mm
Incision length	90°
Depth	100%—60 μm
Energy	1.5 μJ
Angle of incidence	150°
Number of incisions	2

Table 10.8 Refractive cylinder correction for each optical zone

Diam	Preop	1 Month	3 Months	Difference (D)
5.5	−2.95	−1.75	−1.50	1.45
6.0	−2.42	−1.25	−1.40	1.02
6.5	−2.75	−1.50	−1.50	1.25
7.0	−1.18	−0.50	−0.28	0.90
8.0	−1.71	−1.25	−1.10	0.60

Group C

After analyzing the results of the CIRI procedure on the previously treated PK eyes, we decided to examine refractive effect after cutting either Descemet's layer (Fig. 10.11a–c) or Bowman's layer with epithelium (Fig. 10.12a–c) in order to induce more correction. We found that incising Descemet's or Bowman's layer/epithelium considerably increases the amount of cylinder correction (Table 10.9), but also tends to reduce the predictably of effect when compared to the purely intrastromal procedure.

Discussion

With the advent and growth of premium IOL surgery as a refractive procedure, cataract surgeons have been searching for a less invasive approach to improve residual refractive errors, and to diminish corneal surface surgery-related drawbacks [62–64]. At present, limbal relaxing incisions (LRI) are still the preferred approach of many cataract surgeons for managing astigmatism [65, 66]. It is important to mention that the eyes of most cataract patients have <1.25 D of astigmatism [67]. Throughout the 1990s, numerous authors recognized the advantages of moving corneal astigmatic relaxing incisions peripherally towards the limbus. LRI's evolved by creating paired-incisions at the corneal limbus just anterior to the vascular arcade. By adjusting the depth, length and location of the incisions, one can induce changes in the corneal astigmatism. With peripheral corneal relaxing incisions, the coupling ratio is approximately 1:1, which means that a decrease/flattening in corneal power by 1 D at the incision will result in an increase/steepening of the corneal power in the meridian 90° away, without changing the spherical equivalent (Sph. Equiv.) refraction. Professor Lans first described this property, called the coupling effect in 1897. Despite the merits of LRI's, they do show certain disadvantages, in comparison to laser vision correction surgery, such as low predictability and stability, as well as an increased incidence of epithelial ingrowth. Other potential complications are biomechanical corneal weakening due to the cutting of the anterior most corneal fibers, corneal perforation, worsening of astigmatism, incorrect incisional placement, and corneal hypoesthesia [68].

The laser vision correction approach, however, is not without its own problems secondary to dry eyes, folds, irregular cuts, and epithelial ingrowth in LASIK cases [69–72] as well as haze, postoperative pain, and regression following PRK procedures. These procedures, when performed in an older cataract patient population, have a much greater likelihood of precipitating dryness-related compromises in visual function than the

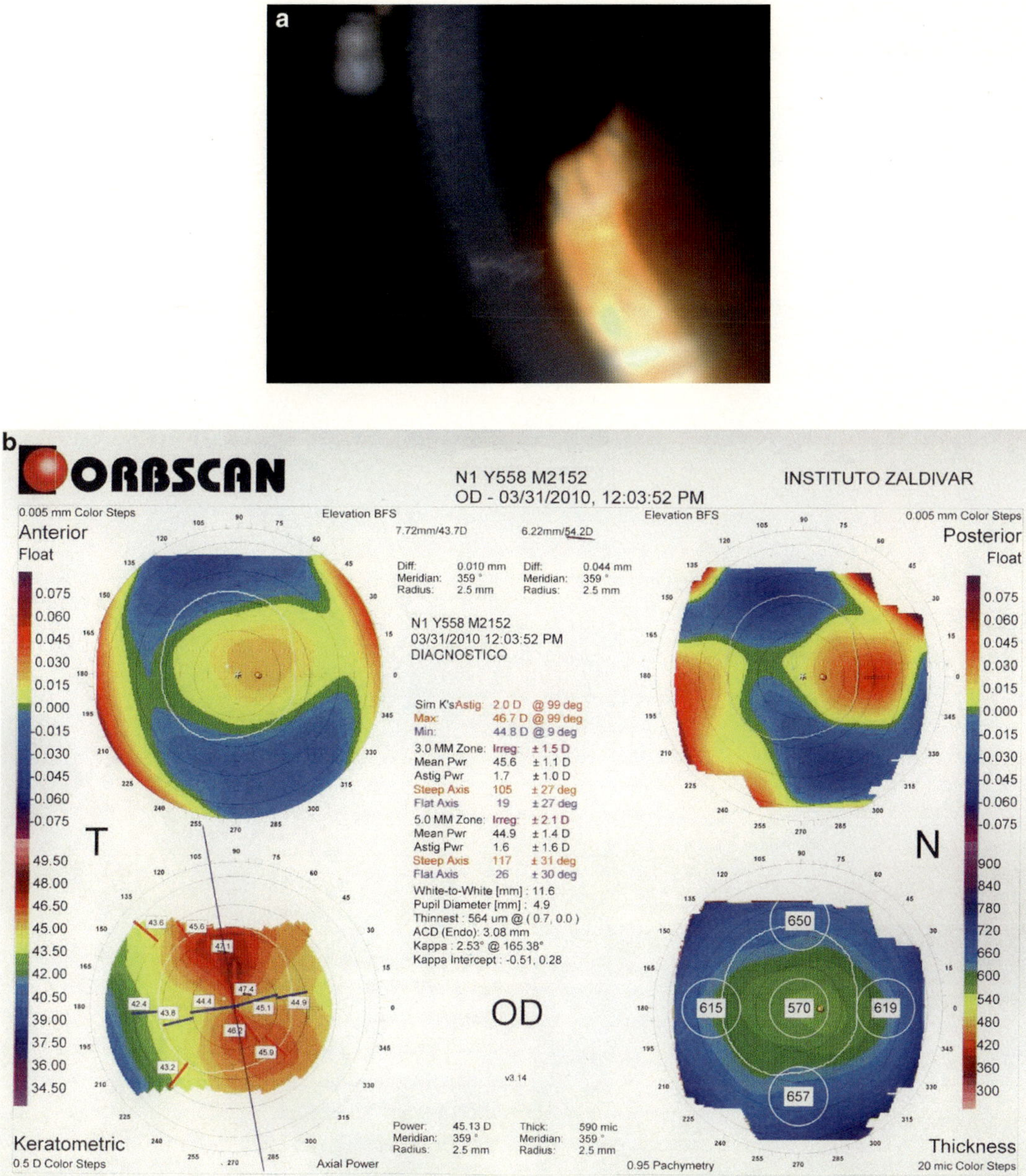

Fig. 10.11 (**a**) Slit lamp image reveals that Descemet's membrane has been cut. (**b**) Topographic image obtained with a Orbscan II that shows a preoperative cylinder of 2.0 D at 99°. (**c**) Topographic image obtained with a Orbscan II that shows a postoperative (6 months) cylinder of 0.9 D at 143°. Also note overall steepening of mean keratometry readings for the central three optical zone

typically younger, healthier refractive surgery patient cohort. Optical problems caused by an unstable ocular surface can usually be tolerated in a monofocal optical system, where all the light is sent to the same focus, but can more easily impair visual performance in the multifocal optical system present after implantation of diffractive multifocal IOLs, where any compromise of the path of light, can significantly impact visual quality.

c
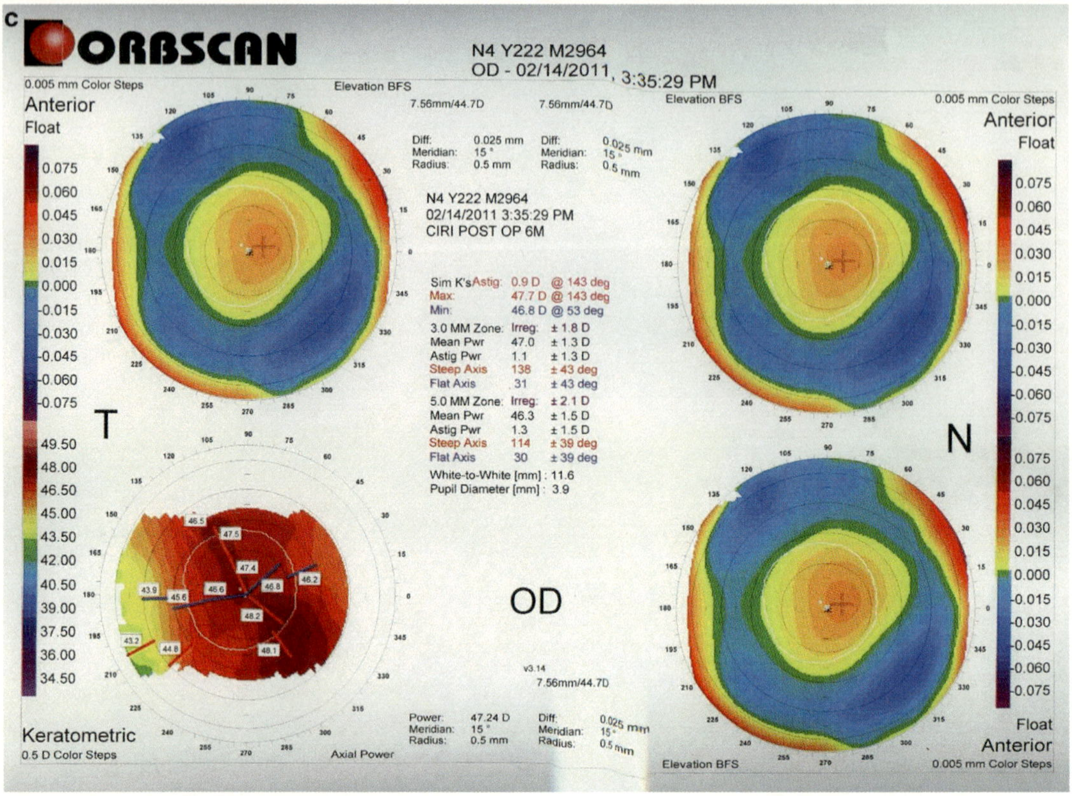

Fig. 10.11 (continued)

a
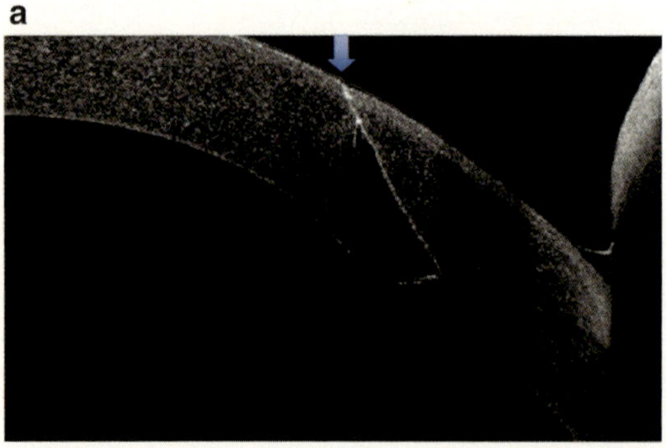

Fig. 10.12 (**a**) Immediate postoperative OCT image (Optovue) reveals a cut in the epithelium. (**b**) Topographic image obtained with a Orbscan II that shows a preoperative cylinder of 2.2 D at 103°. (**c**) Topographic image obtained with a Orbscan II that shows a postoperative (18 months) cylinder of 1.1 D at 170°

Diffractive multifocal lenses need a perfect optical system to perform accurately because they function with constructive interference and in theory any disturbance in the light path through the optical media will result in destructive interference with a critical decrease in modulation transfer function (MTF) or contrast sensitivity (CS) [73, 74] (Figs. 10.13 and 10.14) and resultant increase in the incidence of dysphotopsias. Therefore, treatment of low residual refractive errors (as illustrated by the case outlined in Tables 10.10 and Figs. 10.15 and 10.16) or early posterior capsular opacification may have an important impact on visual outcomes (again, see effect of PCO on contrast sensitivity in Fig. 10.14). As noted above, another important component of the ocular refractive media is the tear film. Recent work has strongly suggested that the tear film needs to be preserved in these complex diffractive multifocal IOL systems, as the appearance of new micro-aberrations caused by dry eye could result in decreased optical performance [75–78].

b

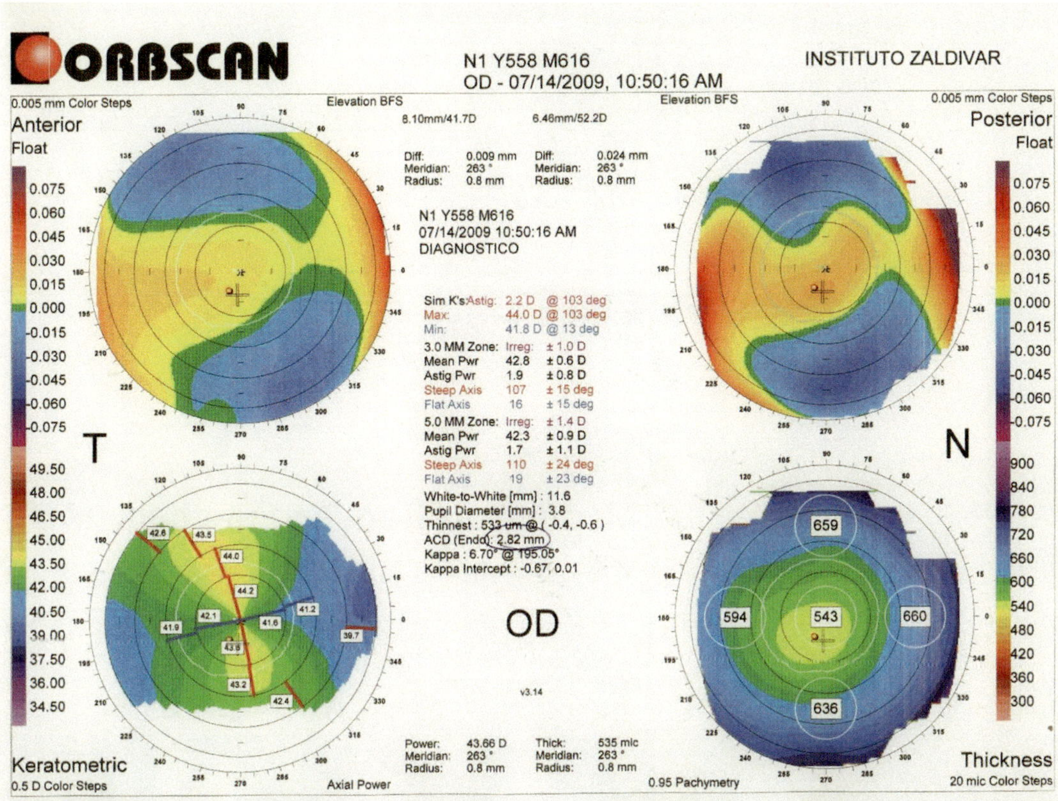

c

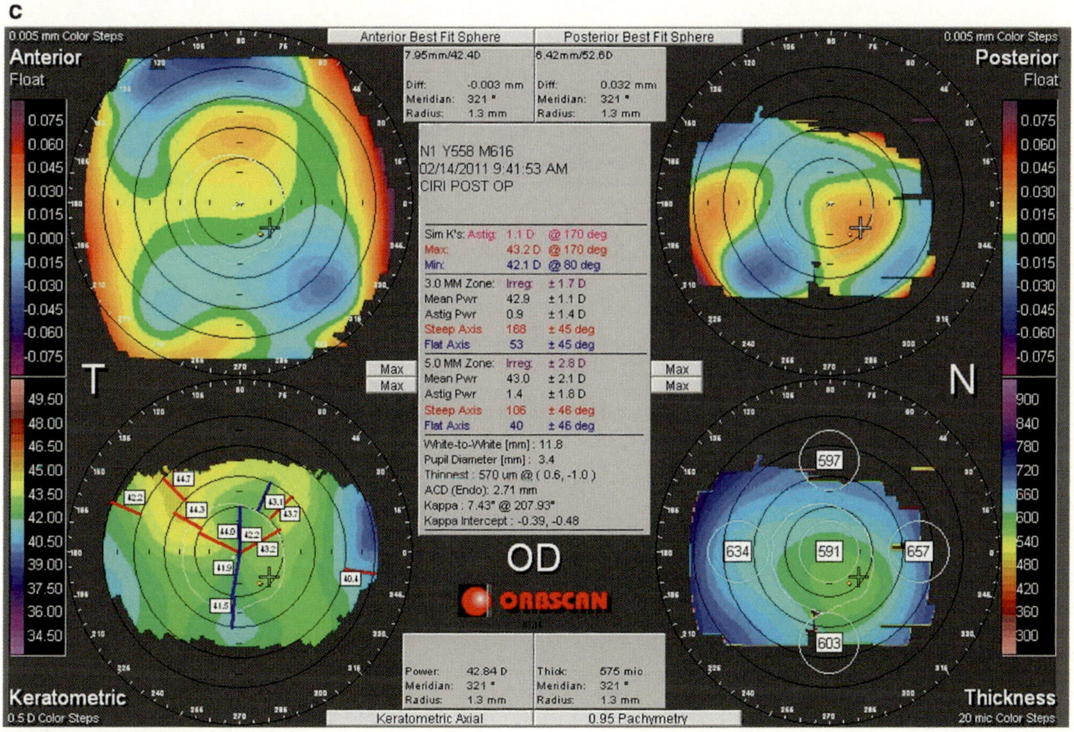

Fig. 10.12 (continued)

Table 10.9 Refractive cylinder correction achieved by cutting the epithelium or Descemet's membrane

	Visual acuity	BMC	Patient satisfaction	Plan
Pre-op	UCVA: OD: 20/20			
	UCNVA: OD: 20/16 OS: 20/16	Pseudophakia 3 Months follow-up (IOL restor +3)	Unhappy with OD	CIRI
	OD: Sph: +.50 Cyl: −0.75 × 95°			
1 Day post-op	UCVA: OD: 20/20 OS: 20/20 UCNVA: OD: 20/16 OS: 20/16	Pseudophakia 3 Months follow-up (IOL restor +3)	Extremely happy	–

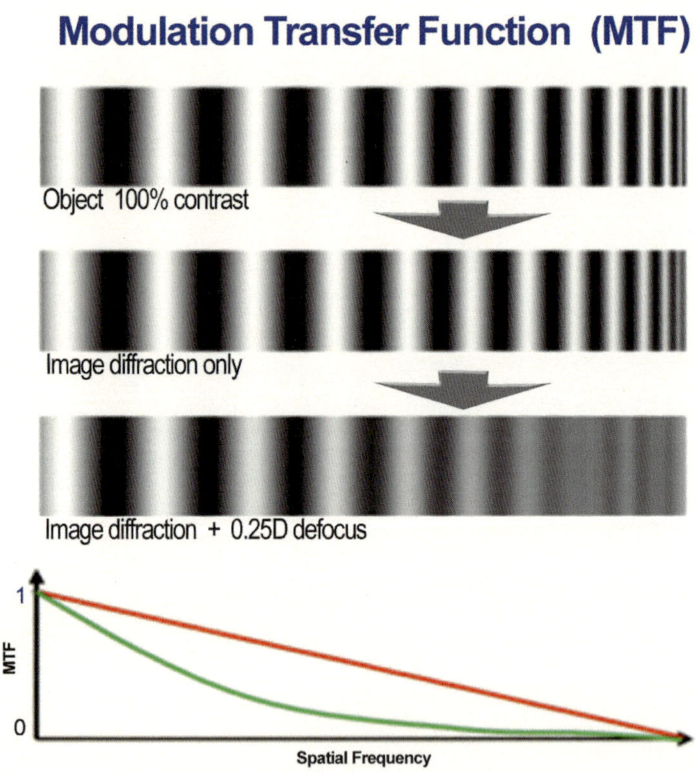

Fig. 10.13 MTF representing the high impact of defocus in a diffractive multifocal system

With these concerns in mind we designed CIRI as an intrastromal corneal surgery technique that leverages FS laser technology to safely address low amounts of cylinder (≤1.50 D), by avoiding epithelial ingrowth, and considerably decreasing dry eye symptoms when compared to a surface ablation treatment.

As described in our results, the CIRI technique can be used with other corneal or intraocular surgical procedures to achieve an emmetropic outcome. We found that the highest degree of cylinder correction with CIRI was achieved using the smallest optical zone. Although the difference in the amount of correction observed with CIRI

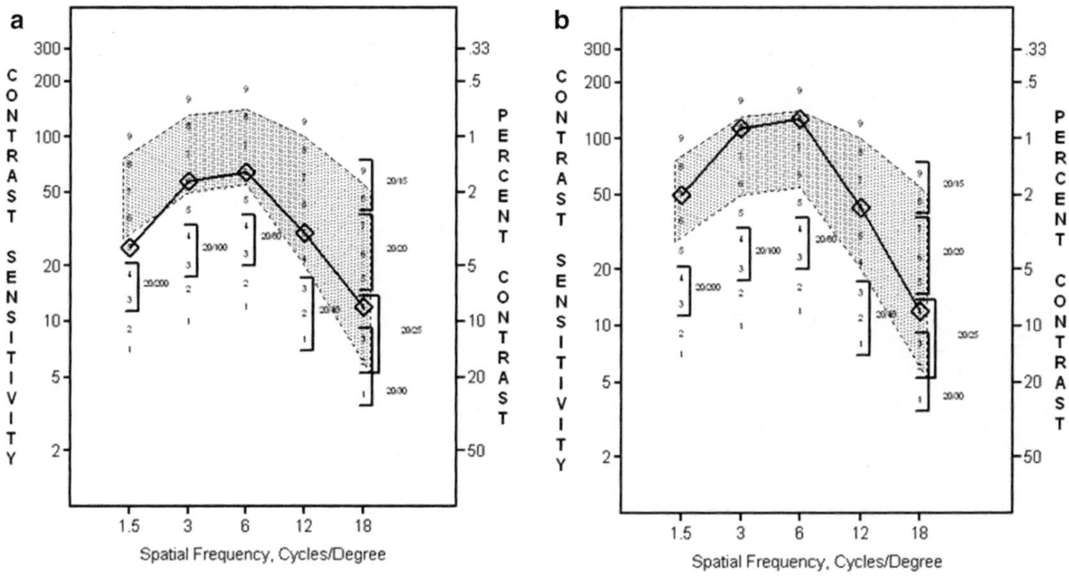

Fig. 10.14 (**a**) Preoperative CS examination of OD prior to YAG laser capsulotomy (Optec 5600). (**b**) Postoperative (1 day) CS examination of OD (Optec 5600)

Table 10.10 Treatment result following CIRI (patient complained of suboptimal visual acuity following multifocal IOL implantation)

	Visual acuity	BMC	Patient satisfaction	Plan
Pre-op	UCVA: OD: 20/20 OS: 20/20			
	UCNVA: OD: 20/16 OS: 20/16	Pseudaophakia 3 Months follow-up (IOL restor +3)	Unhappy with OD	CIRI
	OD: Sph: +0.50 Cyl: −0.75 × 95°			
1 Day post-op	UCVA: OD: 20/20 OS: 20/20	Pseudophakia	Extremely happy	–
	UCNVA: OD: 20/16 OS: 20/16	3 Months follow-up (IOL restor +3)		

appeared to be less than after traditional AK and LRI incisions, the stability with different optical zones between 1 and 6 months post-op (excepting the post-PK cases described below) was acceptable and no eye losing BDVA. After analyzing the results of the CIRI procedure in eyes having undergone PK, we realized that cutting either the Descemet membrane or the epithelium induced more correction. This, however, was not without a diminished predictability and stability when compared to CIRI procedures where the Descemet's and epithelial structures are preserved.

While these preliminary results are quite promising, further studies in untreated eyes are needed to better understand the full effects of the CIRI procedure and develop standard nomo-

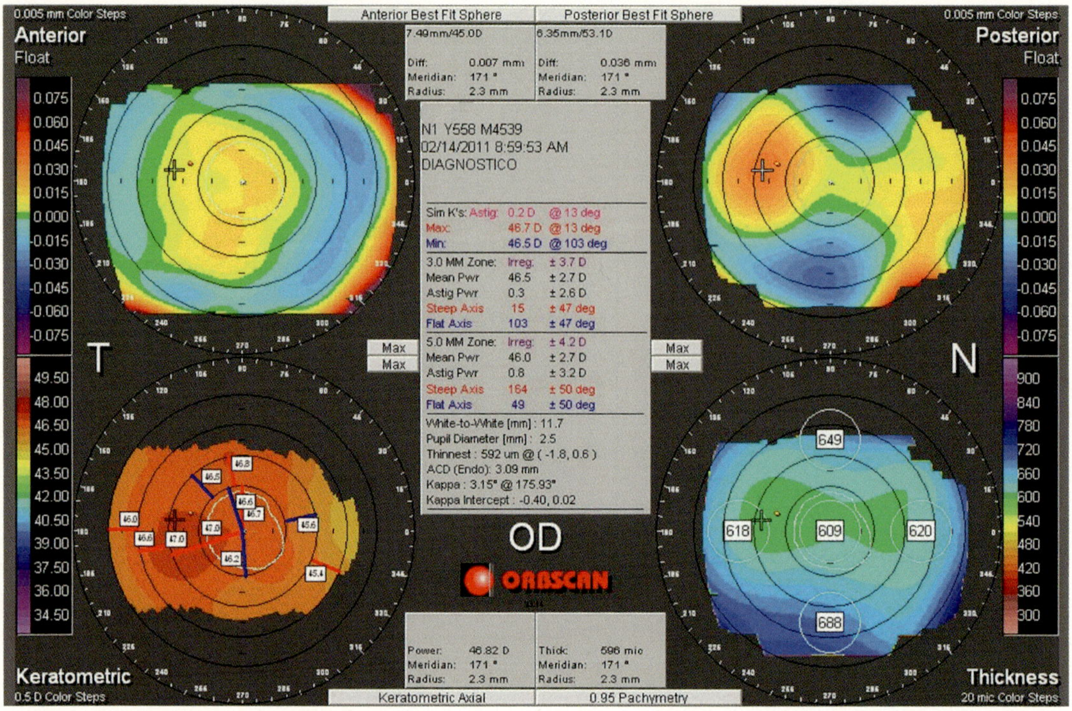

Fig. 10.15 Topographic image obtained with a Orbscan II that shows a preoperative cylinder of 0.2 D at 13°. Considering the manifest refraction was +0.50–0.75 × 95 we inferred that intraocular lens had a small tilt

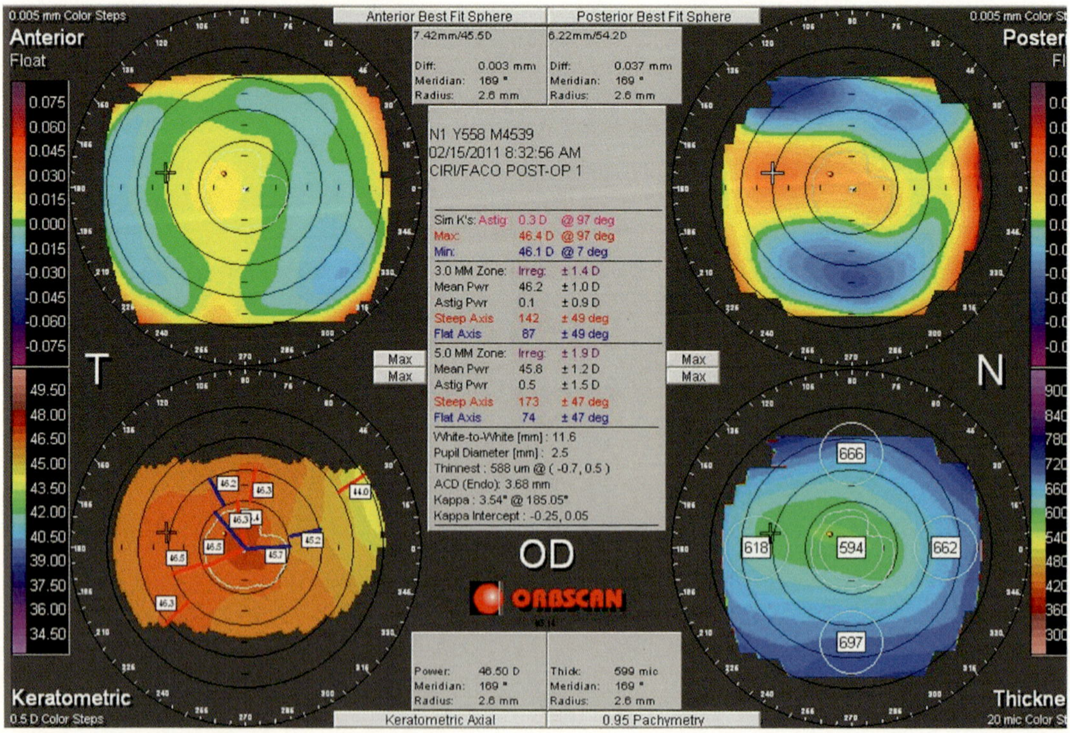

Fig. 10.16 Topographic image obtained with a Orbscan II that shows a postoperative cylinder of 0.3D at 97°

grams. We consider the CIRI procedure a great step forward towards achieving better optical quality for all patients with astigmatic error and look forward to seeing this new procedure evolve to assume its place in refractive laser assisted cataract surgery and beyond.

Key Points

1. Proper centering of the laser suction ring on the cornea is mandatory.
2. It is better to use a different microscope (not the one included in the Intralase) for marking the cornea intercept of the center of the entrance pupil.
3. Carefully align the axis from the suction ring with the 180° axis previously marked at the slit lamp in order to avoid cyclotorsion's induced error.
4. With CIRI, respect a 100 µm distance from the epithelium and 60 um from Descemet's membrane to avoid unpredictable results.

References

1. Ferrer-Blasco T, Montés-Micó R, Peixoto-de-Matos SC, González-Méijome JM, Cerviño A. Prevalence of corneal astigmatism before cataract surgery. J Cataract Refract Surg. 2009;35(1):70–5.
2. Snellen H. Die Richtung der Hauptmeridiane des astigmatischen Auges. Albrecht Von Graefes Arch Klin Exp Ophthalmol. 1869;15:199–207.
3. Shiøtz H. Ein Fall von hochgradigem Hornhautastigmatismus nach Starextraction, Besserung auf operative Wege. Arch f Augenheilk. 1885;15:178–81.
4. Bates WH. A suggestion of an operation to correct astigmatism. Arch Ophthalmol. 1894;23:9–13.
5. Faber E. Operatative behandeling von astigmatisme. Ned Tijdschr Geneeskd. 1895;31:495–6.
6. Lucciola J. Traitement chirurgicale de l'astigmatisme. Arch d'Ophthalmol. 1896;16:630.
7. Lans LJ. Experimentelle Untersuchugen fiber Entstehungvon Astigmatismus durch nich-perforirende Corneawunden. Albrect Von Graefe's Archiv Fur Ophthalmologre. 1898;45:117–52.
8. Akiyama K, Shibata H, Kanai A, et al. Development of radial keratotomy in Japan, 1939–1960. In: Waring III GO, editor. Refractive keratotomy for myopia and astigmatism. St Louis, MO: Mosby Year Book; 1992. p. 179–219.
9. Sato T. Posterior incision of the cornea. Am J Ophthalmol. 1950;33:943–8.
10. Waring III GO. Development of radial keratotomy in the Soviet Union, 1960–1990. In: Waring III GO, editor. Refractive keratotomy for myopia and astigmatism. St Louis, MO: Mosby Year Book; 1992. p. 221–35.
11. Troutman RC. Microsurgical control of corneal astigmatism in cataract and keratoplasty. Trans Am Acad Ophthalmol Otolaryngol. 1973;77:563–72.
12. Osher RH. Paired transverse relaxing keratotomy: a combined technique for reducing astigmatism. J Cataract Refract Surg. 1989;15(1):32–7.
13. Nordan LT. Quantifiable astigmatism correction: concepts and suggestions. J Cataract Refract Surg. 1986;12(5):507–18.
14. Lindstrom RL. The surgical correction of astigmatism: a clinician's perspective. Refract Corneal Surg. 1990;6(6):441–54.
15. Thornton ST. Astigmatic keratotomy: a review of basic concepts with case reports. J Cataract Refract Surg. 1990;16:430–5.
16. Nichamin LD. Astigmatism management for modern phaco surgery. Int Ophthalmol Clin. 2003;43(3):53–63.
17. Shepherd JR. Correction of preexisting astigmatism at the time of small incision cataract surgery. J Cataract Refract Surg. 1989;15:55–7.
18. Davison JA. Transverse astigmatic keratotomy combined with phacoemulsification and intraocular lens implantation. J Cataract Refract Surg. 1989;15:38–44.
19. Maloney WF, Sanders DR, Pearcy DE. Astigmatic keratotomy to correct preexisting astigmatism in cataract patients. J Cataract Refract Surg. 1990;16:297–304.
20. Hall GW, Campion M, Sorenson CM, Monthofer S. Reduction of corneal astigmatism at cataract surgery. J Cataract Refract Surg. 1991;17:407–14.
21. Lindstrom RL, Agapitos PJ, Koch DD. Cataract surgery and astigmatic keratotomy. Int Ophthalmol Clin. 1994;34(2):145–64.
22. Kershner RM. Keratolenticuloplasty: arcuate keratotomy for cataract surgery and astigmatism. J Cataract Refract Surg. 1995;21:274–7.
23. Akura J, Matsuura K, Hatta S, et al. A new concept for the correction of astigmatism: full-arc, depth-dependent astigmatic keratotomy. Ophthalmology. 2000;107:95–104.
24. Wang L, Misra M, Koch DD. Peripheral corneal relaxing incisions combined with cataract surgery. J Cataract Refract Surg. 2003;29(4):712–22.
25. Gills JP. Cataract surgery with a single relaxing incision at the steep meridian [letter]. J Cataract Refract Surg. 1994;20:368–9.
26. Budak K, Friedman NJ, Koch DD. Limbal relaxing incisions with cataract surgery. J Cataract Refract Surg. 1998;24:503–8.
27. Müller-Jensen K, Fischer P, Slepe U. Limbal relaxing incisions to correct astigmatism in clear corneal cataract surgery. J Refract Surg. 1999;15:586–9.

28. Carvalho MJ, Suzuki SH, Freitas LL, Branco BC, Schor P, Lima AL. Limbal relaxing incisions to correct corneal astigmatism during phacoemulsification. J Refract Surg. 2007;23(5):499–504.
29. Kulkarni A, Mataftsi A, Sharma A, Kalhoro A, Horgan S. Long-term refractive stability following combined astigmatic keratotomy and phakoemulsification. Int Ophthalmol. 2009;29(2):109–15.
30. Ouchi M, Kinoshita S. Prospective randomized trial of limbal relaxing incisions combined with microincision cataract surgery. J Refract Surg. 2010;26(8):594–9.
31. Nichamin LD. Management of astigmatism in conjunction with lens surgery. In: Tasman W, Jaeger EA, editors. Duane's ophthalmology on CD-ROM. Philadelphia, PA: Lippincott Williams & Wilkins; 2006.
32. Gills JP. Treating astigmatism at the time of cataract surgery. Curr Opin Ophthalmol. 2002;13:2–6.
33. Amesbury EC, Miller KM. Correction of astigmatism at the time of cataract surgery. Curr Opin Ophthalmol. 2009;20(1):19–24.
34. Donnenfeld ED. Redeeming the reputation of LRIs. Cataract Refract Surg Today 2007;48–49. Available at: http://www.crstoday.com/PDF%20Articles/0307/CRST0307_07.php. Accessed 14 June 2011.
35. Nichamin LD. Modified astigmatism correction nomogram. J Refract Surg. 2008;24(6):562–3.
36. Lindstrom RL, Lindquist TD. Surgical correction of postoperative astigmatism. Cornea. 1988;7(2):138–48.
37. Thornton SP. Transverse astigmatic keratotomy. J Cataract Refract Surg. 1991;17(6):861.
38. Price Jr FW, Grene RB, Marks RG, Gonzales JS. Arcuate transverse keratotomy for astigmatism followed by subsequent radial or transverse keratotomy. ARC-T Study Group. Astigmatism Reduction Clinical Trial. J Refract Surg. 1996;12(1):68–76.
39. Raju LV, Wang L, Weikert M, Koch DD. Incisional keratotomy. In: Krachmer JH, Manis MJ, Holland EJ, editors. Cornea, vol. 2. 3rd ed. Philadelphia, PA: Elselvier; 2011. p. 1899–908.
40. Kymionis GD, Yoo SH, Ide T, et al. Femtosecond-assisted astigmatic keratotomy for post-keratoplasty irregular astigmatism. J Cataract Refract Surg. 2009;35:11–3.
41. Nubile M, et al. Femtosecond laser arcuate keratotomy for the correction of high astigmatism after keratoplasty. Ophthalmology. 2009;116(6):1083–92.
42. Kumar NL, et al. IntraLase-enabled astigmatic keratotomy for post-keratoplasty astigmatism: on-axis vector analysis. Ophthalmology. 2010;117(6):1228–35.
43. Bahar I, et al. IntraLase-enabled astigmatic keratotomy for postkeratoplasty astigmatism. Am J Ophthalmol. 2008;146(6):897–904.
44. Thornton SP. Theory behind corneal relaxing incisions/Thornton nomogram. In: Gills JP, Martin RG, Sanders DR, editors. Sutureless cataract surgery. Thorofare, NJ: SLACK Incorporated; 1992. p. 124–43.
45. Faktorovich EG, Maloney RK, Price Jr FW. Effect of astigmatic keratotomy on spherical equivalent: results of the Astigmatism Reduction Clinical Trial. Am J Ophthalmol. 1999;127(3):260–9.
46. Krader CG, Nichamin LD. Computer model harnessed for femtosecond-induced incisions. Ophthalmology Times 2010;30. Available at: http://digital.healthcaregroup.advanstar.com/nxtbooks/advanstar/ot_20100915/index.php?startid=30#/38. Accessed 14 June 2011.
47. Clinical trials feeds website. Available at: http://clinicaltrialsfeeds.org/clinical-trials/show/NCT01210820. Accessed 14 June 2011.
48. Bethke W. New approach to femtosecond AK. Rev Ophthalmol. Available at: http://www.revophth.com/content/d/refractive_surgery/c/26705/. Accessed 14 June 2011.
49. Abbey A, et al. Femtosecond laser-assisted astigmatic keratotomy in naturally occurring high astigmatism. Br J Ophthalmol. 2009;93(12):1566–9.
50. Hurmeric V, Yoo SH. Femtosecond-assisted astigmatic keratotomy: enabling precise and predictable corneal incisions. Cataract Refract Surg Today Eur. 2010;5:31–3.
51. Hoffart L, et al. Correction of postkeratoplasty astigmatism by femtosecond laser compared with mechanized astigmatic keratotomy. Am J Ophthalmol. 2009;147(5):779–87.
52. Poll JT, et al. Correction of astigmatism during cataract surgery: toric intraocular lens compared to peripheral corneal relaxing incisions. J Refract Surg. 2010;28:1–7.
53. Knorz MC, Vossmerbaeumer U. Comparison of flap adhesion strength using the Amadeus microkeratome and the IntraLase iFS femtosecond laser in rabbits. J Refract Surg. 2008;24:875–8.
54. Mullin DW, Altersitz K, Boyle EL, Cimberle M. Modified depth, incisions for LASIK flap increase strength, prevent strain on cornea. Ocular Surgery News U.S. Edition. 10 October 2008.
55. Chang J. Cyclotorsion during laser in situ keratomileusis. J Cataract Refract Surg. 2008;34(10):1720–6.
56. Kim H, Joo CK. Ocular cyclotorsion according to body position and flap creation before laser in situ keratomileusis. J Cataract Refract Surg. 2008;34(4):557–61.
57. Ciccio AE, Durrie DS, Stahl JE, Schwendeman F. Ocular cyclotorsion during customized laser ablation. J Refract Surg. 2005;21(6):S772–4.
58. Park SH, Kim M, Joo CK. Measurement of pupil centroid shift and cyclotorsional displacement using iris registration. Ophthalmologica. 2009;223(3):166–71 [Epub 2009 Jan 22].
59. Bharti S, Bains HS. Active cyclotorsion error correction during LASIK for myopia and myopic astigmatism with the NIDEK EC-5000 CX III laser. J Refract Surg. 2007;23(9 Suppl):S1041–5.

60. Hori-Komai Y, Sakai C, Toda I, Ito M, Yamamoto T, Tsubota K. Detection of cyclotorsional rotation during excimer laser ablation in LASIK. J Refract Surg. 2007;23(9):911–5.
61. Arba-Mosquera S, Merayo-Lloves J, de Ortueta D. Clinical effects of pure cyclotorsional errors during refractive surgery. Invest Ophthalmol Vis Sci. 2008;49(11):4828–36 [Epub 2008 Jun 27].
62. Hovanesian JA, Shah SS, Maloney RK. Symptoms of dry eye and recurrent corneal erosion syndrome after refractive surgery. J Cataract Refract Surg. 2001;27:577–84.
63. Jabbur NS, Sakatani K, O'Brien TP. Survey of complications and recommendations for management in dissatisfied patients seeking a consultation after refractive surgery. J Cataract Refract Surg. 2004;30:1867–74.
64. Ambrósio Jr R, Trevo T, Wilson SE. LASIK-associated dry eye and neurotrophicepitheliophaty: pathophysiology and strategies for prevention and treatment. J Refract Surg. 2008;24:396–407.
65. Miyata K, Miyai T, Minami K, Bissen-Miyajima H, Maeda N, Amano S. Limbal relaxing incisions using a reference point and corneal topography for intraoperative identification of the steepest meridian. J Refract Surg. 2010;15:1–6.
66. Roman S, Auclin F, Baudouin C. Limbal relaxing incisions to correct preexisting astigmatism during cataract surgery. J Fr Ophtalmol. 2009;32(6):390–5.
67. Ferrer-Blasco T, Montés-Micó R, Peixoto-de-Matos SC, González-Méijome JM, Cerviño A. Prevalence of corneal astigmatismo befote cataract surgery. J Cataract Refract Surg. 2009;35(1):70–5.
68. Louis D. Nichamin, Corneal Relaxing Incisions: AdvancedPearls *MD* Ophthalmic Hyperguide May 30, 2008
69. Kuo IC, Jabbur NS, O'Brien TP. Photorefractive keratectomy for refractory laser in situ keratomileusis flap striae. J Cataract Refract Surg. 2008;34:330–3.
70. Latvala T, Linna T, Trevo T. Corneal nerve recovery after photorefractive keratectomy and laser in situ keratomileusis. Int Ophthalmol Clin. 1996;36(4):21–7.
71. Agarwal A. Tips for preventing and treating epithelial ingrowth after LASIK. Ocular Surgery News Europe/Asia-Pasific Edition. 1 June 2007.
72. Elderkin SJ, Epstein RJ, Seldomridge DL. Successful treatment of recurrent epithelial ingrowth associated with interface fluid syndrome, flap necrosis, and epithelial defects following LASIK. J Refract Surg. 2011;27(1):70–73.
73. Ravalico G, Baccara F, Rinaldi G. Contrast sensitivity in multifocal intraocular lenses. J Cataract Refract Surg. 1993;19(1):22–5.
74. Leyland M, Zinicola E. Multifocal versus monofocal intraocular lenses in cataract surgery: a systematic review. Ophthalmology. 2003;110(9):1789–98.
75. Thibos LN, Nam J, Himebaugh N, Liu H, Bradley A. Measuring light scatter during tear break-up with Shack-Hartmann Wave front aberrometer. Bloomington, IN: School of Optometry, Indiana University; 2010.
76. Thibos LN. Measuring the optical effects of tear film instability. Bloomington, IN: School of Optometry, Indiana University; 2010.
77. Himebaugh N, Bradley A, Begley C, Thibos L. The effect of tear film break-up on the optical aberrations and light scatter of the eye. Invest Ophthalmol Vis Sci, submitted for publication.
78. Tear film aberration and vison-related quality of life in patients with dry eye disease. Denoyer A, Rabut G, Baudouin C. Ophthalmol. 2012;119(9):1811–1818.

Femtosecond Laser Versus Phacoemulsification

11

Zoltan Z. Nagy and Robert Cionni

Small incision cataract surgery performed using the latest generation of phacoemulsification technology and with implantation of a foldable IOL is highly successful in restoring good levels of best-corrected visual acuity with an acceptable safety profile. However, a comparison of the refractive predictability and complication rates of cataract surgery and laser vision correction procedures indicates there is room for significant improvement in cataract surgery outcomes. Furthermore, the bar for judging cataract surgery success in the modern era has been raised as patients today are presenting with higher expectations for good uncorrected vision. In addition, advances in premium IOL technology are driving increased consumer interest in presbyopia-correcting IOL implantation after cataract surgery as well as in refractive lens exchange. The ability to consistently deliver successful outcomes and achieve satisfaction among patients with multifocal and accommodating IOLs depends on performing uncomplicated surgery with excellent refractive predictability.

With advantages for increasing the precision of multiple surgical steps, the femtosecond (FS) laser holds the potential to create a major paradigm shift in cataract surgery and to become an essential tool for refractive lens procedures. Understanding of the capabilities and limitations of the FS laser, its clinical advantages relative to standard phacoemulsification, and the pragmatic issues associated with integrating this technology is critical as surgeons contemplate adopting refractive laser assisted cataract surgery (ReLACS) into clinical practice.

Z.Z. Nagy (✉)
Department of Ophthalmology, Semmelweis University, Maria u. 39, Budapest 1085, Hungary
e-mail: zoltan.nagy100@gmail.com; nz@szem1.sote.hu

R. Cionni
The Eye Institute of Utah, Salt Lake City, UT, USA

Sequence of Steps in Phacoemulsification

1. Patient Selection and Preparation
2. Transcorneal Incisions and Viscoelastic Filling
3. Capsulotomy
4. Hydrodissection and Hydrodelineation
5. Nucleus Fragmentation and Emulsification
6. Cortex Removal and Capsular Polishing
7. Viscoelastic Filling and IOL Insertion/Centration
8. Viscoelastic Removal and Wound Hydration/Closure

Refractive Laser Assisted Cataract Surgery (ReLACS)

The FS laser can be used for capsulotomy, crystalline lens fragmentation/liquefaction, and to create clear corneal incisions, including the main and side port incisions for phacoemulsification

R.R. Krueger et al. (eds.), *Textbook of Refractive Laser Assisted Cataract Surgery (ReLACS)*,
DOI 10.1007/978-1-4614-1010-2_11, © Springer Science+Business Media, LLC 2013

and relaxing incisions for astigmatic correction. In contrast to other lasers used previously for lens fragmentation, lens treatment with the FS laser is performed without physically entering the eye, and the corneal incisions remain sealed until manually opened by the surgeon. Therefore, all the FS laser treatments can be performed in a clean (rather than sterile) laser room before the patient is brought into the OR.

Personal Experience with the LenSx Laser

Our experience with ReLACS is with the LenSx laser (Alcon LenSx Inc., Aliso Viejo, CA). The following is a summary of the steps involved in its setup and considerations for use in its various indications.

Calibration

The LenSx FS laser performs an automated self-check and calibration at start-up and during designated stages of the procedure to assure safety. This is in contrast to excimer lasers that require manual calibration.

Patient Preparation

Excellent pupil dilation (optimally to 8.0-mm) should be sought. In addition to dilating drops, patients receive a topical anesthetic and non-steroidal anti-inflammatory drops (topical diclofenac is our preference) as part of the preoperative regimen.

Planning and treatment with the FS laser is performed with the patient resting supine and positioned so that the target eye lies approximately at the midline of the table. Use of a rigid head rest is recommended instead of a soft pillow to avoid any downward movement of the patient's head position.

Prior to surgery, the surgeon should record the details of the FS laser treatment (i.e., corneal incision size and location, capsulotomy size, and lens fragmentation pattern) into the patient's chart. Then, the technician can use this information to preprogram the treatment into the laser so that the surgeon needs only to verify the settings, and position the patient and the patient interface (PI). Imaging and treatment can be started immediately after administering the topical anesthesia.

Laser Docking and Coupling

The LenSx laser docks and couples the eye to the optical system using a single-piece PI with an onboard vacuum system. Care must be taken to assure proper positioning of the PI as it is essential for achieving a centered and regular capsulotomy, complete lens fragmentation, and proper location of the corneal incisions. Docking can be more difficult if the patient has a large nose, but this anatomic interference can be overcome by turning the patient's head slightly so that the tip of the nose is pointing away from the PI.

Once the PI is properly fitted, suction is applied to engage and stabilize the eye, and the surgeon can proceed with the OCT imaging and pattern positioning. The LenSx laser PI features a curved contact lens that follows the surface contour of the eye and allows fixation to be achieved with less suction compared with mechanical microkeratomes and PI's with a flat contact lens. The lower suction level minimizes distortions of the globe as well as IOP increase. The Technolas system also uses a curved contact lens applannation system, while both LensAR and OptiMedica use a fluid interface, as specified in more detail in Chap. 6.

Image-Guided Alignment

Integrated, real-time imaging systems in commercially available FS lasers developed for cataract surgery are a critical component in assuring accuracy and safety in performing the various surgical steps. The LenSx laser features a high-resolution Fourier-domain OCT imaging system to guide treatment planning and delivery (see Fig. 11.1a–d).

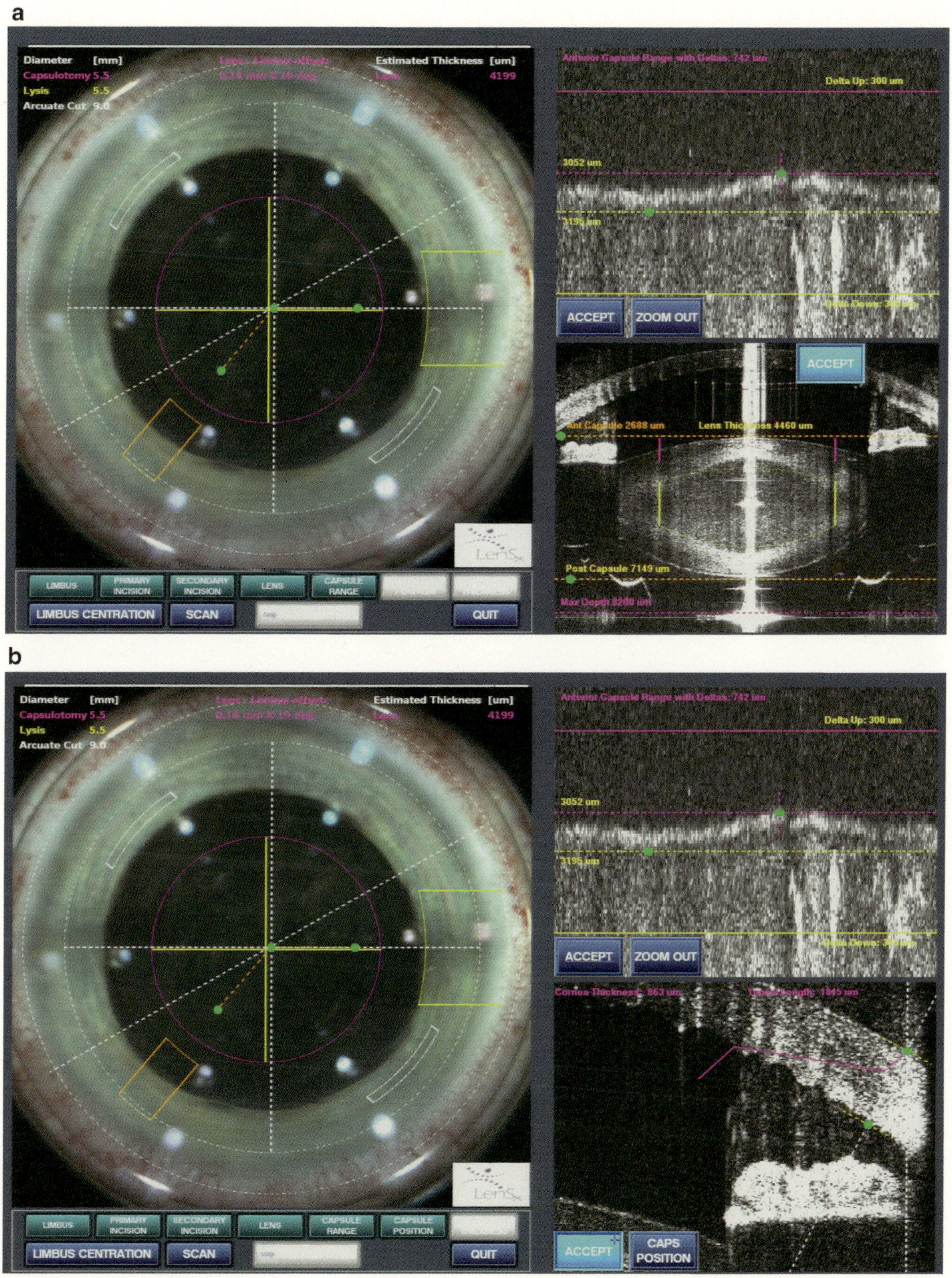

Fig. 11.1 The surgeon observes all activities on the high definition surgical monitor. After the eye is docked, graphical overlays for each programmed incision are automatically pre-positioned over their respective anatomical structures. Panel (**a**) shows lens 4-quadrant chop, 5.5 mm capsulotomy, primary, secondary, and paired arcuate incisions positioned on the fixated eye. OCT image on the *top right* shows a circle scan of the anterior capsule

c

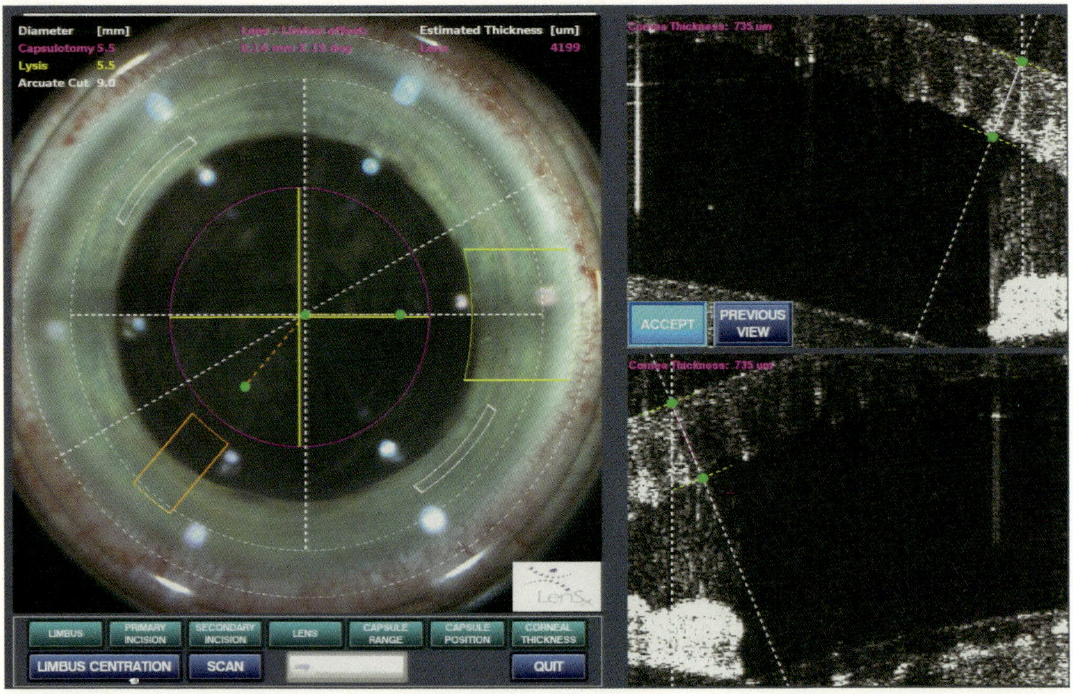

d

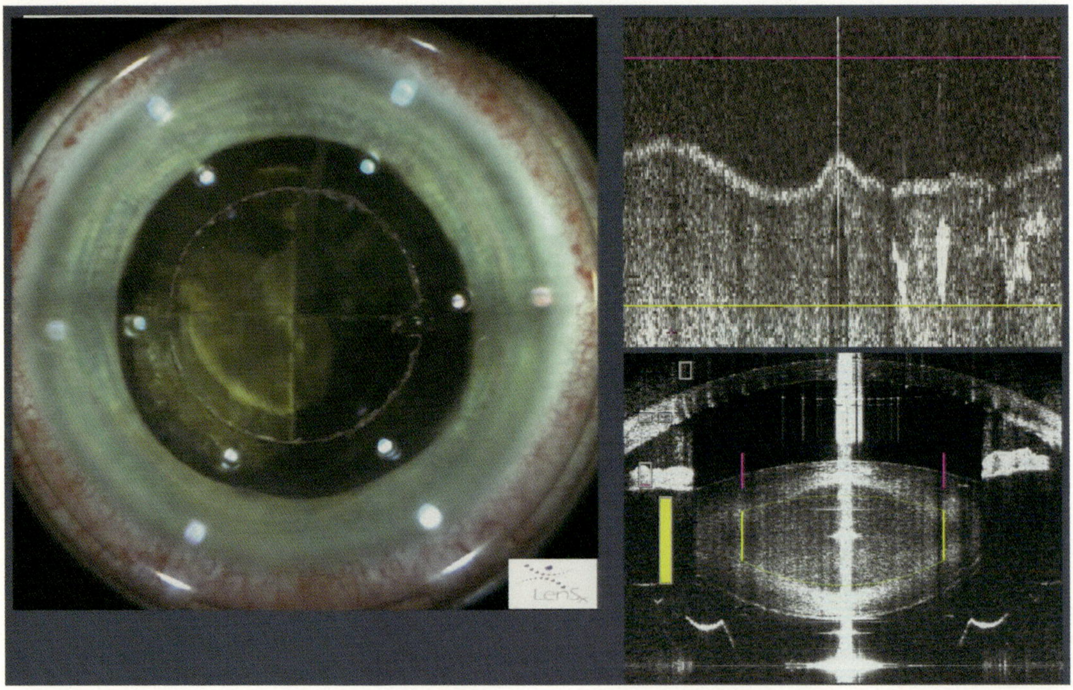

Fig. 11.1 (continued) to determine the depth. Image on the *bottom right* shows a cross section of the anterior segment and placement of the lens fragmentation pattern. Panel (**b**) shows a cross section of the cornea with the planned multiplane incision pattern. In panel (**c**), the cornea thickness for each area of the planned partial thickness arcuate incision is accurately measured. After the surgeon verifies that all pre-positioned patterns are in the correct location, treatment is initiated. Panel (**d**) shows lens fragmentation and capsulotomy being performed

OCT imaging is begun after the eye is fixated with the PI, and the planning is done by surgeon-guided alignment of the treatment patterns for capsulotomy, lens fragmentation, and corneal incisions on the OCT images.

The treatment patterns are computer-projected onto the OCT image of the eye on a high-definition video display screen, and the surgeon controls the position of the projected circles and lines. Three separate OCT images are taken:

1. The first OCT measurement identifies the anterior capsule and then the distance above and below the capsule where the laser shots will be delivered to create the capsulotomy. The OCT image also identifies the axis of the eye with the maximum tilt to enhance the safety during lens fragmentation pattern positioning.
2. Next, the surgeon identifies the relative positions of the anterior and posterior capsules: the lens fragmentation pattern is positioned at the preprogrammed distance away from the capsules.
3. During the third OCT measurement, corneal thickness is measured to assure accurate depth of the laser incisions. Once the treatment parameters are verified and accepted, all data are transferred to the FS laser computer.

Within just seconds, the treatment can be initiated by depressing the footswitch. Capsulotomy is performed first, followed by lens fragmentation/liquefaction, the corneal incisions, and last, any incisions for astigmatic correction.

Laser Treatment Steps

Capsulotomy

Capsulotomy is performed prior to lens treatment in order to maximize accuracy of the capsular cut. If the procedure starts with the lens treatment, gas bubbles created within the lens can expand the capsular bag, thereby invalidating the previously obtained measurements for guiding the capsulotomy cut. Performing capsulotomy first avoids the inefficiency of having to repeat the OCT measurements and modify the capsulotomy treatment parameters.

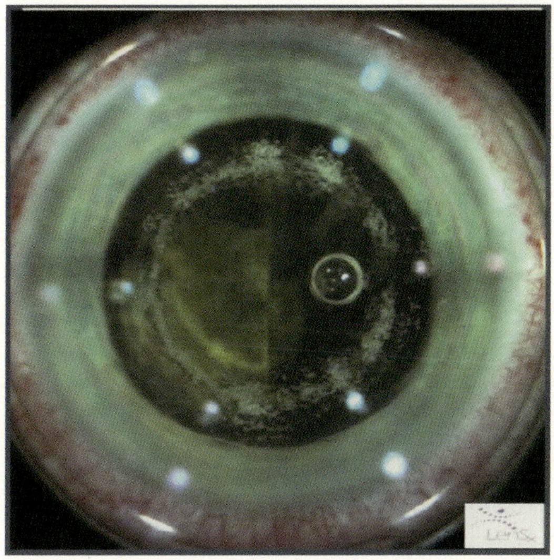

Fig. 11.2 Intraoperative image while performing laser lens fragmentation and capsulotomy. A chop pattern is performed within the lens nucleus and a cylindrical cut to create an anterior capsulotomy. *Bubbles* in the anterior chamber indicate that the capsule has been completely incised allowing gas to escape

The capsulotomy is performed by aiming the laser beam in a circular pattern starting at approximately 100 μm below the anterior capsule and ending at about 100 μm above it. As the capsulotomy is made, a circular line will appear on the platform's video screen, and then small bubbles will be visible in the anterior chamber. Bubble breakthrough indicates that the laser has cut through the anterior capsule (see Fig. 11.2).

Using the femtolaser provides surgeons the advantage of being able to precisely vary the diameter of the capsulotomy according to the posterior chamber lens being implanted. For the usual 6.0 mm diameter posterior chamber lenses, a 4.75 or 5.00 mm capsulotomy is recommended, whereas a 5.5 mm capsulotomy is preferred when implanting the CrystaLens accommodating IOL (Bausch+Lomb Surgical, Aliso Viejo, CA). However, it is important that the laser treatment not be placed too close to the dilated pupil margin, as miosis or bleeding can result. To avoid these complications, we recommend that whenever possible a clearance zone of 1.5 mm between the iris margin and the laser capsulotomy treatment be maintained. It should be noted that the magnifying effect of the cornea (~1.15×), which creates a perception to the surgeon that the pupil is larger than it actually is, has no effect on the performance of the laser system. This is confirmed by our clinical results with the femtolaser that demonstrate excellent accuracy in achieving intended capsulotomy diameter [1].

Nucleus Fragmentation

Patterns for treating the crystalline lens with the FS laser are designed for either liquefaction or chopping. A liquefaction ablation pattern is recommended for use only in cataracts with density up to LOCS III grade 2.0 and is well suited for cases of refractive lens exchange, especially in younger patients with high myopia and hyperopia or in patients where restoration of accommodation is needed. For liquefaction, concentric rings are created within the nucleus, starting posteriorly (about 800 μm from the posterior capsule) and progressing toward the anterior capsule. The surgeon maintains micron-precision control of the position of the laser beam within the crystalline lens during the treatment. After effective liquefaction of the central nucleus, the lens material can usually be removed simply by aspiration.

The chop pattern facilitates removal of harder cataracts and can be used in nuclei up to LOCS III grade +4.0. Chopping or cracking the nucleus with the femtolaser improves efficiency of phacoemulsification for lens removal while reducing or eliminating any need for challenging manual maneuvers and use of phaco energy for nucleus fracture. Creating at least four quadrants is compulsory and can be achieved using the FS laser to create a cross-pattern, in which two intersecting ellipsoidal planes are made, dividing the lens into four equal segments. However, the surgeon may choose to make six or eight cuts in a pie pattern, if desired.

Corneal Incisions

The femtolaser can also be used to create corneal incisions for coaxial or bimanual microincisional surgery. Incisions can be customized with respect to architecture (uniplanar, biplanar, multiplanar), length, width, and location (e.g., superior, temporal) according to the preference of the surgeon (see Fig. 11.3). My usual technique is to create a biplanar incision with a 2.0-mm tunnel located at 11:30 and a sideport incision at 1:30.

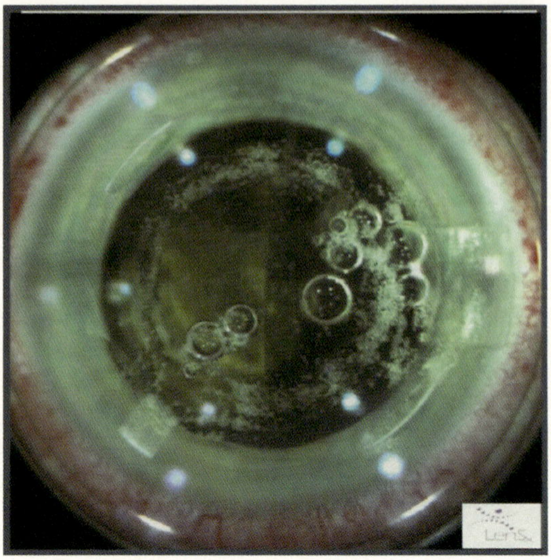

Fig. 11.3 Intraoperative image while performing penetrating primary and secondary corneal incisions. A pair of non-penetrating arcuate incisions at 9 mm optical zone is also performed

Positioning the corneal incision on the limbus is of utmost importance to minimize surgically induced astigmatism. Therefore, during docking and fixation of the eye, the surgeon must be certain that the limbus is within the 12 mm surgical field of view as anything outside of this area cannot be treated by the laser.

Phacoemulsification After Femtosecond Laser Treatment

It is worthwhile to reiterate that the corneal incision made with the femtolaser remains sealed until it is opened manually with another instrument. Therefore, all of the femtolaser treatment steps can be done in a dedicated laser room outside of the OR and even a few hours prior to the lens removal surgery. Care must be taken to make sure that the laser pretreatment does not cause an elevation of intraocular pressure from a lengthy exposure to liberated lens proteins If the time elapsed is more than 2 h after femtolaser pretreatment miosis can be a problem. Elevated intraocular pressure is also a potential concern, but we have not encountered this complication. Installation of the FS laser outside of the OR and the opportunity to wait before the patient is brought into the OR has economic and efficiency implications in terms of facilitating patient flow, allowing one device to be shared by multiple surgeons operating in different rooms, and minimizing OR time per case.

Ease of Entry, Capsule Removal and Nucleus Emulsification

After the eye is prepped and draped, the surgeon identifies the cut lines in the epithelium from the laser and then can easily open the incisions with a blunt spatula. A gentle maneuver should be used, taking care to avoid scratching the epithelium, which can lead to delayed incision healing, dehiscence, infection, and, in the worst case scenario, endophthalmitis.

Once the corneal incisions are opened, the anterior chamber is filled with viscoelastic material and the capsule disk can be removed. After verifying the FS laser has made a complete, 360° incision, I usually identify one edge of the capsulotomy with a cystotome and then use a rhexis forceps to grasp around the edge of the cut capsule, removing the disk with a circular movement. Sometimes the cut portion of the capsule may be displaced upon injection of the viscoelastic material. In that situation, the surgeon may simply grasp and remove the whole cut capsule from the eye.

Surgeons may be tempted to remove the capsule disk using a capsule forceps to grasp the tissue in the middle and pull anteriorly with a single motion. However, this should be avoided, as the presence of small capsular tags can lead to an anterior capsular tear that increases the risk of complications intra- and postoperatively.

Lens removal is very easy in soft lenses pretreated with the liquefaction pattern and can often be done without the need to fragment the lens using phaco energy. With the I/A tip, the surgeon may simply aspirate the nucleus and also the equatorial part of the lens. The removal of the liquefied nucleus is usually simple. We have observed a thicker epinucleus after removing the nucleus in some cases, but it should be treated the same way as during standard phacoemulsification.

In harder cataracts that have been treated with the chop pattern, it is recommended to first split the nucleus in half and then into quadrants before beginning phacoemulsification of the fragmented parts. Completing nucleus fragmentation in harder nuclei is easily done using a slim, slightly sharp second instrument. I recommend grabbing the lens using only aspiration force with the phaco tip (about 200–300 mmHg) and then entering the eye with the second instrument to divide the lower part of the lens. Next, the nucleus is rotated and the remaining areas are divided using a similar technique. The resulting quadrants (or smaller segments if more cuts are made) are easy to remove with the traditional phacoemulsification technique.

If the fragmentation pattern was used in a softer nucleus, it is better to use a drop type chopper (blunt chopper) to go underneath the quadrants and lift them toward the phaco tip. With this technique, the surgeon can avoid using any phaco energy for lens fragmentation.

After finishing the lens and cortex removal, cleaning of the anterior capsule inner surface in a 1.0 mm zone is advised to prevent subsequent fibrosis around the capsular edge.

Proper Patient Selection and Counseling

Optimizing outcomes of ReLACS depends on appropriate patient selection and counseling. Patients should have a positive attitude, understand the importance and benefits of the laser treatment, and be expected to tolerate a feeling of pressure on the eye during the treatment and to accept the possible problems that can occur using the FS laser technology.

In the preoperative consultation, the details of the FS laser procedure, its benefits, and its extra costs are reviewed. The importance of cooperation during the treatment is also emphasized, as it is necessary for patients to rest still and look into a fixation light during the procedure. Consent is obtained prior to surgery after providing the patient with a brief review of the procedure and its possible risks.

There are just a few clinical features to consider when selecting patients for ReLACS. Deep set orbits can make docking a challenge, although there is usually no problem if the lid fissure is wide enough. Patients receiving anticoagulant therapy should be excluded because the suction force from the PI may cause conjunctival hemorrhage.

Performing capsulotomy and lens fragmentation safely requires that the pupil dilate well, optimally to approximately 8.0 mm, and so patients with poorly dilating pupils, such as those with anterior or posterior synechiae, may not be good candidates for this femtolaser treatment. However, the procedure can be performed in eyes at risk for intraoperative floppy iris syndrome (IFIS), as long as adequate dilation of the pupil can be achieved.

Dense nuclei (up to LOCS III grade +4.0) can be treated with the FS laser, but the laser energy is not absorbed by white or brunescent nuclei so that lens fragmentation cannot be performed in the latter eyes. However, they can still receive FS laser treatment for capsulotomy and corneal incisions. In fact, capsulotomy with the femtolaser has a safety advantage in white cataracts since it avoids the expulsion of white material from the lens that occurs just after starting a manual rhexis.

Corneal opacities do not affect OCT imaging but can interfere with laser beam delivery into the eye. However, mild opacity is usually not a problem and should not be considered a contraindication to a FS laser procedure.

Advantages of Femtosecond Laser Surgery

There has been little change in surgical technique for phacoemulsification in the past 20 years, so the procedure remains manually based with outcomes highly dependent on surgeon skill. However, complications and unexpected outcomes also occur in expert hands. By bringing precision and reproducibility to the procedure, the FS laser laser can provide a host of efficacy and safety advantages relative to traditional phacoemulsification. In addition, the FS laser may be a powerful marketing tool and have practice-building potential. Some of the benefits of using the femtolaser have already been proven, while others are intuitive, but remain theoretical.

Safety

Use of the femtolaser in cataract surgery has the potential to reduce or eliminate the most common and serious complications of cataract surgery, which include irregular capsulotomy, anterior and posterior capsular tears, endothelial damage, cystoid macular edema (CME), dropped nucleus with its sequelae, and endophthalmitis.

Capsulotomy

With proper technique, the FS laser can predictably create a capsulotomy that is perfectly regular, accurately sized, and well centered and also without risk of causing inadvertent anterior capsule tears that can lead to posterior capsule rupture, vitreous loss, need for vitrectomy, and retinal detachment [2, 3]. Avoidance of anterior capsule tears using the FS laser suggests it may have a particular role in pediatric cataract surgery, considering that the thin, elastic capsule in these young eyes is particularly susceptible to radialization of the tear during manual capsulotomy.

Nucleus Fragmentation

Since application of the FS laser for lens fragmentation and liquefaction would obviate the need for sculpting and other manual nucleus fracture manuevers (e.g., divided and conquer, quick chop, stop and chop, nucleus flip), and reduce the need for phacoemulsification prior to I&A, its use could also reduce the occurrence of posterior capsular tears. In sculpting the lens, surgeons face the challenge of aiming to create a deep grove without knowing the exact location of the posterior capsule. During the FS laser procedure, the entire anterior segment is imaged with the aid of the built-in OCT. The surgeon maintains control in positioning the lens treatment, so that it remains at a safe distance away from from the posterior capsule. In our clinical experience to date, we have encountered no cases of FS laser-induced posterior capsule damage after using the FS laser for nucleus fragmentation/liquefaction in hundreds of eyes.

In a clinical study, we documented that use of femtolaser technology for lens pretreatment decreased average phaco power by 43% and average effective phaco time by 51% compared with traditional phacoemulsification [1]. Use of less ultrasound energy in the eye minimizes heating of the aqueous and subsequent thermal damage to the endothelium so that a FS laser-assisted procedure would be expected to result in less endothelial cell loss. Shorter, more efficient surgery could also decrease CME, and in a clinical study we demonstrated less macular thickening and volume increase postoperatively in eyes that underwent ReLACS compared with a control group having traditional phacoemulsification [4]. Moreover, since the need for manual maneuvers to remove the cataract is also decreased after using the FS laser for fragmentation or liquefaction, the FS laser-assisted procedure should result in less distortion and folds on the cornea.

Corneal Incisions

There are also potential safety benefits accompanying femtolaser creation of corneal incisions. Since the risk of iris prolapse through the incision is affected by incision shape and length, predictable incision creation using the laser should mitigate these events.

Use of the femtolaser also enables the surgeon to reproducibly create incisions with geometry that promotes self-sealing compared with a manual technique using an ultra-sharp blade. Furthermore, because the FS laser corneal cut is so precise, the incision it creates has a finer channel compared to blade-made wounds, which further enhances self-sealing. Incision integrity has implications for reducing the risk of endophthalmitis, and consistent creation of a well-constructed incision also helps control surgically induced astigmatism.

Efficacy

The ability of the FS laser to create capsulotomies that are accurately centered, symmetrically shaped, and of predictable size has a number of implications for improving visual function outcomes after cataract/refractive lens surgery. We have reported that eyes with a FS laser capsulotomy achieved better IOL centration, better anterior capsule/IOL overlap, significantly less higher order aberrations and better quality of vision relative to a comparator group with manual capsulotomies [5]. In addition, consistency in capsulotomy size, shape and centration is believed to account for reduced variability in the effective lens position (ELPo) after FS laser capsulotomy compared with manual capsulotomy [6]. In the latter study, decreased variability in refractive outcome was also demonstrated in the eyes that had the FS laser pretreatment for capsulotomy, which is what would be expected considering that the effective power of the IOL depends on its position in the eye.

Faster visual recovery can also be expected with the use of a better surgical technique that guarantees capsulotomy size and centration, minimizes the amount of phaco energy used for lens removal, and assures creation of corneal incisions with proper structure for enabling self-sealing and minimizing surgically induced astigmatism.

The efficacy benefits derived from using the FS laser in cataract/refractive lens surgery would have relevance to all patients. However, they are of particular importance for two groups—(1) *premium lens patients*, who are generally younger and have high expectations for undergoing surgery that will allow them to return quickly to their normal daily activities with excellent optical results and spectacle-independent vision, and (2) *high myopes*, because surgeons often tend to make the capsulotomy larger than required in these relatively large eyes, resulting in uneven overlap of the anterior capsule rim over the IOL optic, forward shifting of the IOL, and a refractive outcome that is more myopic than planned.

Advantages After the Learning Curve

Once the surgeon has overcome the learning curve for using the FS laser and the details of patient flow and work tasks for the OR staff have been fine-tuned, surgeons should find efficiency advantages for using the FS laser. As with the adoption of any new surgical technique, ReLACS is more time consuming initially. However, as all of the personnel become familiar and comfortable with their roles, case time will decrease. OR time is costly, but the OR time per case is reduced for a procedure performed with FS laser pretreatment. As less OR time is needed per case, productivity can be increased in terms of the total number of cases performed each day.

The availability of ReLACS can also be a powerful marketing tool that sets a practice apart from others in the community and draws patients. Safety is always foremost in the minds of consumers, but receiving state-of-the art health care is also valued. Although not necessarily true, some patients may believe that surgeons using cutting edge technology, such as the femtolaser, are better surgeons than those using older techniques. In addition, the public has tremendous trust in laser technology. The average layperson seems to appreciate that the laser is an advanced and precise surgical tool and many people assume that a laser procedure has safety advantages relative to one that depends on a surgeon's manual skills. Since the introduction of the FS laser for LASIK, patients undergoing cataract or refractive lens surgery have been asking if their procedure will be performed with a laser. Now, this surgery is a reality, and we can expect that word of its benefits will be spread rapidly by satisified patients. Patient demand for FS laser surgery will increase and its availability may causes patients to choose one practice over another.

Making the Transition: Will it be Worth it?

One of us (Z.Z. Nagy) began working with an early prototype of the LenSx laser in 2008, using it first in animal studies, and then to perform the first treatments in human eyes. Over a relatively short period of development, a number of upgrades in the hardware and software have already been introduced and have made the technology easier to use.

Role of Standard Phacoemulsification

We have not abandoned standard phacoemulsification, mainly because there are some patients who are unable to pay the extra cost of a FS laser procedure. Therefore, our surgical schedule dedicates certain days during the week to the FS laser cases, while standard phacoemulsification and other procedures (e.g., corneal transplantation, glaucoma surgery, etc.) are performed on the remaining days.

What About the Learning Curve?

Surgeons should be prepared to face a learning curve before mastering ReLACS, just as for any new intraocular microsurgery technique. However, the learning curve is much shorter than that required when transitioning from extracapsular cataract extraction to phacoemulsification.

What Will it Cost and Will Patients pay?

There are definitely costs associated with integrating FS laser technology into cataract and refractive lens surgery that are related to the cost of the equipment, its maintenance, cost of the PI, and any changes that must be made to the physical space to accommodate the device. While surgeons may be convinced that the benefits of safer and more predictable surgical outcomes justify the increased procedure cost, it is reasonable to wonder whether consumers will be willing to pay a higher fee for a FS laser refractive cataract procedure. Using experience with LASIK as a reference, we can expect that the answer will be "yes" for patients in many countries, including the U.S. and for those living in most Western and Central European nations.

The refractive FS lasers first became commercially available for LASIK flap creation in 2001. Data from surveys of refractive surgeon practice patterns show adoption of the FS laser increased steadily after its introduction [7]. By 2008–2009, it became the dominant technology for LASIK flap creation, replacing the mechanical microkeratome for a majority of surgeons because they recognized the laser brought greater predictability and safety in flap creation along with better functional outcomes, and patients were willing to pay for those benefits.

Although there are risks for trying to predict the future, there is good reason to expect there will be similar acceptance of the premium cost of FS laser refractive cataract (and refractive lens) surgery. Whether in ocular surgery or other medical fields, patients generally show a willingness to pay for advanced interventions that improve quality of life.

Introduction of the FS laser also coincides with the beginning of a decade when there will be a tremendous growth in cataract surgery procedures and anticipated growth in premium IOL implantations. The first baby boomers turned 65 in January, 2011, and the aging of the baby boomer generation is expected to contribute to a more than 30% increase in the annual number of cataract procedures performed between 2010 and 2020. The baby boomers will represent the first main group of patients who have the option of ReLACS, and they are ideal candidates for premium IOL surgery with a FS laser, because they enjoy an active lifestyle that is compatible with spectacle-independence, have a high level of disposable income, and want the best surgical outcomes their money can buy.

Conclusion

Improving outcomes after cataract/refractive lens surgery is a multifaceted challenge because of the variety of factors that affect safety, efficacy, and predictability. Progress has occurred in the past several years thanks to a number of developments. Recently, there have been advances in diagnostic instrumentation used for measuring keratometry and axial length, new IOL power calculation formulae have been introduced that are particularly helpful for improving refractive accuracy in challenging cases (e.g., high ametropes and eyes with a history of refractive surgery), and various manufacturers have developed new ultrasound modes that have enabled further reduction in incision size and improved surgical safety and efficiency. However, the FS laser stands apart from all of these innovations because of its broad potential impact. Use of the FS laser for capsulotomy, lens treatment, and corneal incisions addresses many of the current issues that limit success of cataract/refractive lens surgery. Acting through a variety of mechanisms to deliver multiple benefits, the FS laser can vastly improve both safety and efficacy to revolutionize lens removal surgery and maximize patient satisfaction.

Key Points

1. The FS laser portion of cataract surgery can be performed in a clean rather than sterile environment, as the corneal incisions remain intact until they are opened by manual blunt dissection.
2. Dilation should be as maximal as possible, and at least 8.0 mm.
3. Minimize the interval between laser treatment and surgery in the OR: miosis and IOP elevation can if hours are allowed to elapse.
4. Recommended capsulotomy sizes are 4.75–5.0 mm for standard IOLs and 5.5 mm for the Crystalens.
5. The primary corneal incision must be positioned at the limbus. If docking does not permit this, do not proceed with the incision.
6. Soft lenses are best treated with a liquefaction pattern and use of a blunt, wide edged chopper to lift segments into the phaco or I/A tip.
7. Hard lenses are best treated with a fragmentation pattern which creates four or more segments. Use of a thin, sharp tipped chopper facilitates segment separation.

References

1. Nagy Z, Takacs A, Filkorn T, Sarayba M. Initial clinical evaluation of an intraocular femtosecond laser in cataract surgery. J Refract Surg. 2009;25: 1053–60.
2. Nagy ZZ, Kranitz K, Takacs A, Mihaltz K, Kovacs I, Knorz MC. Comparison of intraocular lens decentration parameters after femtosecond and manual capsulotomies. J Refract Surg. 2011;27:564–9.
3. Marques FF, Marques DM, Osher RH, Osher JM. Fate of anterior capsular tears during cataract surgery. J Cataract Refract Surg. 2006;32:1638–42.
4. Unal M, Yucel I, Sarici A, Artunay O, Devranoglu K, Akar Y, Altin M. Phacoemulsification with topical anesthesia: resident experience. J Cataract Refract Surg. 2006;32:1361–5.
5. Knorz MC, Nagy ZZ (2011) Comparison of conventional and femtosecond laser-assisted phacoemulsification cataract surgery on the macula. In: Program and abstracts of american society of cataract and refractive surgeons symposium on cataract, IOL, and refractive surgery, San Diego, CA, 25–29 Mar 2011
6. Ecsedy M, Mihaltz K, Kovacs I, Takacs A, Filkorn T, Nagy ZZ. Effect of femtosecond laser cataract surgery on the macula. J Refract Surg. 2011;27:717–22.
7. Nagy ZZ Comparison of femtosecond laser and manual capsulotomy on postoperative quality of vision. In: Program and abstracts of american society of cataract and refractive surgeons symposium on cataract, IOL, and refractive surgery, San Diego, CA, 25–29 Mar 2010

Economics of ReLACS: Marketing a New Technology to Your Patients

12

Richard L. Lindstrom and Shareef Mahdavi

Merriam-Webster's Dictionary defines marketing as "the process or technique of promoting, selling, and distributing a product or service" [1]. In this chapter, we aim to put this definition in the context of modern surgery and elective medicine. We also strive to help surgeons understand that marketing is a much broader term than what is typically thought of as advertising and promotion.

Introduction

A quick review of recent postings by surgeons on the chat boards shows that Refractive Laser-Assisted Cataract Surgery (ReLACS) is indeed controversial, with surgeons questioning its value in a procedure that is already deemed excellent, especially when it is being offered in an environment where cost pressures are likely to drive reimbursement down rather than allow it to expand to accommodate even more technology. In a recent audience poll of surgeons, only 5% believed that "increased reimbursement" was how they would recoup costs for the investment in ReLACS technology [2].

R.L. Lindstrom (✉)
Minnesota Eye Consultants &, Department of Ophthalmology, University of Minnesota, Minneapolis, Minnesota 55431, USA
e-mail: rllindstrom@mneye.com

S. Mahdavi
SM2 Strategic, Inc.,
555 Peters Avenue, Pleasanton, CA 94566, USA
e-mail: Shareef@sm2strategic.com

The authors agree with the unlikely scenario of increased reimbursement, and believe this will be a patient-funded offering, one that builds upon the consumer awareness and success of both refractive surgery (with LASIK being the most widely performed elective surgical procedure both in the USA and worldwide) and cataract surgery (the most widely performed surgical procedure on a global basis, with over 20 million procedures forecast for 2012.) [2].

Within the term "marketing" is the word "market," and the evolving market dynamics—demographics, technology, and consumer-driven healthcare spending—support the thesis that ReLACS will have a strong opportunity to succeed on a commercial basis. The single biggest variable is neither the technology nor the patient, but rather the surgeon and the "channel of distribution" (one of several key marketing concepts that will be used throughout the chapter). That is, the ultimate success of this procedure will depend upon surgeon behavior in how they think about and promote this offering to their patients. Manufacturer investment and consumer demand need to be connected or "bridged" by surgeons and their staff (and, by extenstion, executives and administrators of hospitals, ASCs and eventually office environments where ReLACS can be performed).

Where to Begin?

There are three key principles that surgeons will need to consider and accept in order to succeed with ReLACS. Each of these principles helps

R.R. Krueger et al. (eds.), *Textbook of Refractive Laser Assisted Cataract Surgery (ReLACS)*,
DOI 10.1007/978-1-4614-1010-2_12, © Springer Science+Business Media, LLC 2013

establish the proper mindset and serves to inform surgeon and team as they develop plans for incorporating ReLACS technology into their well-established cataract surgery system.

Principle #1: ReLACS Is Refractive Surgery, Not Cataract Surgery

Refractive Endpoint

Although ReLACS is performed by cataract surgeons in conjunction with cataract surgery, the technology, by itself, is not cataract surgery. This is a critical distinction from a regulatory as well as a marketing standpoint. In the US healthcare system, CMS regulations clearly state that the government will not pay for a "new and improved" form of cataract surgery (often referred to as the "golden scalpel" rule). Thus, cataract surgery being performed with a laser won't suffice as sufficient justification for offering ReLACS to patients, and would not qualify as an additional covered service by Medicare (and likely all third-party insurance payors).

Cataract surgery is used to remedy a pathologic condition with the replacement of the natural lens (as defined by CPT code 66984) to allow for improved best corrected visual acuity via the use of glasses to function at all distances. In cataract surgery, no special effort is required (or compensated for) to lessen the need for glasses. Today's modern cataract procedure is performed with a series of tools and processes in order to remove a cataractous lens and insert an artificial one and, after healing is complete, prescribe and fit the patient with glasses or contact lenses to restore best corrected functional vision. This is where third party reimbursement for cataract surgery begins and ends; anything else done to improve the refractive outcome should be viewed as refractive surgery.

FS lasers are just one technology out of many used in refractive surgery with a goal of providing the patient with a specific refractive outcome. The goals of refractive surgery in the context of a cataract surgical procedure are twofold: first, to increase the likelihood of functioning without glasses, and second, to reduce the likelihood of secondary treatment to enhance the refractive outcome. These tools include refractive diagnostics performed before, during and after cataract surgery, additional surgical planning, LRI procedures, specialty IOLs designed to correct for presbyopic or astigmatic error, more follow-up visits to insure patient outcome and satisfaction, laser enhancements (post-procedure) as well as a laser that can be used just prior to cataract surgery.

Refractive Balance Billing

For decades, surgeons have been able to perform refraction, LRI enhancements and postsurgical laser enhancements as non-covered services. Surgeons have been able to offer the ability to achieve a refractive outcome post-cataract surgery, and also charge patients directly. In 2005 and again in 2007, CMS issued two rulings that clearly separated refractive components related to the properties and use of intraocular implants themselves. In CMS-0501, the government clearly distinguishes the presbyopia-correcting element of the IOL as non-covered by the global fee for cataract surgery. Approximately 2-years later, CMS provided a similar distinction for the treatment of astigmatism. A careful analysis of these rulings also makes it clear that the government does not pay for these services and also does not mandate how you treat these refractive errors.

Refractive Mindset

What gets confusing is the way surgeons have interpreted this longstanding directive. Some choose to offer and charge patients to perform procedures in addition to the cataract surgery that provide a refractive outcome. Others perform some of them (e.g., LRI) but not all of them (e.g., laser vision correction). Some choose to charge for some methods (e.g., laser vision correction) but not others (e.g., LRI) based on a self-defined notion of what methods are sufficiently accurate to justify an additional fee to patients. And some doctors choose to either do nothing or, if they do a refractive enhancement, do it at no charge. We understand that some surgeons have been "giving it away" for decades and that charging patients for a refractive component of their surgery and perioperative care is a foreign concept. Our view is that surgeons need to avoid the scenarios where they provide these services "free of charge" or where they charge some patients but not others. Providing refractive services at no charge could be considered an inducement to the patient for that surgeon to perform the cataract surgery, which is risky and ill-advised. Charging for some patients (or even for some refractive services but not others) would likely not meet a fairness test and could be considered discriminatory, regardless of the criteria used to justify the specific intervention. Furthermore, performing refractive surgery at no charge, as part of the cataract surgical procedure to grow your practice, could be considered illegal, as it is an "inducement" for the patient to undergo otherwise non-indicated or non-covered surgery.

The solution we propose is that surgeons adopt a mindset that all the tools used to achieve a specific refractive outcome, tools that now include a FS laser used in conjunction with cataract surgery, be viewed as part of a refractive surgery toolkit. No refractive surgeons we know perform LASIK for free. That same rule, applied consistently in the use of ReLACS, will help surgeons develop their offering and educate their patients appropriately.

Implications of Principle #1: The Refractive Conversation

As shown in Table 12.1, there are three-steps that surgeons should use to incorporate ReLACS as part of the refractive surgical component of their existing cataract surgery system. First, document the medical necessity and existing pathology of the cataract and state that insurance and medicare does indeed cover this surgery.

Table 12.1 Surgical counseling for ReLACS should include a consistent protocol that documents both medical necessity for cataract surgery and lifestyle preferences for that patient

3-Step process
Document medical necessity
Establish refractive goals
Determine the tools you will use to meet the patient's refractive goals

Second, discuss and establish the patient's refractive goals following cataract surgery. If the patient is indifferent and does not seek a refractive outcome beyond repairing the pathology, they do not have a goal and therefore you have nothing additional to offer or discuss. However, if they seek to optimize their vision at one or more distances, and state that they want to do so in order meet a specific lifestyle need or quality of life desire, then they are seeking a refractive outcome that enhances their personal lifestyle. The surgeon should document that the management of astigmatism or presbyopia or both are required to meet the patient's personal lifestyle enhancing refractive outcome goal. Relative spectacle independence requires the use of special testing, special planning, advanced technology IOLs, and management of astigmatism to achieve the required target of less than 0.50 diopters residual astigmatism and defocus when fully healed. The surgeon and staff need to clearly distinguish that the government and insurance do not pay for that outcome, and that the patient has the opportunity to reduce his or her use of glasses. The answer to an important question, "are you interested in reducing your dependence on glasses after surgery?" should be documented to establish the patient's motivation. Following that, questions need to be asked to determine more specifically what those goals are.

This leads to the third step, which is where the surgeon decides what tools should be used and makes a specific recommendation to the patient, which the patient is free to accept and pay for.

This three-step process, applied consistently, helps distinguish between cataract surgery and services performed to improve the refractive outcomes of that surgery.

Principle #2: Focus on Developing the Category Rather Than the Brand

Category Building

Once a surgeon and team have clearly established that ReLACS is a form of refractive surgery, the next principle affects how they will communicate with and educate patients, referral sources, and the surrounding community. The single most important strategic marketing decision that has to be made at the outset is how to define ReLACS so that it makes sense and has relevance with the different target audiences that will be learning about it. All of us are surrounded by consumer marketing, with most of it focused on attempting to "brand" the offering in the minds of the consumer. Huge amounts of money are spent on brand-building as a means of differentiation so that the target audience will select the advertised brand rather than a competitor's version of the same product or service.

Each and every brand that exists within a category (e.g., automobile) and subcategory (e.g., hybrid) has been developed to help people make sense of what is being offered. Consumers attempt to make sense of things by categorizing them according to a scheme or relatable context. Surgeons and staff have long used analogies when counseling patients on their surgical options; analogies similarly provide context so that a patient can understand and make sense of what is being discussed.

When a brand new category or subcategory is being formed (as is the case with ReLACS), it is much more important to focus on developing the categorization than it is to build a brand. We need look no further than LASIK and how that market developed to understand the differences between category and brand building. The terms "laser vision correction" and "LASIK" were category and subcategory definitions that emerged and became widely used by surgeons and centers. As surgeons and centers sought to differentiate their version or "brand" of LASIK, they focused on differentiation via their name (and associated experience performing the procedure), the technology employed (e.g., laser manufacturer or specific features of that laser), a branded name of the procedure (i.e., a specific form of customized ablation treatment), or even an entirely made-up name with no inherent consumer meaning (e.g., down-up LASIK). With few exceptions, there have not been sufficient resources available to form and sustain consumer awareness around any of these branding efforts. The lack of sufficient return-on-investment in these forms of brand-building led a significant number of providers to conclude that commoditization had taken place and thus price was the best available means by which to differentiate their offering. The result (seen in Fig. 12.1) was not good, as the industry saw procedure volumes decline rather than increase, as the average fee for LASIK came down in the early 2000s. Brand building in LASIK has largely been a failed experiment that all ophthalmic surgeons should remember as they plan to introduce ReLACS to their practice and community. Instead, surgeons should focus on the common goal of category building.

Category Term Selection

With respect to ReLACS, industry and surgeons will be well served to agree upon a single term or set of terms to use to distinguish this offering (a new subcategory) from traditional cataract surgery (which can be thought of as the broader category). This is important because consumers have come to expect that cataract surgery is "free" in the sense that it is covered by insurance or Medicare. The current penetration of premium IOLs (approximately 15% of all cataract surgery performed in the US) provides a key data point illustrating the importance of properly differentiating the new subcategory. One of the reasons penetration is not higher is that the patient arrives at a cataract consultation with a mindset that the surgery is covered, and attempting to "undo" that preconceived notion is indeed challenging.

While this book contains the term "ReLACS," which stands for "Refractive Laser Assisted Cataract Surgery," some of the other terms being proposed to define this new subcategory are as follows:

- LAser Cataract Surgery (LACS)
- Laser-Assisted Refractive Cataract Surgery (LARCS)
- Femtosecond Laser-Assisted Cataract Surgery (FLACS)
- Femtosecond LAser Refractive Cataract Surgery (FLARCS)
- Femtosecond Laser-Assisted Refractive Cataract Surgery (FLARCS)
- Laser Refractive Lens Surgery (LRLS)
- Laser Refractive Cataract Surgery (LaRCS)

There are pros and cons to each of the terms being offered. The key criterion in term selection

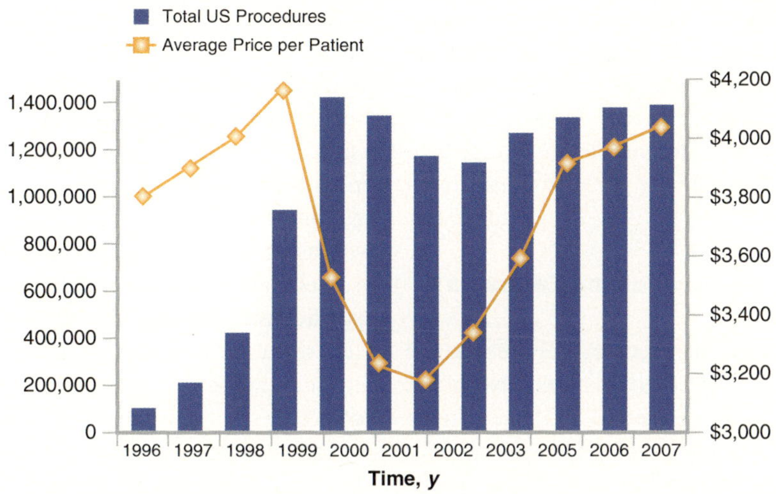

Fig. 12.1 Surgeons' reduction in their LASIK fees proved disastrous to most practices and failed to stimulate increased demand for the procedure. Historical relationships between average price and total procedure volume show that demand for LASIK is inelastic

is to achieve both relevance and memorability. We can use lessons learned from the premium channel IOL market, where categories and subcategories are easily understood and differentiated by surgeons and industry but were confusing to consumers: Premium IOLs for the correction of presbyopia are subcategorized as multifocal and pseudo-accommodating, with a further premium channel subcategory of toric (astigmatism correcting) IOLs. Confusion still exists today when we look at the different ways that doctors and their staff describe premium IOLs to their patients.

The terms we collectively choose to use in FS ReLACS are equally as important because they will help consumers "frame" their perception and understanding of what is being offered. Use of a single term by all providers will help reduce confusion and facilitate decision-making.

Category Building Demographics

Category building is especially critical given the demographic and psychographic shift beyond what has traditionally been described as a "cataract population." With the first wave of 78 million Baby Boomers now entering Medicare, demand for cataract surgery will increase significantly over the next two decades. The purchasing mindset among Baby Boomers has been well documented and will impact how they perceive the ReLACS offering. Hence, some surgeons are proposing that we eliminate the word "cataract" when defining this new category, based on the possible negative connotation (e.g., "that's something that happens to old people, and I am not old!") and/or a redefinition of cataract itself. In reality, for the past 40 years a "cataract" diagnosis has been as much a justification for reimbursement as it has a clinical diagnosis. Evidence of this can be seen in the spike in procedure volume performed on patients at age 65 when compared with those at each year 60–64 years of age. This clearly indicates a regulatory phenomenon rather than a clinical one, as cataracts have not been shown to magically mature once someone reaches their 65th birthday. There is simply economic incentive to wait until that age to have the cataract removed. Thus, eliminating the term "cataract" would help differentiate ReLACS from traditional surgery.

The counter-argument, however, should also be made. Cataract is a phrase that has a strong association with eye surgery. Adding qualifiers before it, such as "laser" or "laser refractive" does signify that there is a new way of performing the procedure. The term laser has strong positive connotations with consumers, so perhaps appending it to the front end of the traditional term is what will create sufficient differentiation in the consumer's mind. (*Note*: regulatory bodies will have significant influence on what terms get used, by the manufacturers of devices). Indeed, "naming the baby" becomes a complex exercise and demonstrates the difficulty faced in marketing a new procedure.

Category Expansion: Putting Cataracts into Context

In our current day, cataracts are rarely seen as the white opacity analogous to a waterfall, but rather are more appropriately viewed as the end-stage of a long-term degradation of the lens and quality of vision that first became noticeable in the patient's forties with the onset of presbyopia. In the future, the word "cataract" will likely evolve toward a better descriptor, such as "dysfunctional lens syndrome" [3]. The explanation in the previous sentence(s) helps the patient frame their current vision in a way that makes the discussion of ReLACS much more appropriate and valuable as a possible alternative.

The description of this advanced method to restore someone's vision, along with the way the condition itself is being described, will make a tremendous difference in establishing the ReLACS category in the years to come. Used consistently among most (or all) surgeons and staff, it will help prevent confusion among consumers and referral sources. It will make the "purchase decision" much easier. It will help this new category to grow and succeed and sustain and create value for patients, surgeons and their practices, facilities, and for manufacturers who have taken the risk to develop the technology.

Implication of Principle #2: Education Based Marketing

With 3.5 million cataract procedures forecast in the USA in 2012, there is already a built-in potential demand for ReLACS, in contrast to the demand for LASIK, which needed to be cultivated as a stand-alone procedure "from scratch" each year. In theory, every patient should be educated on available options, and once a sufficiently large base of lasers are in use, this will occur. While the initial surgeon adopters of ReLACS will want to create awareness in their communities (via advertising and public relations), they should strive to promote the category and not any individual brand or product features. This cannot be over-stated if we want to avoid the risk of commoditization. For example, all promotion should avoid mention of specific lasers or laser features (e.g., liquid interface, real-time tracking), as these have no meaning or relevance to patients, as consumers. All promotion should focus on the lifestyle benefits to the patient, who as a consumer will need to decide upon their discretionary spending for healthcare. Creating awareness and interest is the most that can be achieved by any external marketing efforts. Further consideration by the consumer needs to take place in a one-to-one setting once a patient is associated with the practice, whether this begins via the Web site, telephone, or in-person. Surgeons and staff need intensive and ongoing training in order to understand how to appropriately inform, educate, and counsel patients. We view this as education-based marketing (EBM) rather than pushy, aggressive selling (which is not what we recommend). There is sufficient cache in laser-based approaches to surgery that will generate apparent interest among consumers from the outset. (This is indeed the experience observed within the initial clinics that have access to this technology in the USA and worldwide).

The words and phrases that are used in discussing ReLACS with patients are also key to setting the appropriate framing in the consumers' mind. In Table 12.2 we show the benefits of ReLACS from a surgical perspective on the left. Contrast this list with the benefits of ReLACS from a patient perspective on the right.

Reviewing these two lists side-by-side should serve as an ample reminder that what is important to surgeons is not the same (nor described in the same manner) as what is important to patients.

Surgeons and staff should avoid using words and phrases that, while essential to the surgical process, are not understood or relevant to the patient. Example words to avoid include nucleus,

Table 12.2 Benefit perspectives

Benefits to surgeon	Benefits to patient
Precise reproducible incisions	Will see better after surgery without correction, enhancing their personal lifestyle
More reproducible spherical refractive outcomes	Greatly reduced dependence on glasses
Perfect capsulotomy	Greater precision because it uses laser versus blades/manual method
More reproducible surgery patient to patient and surgeon to surgeon	
Reduced phaco time/energy	

capsulorhexis, primary and secondary incisions, phacoemulsification, aspiration, etc.

Principle #3: ReLACS Is Consumer Driven, Not Doctor Driven

Lesson of Phaco Patients

Some eye surgeons (as observed on the message chat boards that are frequently viewed by ophthalmologists) cannot see the value of adding a laser to an already well-established surgical procedure. This debate is reminiscent of the transition to phacoemulsification, whose inventor Charles Kelman, MD remarked, "while doctors debate, patients decide." With regard to the addition of the FS laser for use with cataract surgery, we add that this technology is "about the needs of the patient, not those of the doctor."

Lesson of LASIK Patients

ReLACS is, by definition, an elective component that is paid for directly by consumers when they appear as cataract patients in the practice. These same patients were responsible for building LASIK into the most widely performed elective surgical procedure, as lifestyle demands drove the popularity of a procedure that could promise reduced or no dependence on glasses or contacts. Baby Boomers will affect refractive cataract surgery in a similar manner, and help ReLACS grow in popularity as an adjunct to the traditional cataract surgery procedure. Their entire mindset is around maintaining an active and healthy lifestyle at each and every stage of life. With vision being the most valued of all the senses, and the one responsible for 80% of sensory input, it makes sense that Baby Boomer patients will seek the best options that are consistent with this active and healthy lifestyle. Their desires have spawned numerous self-improvement industries, from health clubs and cosmetic surgery to nutritional supplements and life coaching.

Lesson of Femto-LASIK Patients

The skepticism surrounding ReLACS is inherently similar to that faced by the FS laser with its first medical application over a decade ago. In 2001, very few LASIK procedures utilized a laser for the first-step flap creation (<1%). One decade later, laser-created flaps account for 70% or more of all LASIK procedures. This transition occurred despite the high cost of capital equipment ($450,000 vs. a $50,000 microkeratome) and the higher per-use fee ($160 per eye vs. $30 for use of the keratome blade). The key reason behind this shift is that consumers readily understood and accepted the value proposition of a safer procedure via use of the laser. Surgeons raised their fees an average of nearly $400 or offered patients a choice of laser or blade, with a similar add-on $400 price for use of the laser. When offered the choice, patients chose the laser 80% of the time [4]. In fact, the increased fees charged to use the FS laser, along with increases to perform more advanced wavefront ablations, helped restore the average price charged for LASIK to its pre-commoditization levels (see Fig. 12.2).

Surgeons will need to similarly define their fees to patients for performing refractive services in conjunction with cataract surgery. The fees for these services are dictated by the surgeon, not by

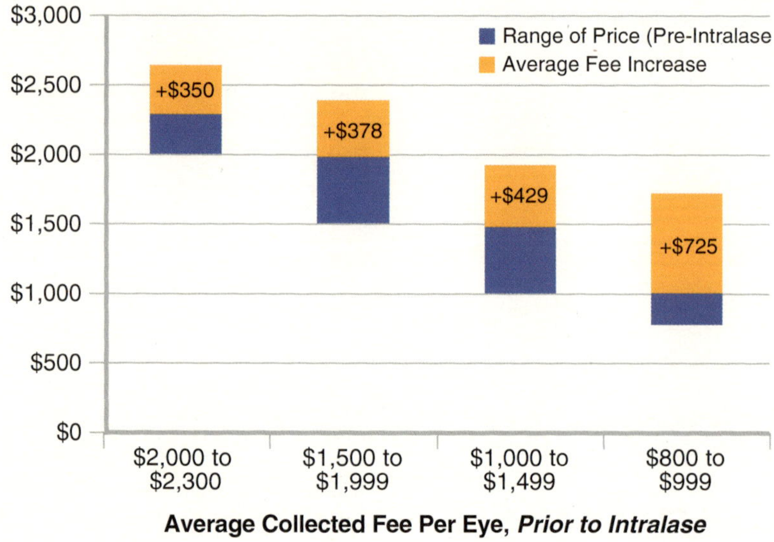

Fig. 12.2 While many surgeons were skeptical that patients would pay an additional fee for the use of a laser to create the flap in LASIK, patients overwhelmingly chose the laser due to a perception of increased safety. Using a laser rather than a blade became also was easy for surgeons and staff to communicate and yielded an obvious benefit to the consumer

Medicare or insurance, and are subject to market forces. While many different models are possible, we predict that several will emerge as the main ways in which ReLACS will be offered:

- One-price for all services, with everything included
- Tiered pricing, with different levels of service and technology
- A la carte, where patients can pick and choose

An example of a tiered pricing model is shown in Table 12.3. The ultimate pricing model used by each provider should be carefully considered and developed. It needs to be both logical and defensible, and providers would be wise to invest in testing proposed pricing models prior to putting them into effect.

Table 12.3 The author's (RLL) approach to a pricing model that incorporates the femtosecond (FS) laser into the already existing set of refractive options that can be added to cataract surgery

How do we charge?
• My model will likely be based on the complexity of the refractive outcome goal
• Tier I ($)=See well at distance without glasses
• Tools: FS laser, monofocal aspheric IOL
• Tier II ($$)=See well at distance w/o glasses (Astigmat)
• Tools: FS laser, toric IOL or LRIs
• Tier III ($$$)=See well at ALL distances w/o glasses
• Tools: FS laser, accommodating or MFIOL, LRIs, corneal surgery enhancement if needed
MINNESOTA EYE CONSULTANTS, P.A.

Different pricing levels are justified by a combination of preoperative refractive error, postoperative refractive goals, and the amount of technology utilized

How Much Will Patients Pay?

"How much to charge?" is a question facing all surgeons who plan to incorporate ReLACS into their surgical practice. The fee should be commensurate with the value derived for the procedure. The ophthalmic community has several reference points established to help guide the decision, as well as a benchmark consumer survey. Laser Vision Correction has typically been priced at $2,000 or more per eye as a global fee, with fees ranging as high as $3,000 per eye and as low as $149 per eye. The premium IOL segment has an average fee for presbyopia-correcting implants of $2,300 per eye [5]. Given that similar technology (e.g., laser) is being used and similar outcomes are being achieved that fall

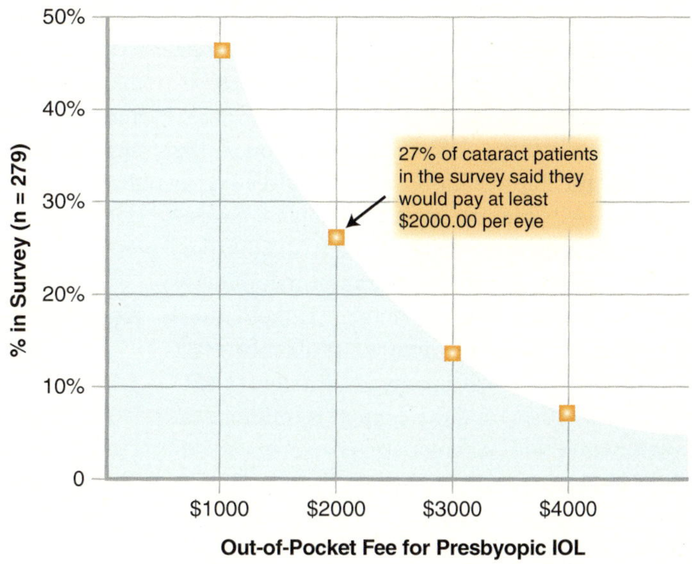

Fig. 12.3 Patients considering cataract surgery in an online survey ($n=279$) show strong interest in paying out-of-pocket to achieve less dependence on spectacles following cataract surgery. This chart shows the price sensitivity when applied to the use of a presbyopic-correcting IOL; the authors believe that ReLACS will show a similar curve given the similar benefits as part of an overall refractive cataract procedure

under refractive improvement of vision, it is reasonable that surgeons will charge in the area of $1,000–$4,000 per eye, depending on what other services are included in the offering.

Consumer interest at these price points was tested in a 2009 online survey of 279 patients who were in the process of deciding to have cataract surgery. More than 80% expressed interest in technology that improved outcomes following cataract surgery [6]. After being given a brief description of the benefit of a presbyopia-correcting implant, they were asked to specify how much they would be willing to pay off their own money to be able to see at all distances without glasses. As shown in Fig. 12.3, 27% said they would pay at least $2,000 per eye and 50% said they would spend at least $1,000 per eye. The study author noted that this came after a very brief statement and without the benefit of in-person counseling and the ability to clarify and answer questions. The results from this survey, while not being a direct reflection of ReLACS, are indicative of consumer interest in advanced technology to improve the refractive outcomes following cataract surgery.

An actual example of the success of ReLACS outside the USA is seen in the practice of Michael Lawless, MD in Sydney, Australia (see Chap. 14). At the time of this writing, Michael had only received his FS Laser for Cataract Surgery (Alcon LenSx, Fort Worth, TX) 2 months prior, and even though he is an early adopter in both laser refractive surgery and premium IOL technology with a practice that is skewed toward this type of patient, he is charging ~$1,000 extra for ReLACS, and is already converting 94% of his cataract surgery patients into this technology!

Implication for Principle #3: It's a Lifestyle Choice

The FS laser technology has the potential to help take the premium surgery channel to an entirely new level, especially as it addresses the fundamental problem with cataract surgery and premium IOLs technology. Namely, we are not generating good enough refractive outcomes. LASIK outcomes are at least twice as good as they are for cataract surgery, and ReLACS will help elevate these outcomes by adding a refractive component (that is LASIK-like in nature) to the traditional cataract surgery that is meant to treat pathology.

Surgeons only need to study the past two decades of refractive surgery in an open marketplace to better understand consumer dynamics as they apply to setting fees that accurately reflect the value of the technology and services being provided. At the top of this list is a recognition that ReLACS is a consumer-driven, lifestyle choice rather than a surgeon-directed, disease-curing choice.

As with both LASIK and the addition of the FS laser for flap creation, surgeons investing in ReLACS will require capital equipment investment, per-use fees, and premium diagnostics. The fact that surgeons have been able to profitably perform corneal refractive surgery is the harbinger that they will be able to profitably offer ReLACS. The environment is different (ASC rather than office) and the context is different (in combination with cataract surgery versus stand-alone procedure) and the patient payment is different (the cataract portion is reimbursed versus none of it is reimbursed). However, the ultimate goal is very much the same: helping patients see well again without glasses. We believe that approximately half of all cataract patients will have sufficient motivation and financial resources for ReLACS, and that in a few short years it will be the standard of care to offer a refractive cataract surgery rather than just cataract surgery.

Summary and Conclusion

There are only three patient desires following cataract surgery:

- See well with glasses
- Drive well without glasses
- See well without glasses

The first desire falls within the realm of traditional cataract surgery. The second and third desire, however, are clearly refractive goals that bring additional value to the consumer, are not covered by third-party reimbursement, and can be charged for by the surgeon to the patient. The availability of the FS laser as part of the armamentarium available to surgeons only enhances the attractiveness of the latter two options to the consumer.

With respect to the controversy surrounding this topic and the unknowns regarding specific regulatory issues, we return to Merriam-Webster's dictionary to highlight an alternative definition for the marketing term promotion: "to contribute to the growth or prosperity of …" [1]. We believe that this definition applies perfectly to surgeons and their patients and the collective goal of helping ReLACS become a successful offering that advances the state of the art in modern ophthalmic surgery.

Key Points

1. Marketing is more than advertising. Patient education and surgeon behavior are very important when medical procedures are involved.
2. Laser technology for refractive cataract surgery will likely be patient funded, and hence consumer driven. Reimbursement by third party payors is unlikely.
3. Marketing a concept or approach is likely to be more successful that promoting a "brand" of equipment.
4. ReLACS and ReLACS are but two of many acronyms which have been proposed to differentiate that fact that refractive services are a principal objective of FS laser technology when used in the context of cataract surgery.
5. Primary goals of ReLACS are refractive in nature: to increase the likelihood of functioning without spectacles and decrease the likelihood of further surgery to enhance the refractive outcome.
6. Balance billing is allowed in the US for refractive services. Adequate explanation to patients and documentation of these discussions and the actions to be taken are essential to justify the charges for these services.
7. Balance billing policies must consistently delineate what refractive services will and will not incur charges, as offering certain refractive services free of charge could be considered an inducement to perform cataract surgery.
8. The elements of the "the refractive conversation" and their written documentation in the medical record create a solid foundation upon which to justify balance billing for the delivery of refractive services related to cataract surgery.

References

1. Merriam-Webster's Collegiate Dictionary. 11th ed. Springfield, MA: Merriam-Webster, Inc.; 2004.
2. Presentation by Richard Lindstrom, MD at 2010 ASCRS Symposium on LenSx and Femtosecond.
3. Credit for this term should be given to Harvey Carter, MD, who first used it when counseling patients on the Crystalens IOL upon commercial approval in 2003.
4. Mahdavi S. The impact of femtosecond laser technology—a three year perspective. www.sm2strategic.com.
5. MarketScope Newsletter, St. Louis, MO. Data from quarterly surveys of ophthalmic surgeons.
6. Mahdavi S. A survey of consumer demand for premium cataract surgery. 2009. www.sm2strategic.com.

Step-By-Step: Starting Your ReLACS Practice

13

Stephen G. Slade

Introduction

Perhaps the most significant advance in Ophthalmology to date in the new twenty-first century is the use of femtosecond (FS) lasers for lens replacement surgery [1]. There are many potential benefits that may arise with FS laser technology. I suspect that patients will benefit from FS laser technology as we anticipate a lower complication rate than currently associated with standard cataract surgery. Current vitreous loss rates range from 2 to 6% of all cases. Wouldn't reducing phaco time with the laser and avoiding a manual capsulorhexis reduce the rate of vitreous loss? Patients want this potentially improved safety as well as freedom from glasses if possible, (the goal of refractive surgery). The FS laser can also contribute to this refractive goal for lens surgery patients. It is time we provided better uncorrected distance visual acuity (UCDVA) to our cataract patients. Results from current IOL studies pale next to LASIK results (40% 20/40 UCDVA compared to 90% with LASIK) [2]. The ability of the laser to make precise, reproducible corneal incisions and capsulotomies will allow surgeons to optimize lens position, more effectively manage preexisting astigmatism, and possibly even reduce induced astigmatism. I believe that the laser will enable us to improve refractive results with such reproducible incisions. We may learn that we are able to improve and quantify the effective lens position of an IOL by controlling the size, centration, and shape of a laser capsulorhexis. Ophthalmologists will be able to make corneal astigmatic incisions with the laser to address preexisting cylinder and further improve postoperative refractive results. We now have the opportunity to learn what we do not know regarding the clinical significance of precisely sized and positioned incisions and capsulotomies. For how are we able to study these steps if we cannot provide a reproducible benchmark? Thus, I believe that this technology represents the perfect marriage of the cataract and refractive subspecialties.

S.G. Slade (✉)
Slade & Baker Vision Center, 3900 Essex Lane, Suite 101, Houston, TX 77027, USA
e-mail: sgs@visiontexas.com

Historical Perspective: My Involvement with the LenSx Laser

The initial clinical evaluation of the LenSx Laser (Alcon) began in 2008 with Professor Dr. Zoltan Nagy of Semmelweis University in Budapest, Hungary [1]. The original work to obtain FDA approval was done by Dr. Nagy as well as the first image-guided ReLACS with the laser in December 2009 [3, 4]. This surgery involved lens fragmentation, the capsulotomy, and corneal incisions. The LenSx laser has obtained four separate 510K clinical approvals from FDA since 2009. These include approvals for the incisions into the eye, the capsulotomy, lens or nuclear cracking

R.R. Krueger et al. (eds.), *Textbook of Refractive Laser Assisted Cataract Surgery (ReLACS)*,
DOI 10.1007/978-1-4614-1010-2_13, © Springer Science+Business Media, LLC 2013

techniques and arcuate incisions in the cornea. In early 2010, a key approval for manufacturing the laser in the USA was granted to LenSx. This complete set of approvals, in such an early timing, was due to the work of the LenSx regulatory team under the guidance of Judy Gordon, DVM.

The manufacturing approval at the beginning of 2010 was key in the ability to place the first laser in the USA, which came to my clinic in Houston, Texas in mid-February of 2010. Since LenSx Lasers delivered the platform to our clinic, we have not been part of an FDA trial or subject to other investigational device restrictions. The laser already had 510(k) clearance for anterior capsulotomy when we received it, and clearance for incisions and lens fragmentation quickly followed. Our first cases, the first ReLACS done in the USA were done on February 28, 2010. Since then, we have been successfully performing ReLACS at our center in Houston.

What excites me the most about ReLACS are the potential benefits that the technology offers to the patient. Safety will be enhanced by reduced phaco time and power, less surgical time in the eye, and finer, more elegant incisions, among other innovations. We have studied whether the precision of lens surgery may be increased by an exactly sized, shaped, and positioned capsulotomy that will better control the IOL's final resting place as well as by precise, reproducible primary incisions and standardized, quantifiable astigmatic keratotomies. FS lasers could also enable and make possible many other technologies, including polymer IOLs that can be injected through a tiny capsulotomy.

Clinical Perspective

The Learning Curve

All new technologies come with a learning curve, and the FS laser is no exception. The procedure does draw heavily on lessons learned from other ophthalmic surgeries including LASIK and Phacoemulsification. There are two parts to the procedure, that of the laser itself and then the intraocular surgery. The laser portion involves planning the surgery and entering patient data and treatment plan. This is of utmost importance, and while no manual skill is needed, the lessons learned from examples of incorrect data entry in LASIK are powerful teachers. Of course, drawing on the experience of other users and a surgeon's own early cases can help with setting the laser parameters such as capsulotomy diameter, incision construction and the lens chop and pattern. Docking is the main technique challenge. The patient interface (PI) is different in design from those used for LASIK, and suction is applied longer, some 45 s at present, but the technique is easily learned. Of course all the typical LASIK techniques to help obtain good exposure and suction and recognize suction breaks and movement become even more critical when intraocular surgery is being done.

The intraocular portion of the surgery requires more learning to recognize what the laser has done in each individual case and tailor the surgery accordingly rather than performing incisions, chops, etc. for all cases. The laser certainly makes the procedure easier in that the incisions, capsulotomy and lens chops are all done. The key is to verify the incisions, make sure that the capsulotomy is complete, and take advantage of the lens chops. For example, the capsulotomy should be verified as complete before the primary incision is opened and the chamber manipulated. Otherwise capsular tags and incomplete cuts could extend in a undesirable fashion. No additional manual skills are typically required, but the more cases one does, the better the surgeon becomes at seeing how best to manage each case. The laser does make the intraocular portion of the case quicker, as fewer steps are required, but as the laser portion is added the total time spent with the patient might increase.

Does the laser allow a less skilled surgeon to do lens surgery, or reduce the skills of a skilled surgeon? Good surgery is the sum of one's manual skill, practice, experience and judgment. The laser, for example, will reduce the number of manual capsulotomies the surgeon does. But the less frequently he or she does capsulotomies, the less practiced one will be for difficult cases such as small pupils or scarred corneas, so the skill level required for these cases is increased in this sense. Try going for several weeks without doing a manual capsulotomy then doing a complex case. One will have to maintain or increase skill level to compensate for the lack of practice.

How does the aspiring laser lens surgeon learn the technique? Is travel, a course or fellowship required? In general, travel to observe the surgery with an experienced surgeon is always a good idea. Not only is the technique with the laser and the intraocular portion of the surgery introduced but patient flow, counseling, preoperative and postoperative aspects can be observed and learned as well. In the case of LenSx, new surgeons observe established ones, and then are fully supported by experienced laser and surgical specialists for their initial cases. Additionally, Web resources, chat lines, and videos are available for reference.

Patient Selection and Indications/ Contraindications

Some cases may not be indicated for ReLACS. The laser cannot pass through opaque media. Thus, in cases with small pupils, or misshapen ones like pictured in this heart shaped pupil (Fig. 13.1), the laser will not be able to make an effective capsulotomy or treat the lens. Of course, the laser can still be used in such cases to make the corneal incisions, including astigmatic cuts.

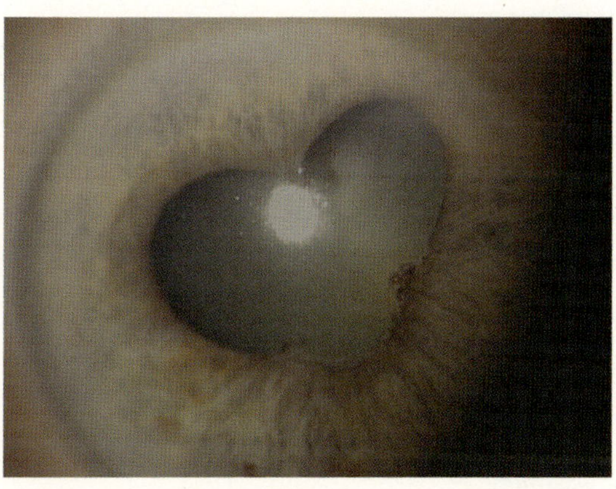

Fig. 13.1 Small pupil and posterior synechiae

In our practice, the vast majority of our lens replacement surgeries are done primarily for cataract. We select patients whose activities of daily living are reduced or impaired, in our findings and their opinion, due to the cataract. While we strive to provide the best possible refractive result and relative freedom from glasses postoperatively, safety and the health of the eye are our primary concerns and drive our patient selection. Not all patients are candidates for ReLACS, and there are additional criteria for patient selection that are dictated by the laser.

The suction ring requires reasonable exposure and patient cooperation, as well as a healthy cornea and conjunctiva. The surgeon should remember that docking the eye raises the pressure in the eye as in LASIK, which may stay elevated for three or more minutes in some cases. As such, patients with advanced glaucomatous optic neuropathy or retinal vaso-occlusive disease are not good candidates. The LenSx applanation lens is curved, so typically the intraocular pressure will increase less than LASIK, but patients with filtering blebs, compromised optic nerves, and extensive corneal scarring or previous surgery may not be good candidates for a suction ring. Some other ReLACS laser systems have non-applanating PIs and induce much less IOP rise, but one can still sees IOP readings go as high as 45 mmHg when in vitro testing is performed. The laser cannot pass through the iris, so patients that dilate poorly or have misshapen or decentered pupils may not be the best candidates for laser lens surgery. The laser likewise cannot pass through a white cataract. In cases of white cataracts, we use the laser to make the corneal incisions, including any astigmatic cuts, and the capsulotomy. The laser does an excellent job with what would otherwise be a difficult capsulotomy. We will often still use capsular dye in the eye to make sure that the capsule is completely free before we remove it. While the laser cannot penetrate a white cataract, it is able to penetrate dark, hard nuclei, the "root beer" cataracts in an impressive fashion. If the surgeon is able to see some retinal detail through the lens at the pre-op exam, even if highly colored, the laser can typically cut the nucleus.

Patient Acceptance and Counseling

I believe that ReLACS will become the preferred method of cataract surgery. Patients are extremely excited about ReLACS, and surgeons will find the procedure more precise and reproducible as well as add new dimensions to their surgery. One of the first things I noticed was how rapidly patients accepted ReLACS. All of us have been in the position where we have counseled a patient for our own "first procedure." We can all remember the first time we used a new technology with our own patients—our first LASIK procedure, wavefront-guided ablation, presbyopia correcting IOL. I was counseling these patients to be the first in the USA to have part of their surgery done with a new laser with no reference for them. Immediately, I saw that this procedure needed less explaining, education, or counseling than any other new technology we have introduced into our clinic.

All new technologies require a different amount of education for the patient to be able to make an informed choice. Why is ReLACS such an easy concept for them? As impressive as the performance of the laser was, the overwhelmingly positive response from the patients was even more exciting. Patients readily appreciate and choose "laser cataract surgery." Then again, many patients have always thought that cataract surgery was performed using a laser, which may have helped overcome any concerns they had about being the first US patients to undergo surgery with this new technology. How patients perceive a particular procedure is vital to how well it is accepted. I learned this with LASIK and FS laser flaps. LASIK results were never proven to be significantly better than PRK, but patients recognized the benefits of quicker recovery and a laser flap rather than one created by a metal keratome. ReLACS is much the same. While most of us are proud of how well we can make an incision with a blade or diamond knife and open a capsule with a bent needle, patients will perceive such steps done as more precise and safer if done by a laser. I believe that their perceptions will drive them to this technology. As with all of our surgeries, we try to avoid over promising any results. As exciting as a laser for cataract surgery is, we make sure that the patient understands there are no promises made as to superior results or safety with the laser. We stress to the patient that the procedure is still surgery, with many manual steps, and the potential for a wide range of complications, including vision loss. Finally, we make sure that every question is answered before the consent is signed.

Patient Preparation of the Day of Surgery

My experience with hundreds of cases with the LenSx laser thus far has helped me develop the surgical strategies for the entire case. We perform the surgery at our office based ambulatory surgery center in Houston, Texas. We examine and counsel each patient in the clinic area one last time, just before his or her surgery. This gives us a chance to further counsel the patient, perform a last slit lamp examination to aid in surgical planning, review the numbers of the laser parameters, and answer any final questions the patients or their families might have. Patients are then brought into the surgery center and placed on a rolling, electronic gurney (IFSK, Germany) in the preoperative area. This area is next to the laser itself. In the gurney, the patient is prepared in the usual fashion, with particular attention to dilation. When we are satisfied that maximal dilation is achieved, we move the patient, on the gurney to the laser area. The data for the corneal incisions, any astigmatic cuts, and the capsulotomy and lens cuts are reviewed and entered. The patient is then placed under the laser and the eye is docked, where the incisions, capsulotomy and nucleus fragmentation are performed then taken to the OR for the remainder of the procedure. We try to minimize the movement of the patient during the entire process, especially between the laser and the operating room, by keeping the patient in the gurney. If there is an incomplete capsulotomy, the capsulorhexis is at risk during any movement.

Preoperative Medications

Preoperative medications are quite similar to what we use for standard lens surgery. We sedate each patient, unless they decline, with oral sedatives including Valium or Versed. We also premedicate with antibiotics, steroids, and NSAIDS. We do pay more attention to the patient's dilation. The application of the suction ring and the deposition of laser energy inside the eye tend to bring the dilated pupil down. I believe that most of this effect is related to the energy used for the capsulotomy, as this is the energy delivered nearest to the pupil. To counteract this, we use Ocufen preoperatively, as well as 10% Neo and 1% Mydriacyl on every case. I also use SugharCaine every case routinely. I use a 5.5 or 6.0 mm capsulotomy, but the pupil does come down on occasion and may require "fishing" under the iris to get the cortex.

The Laser Portion of ReLACS

See Fig. 13.2.

Docking and Laser Treatment

The key to docking is to avoid tilt and have a flat, planar iris that is perpendicular to the laser beam. Furthermore, the PI needs to be well centered on the limbus. A tilted anterior segment, or decentered PI, will limit the surgical options, the placement of the primary incision at the limbus, affect the capsulotomy and may require the lens cuts to be repositioned. If there is any question to placement or design of any of the cuts, they can simply be left off of course and done manually. The LenSx laser does have a very useful fixation light that helps with positioning. Each laser will have

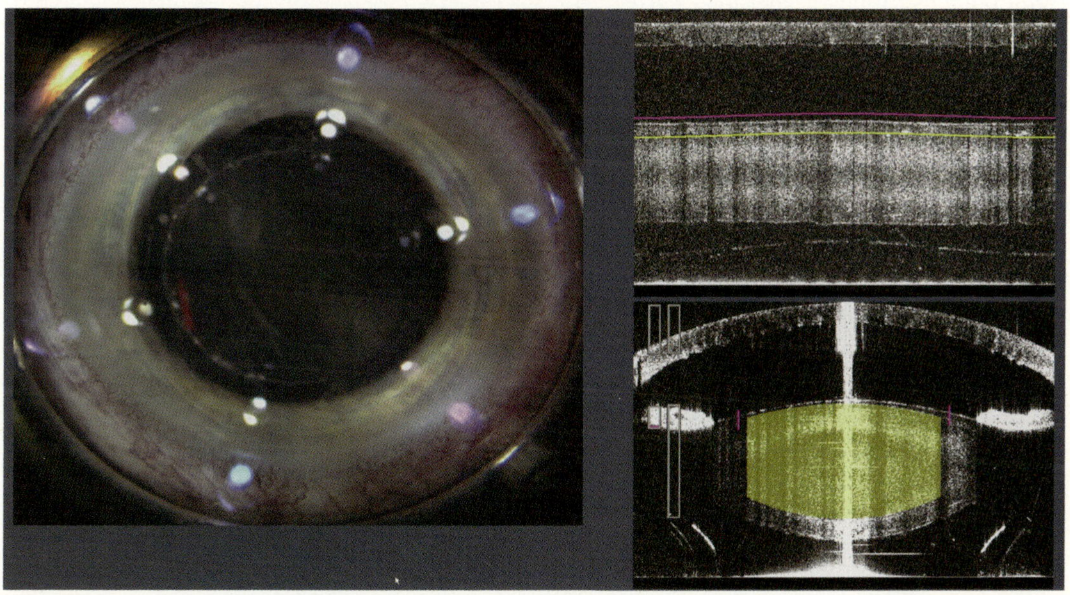

Fig. 13.2 The laser uses a real time OCT imaging system to map the eye and place the incisions, capsulotomy and nucleus cuts. On the *left*, a video image of the surgeon's view is overlaid with "drag and drop" incisions and the capsulotomy parameters. *Top right* is an OCT section of the cornea in which a multi-plane incision is planned and positioned. The *bottom right* image is a section through the anterior segment showing the lens for planning and placement of the nucleus cuts

its own tips and techniques to maximize the efficacy and safety of docking and the surgeon should familiarize themselves with them and practice with the laser before their first cases.

During the laser treatment it is important for the surgeon to carefully monitor the treatment as it progresses. Any poor placement or execution of laser cuts will affect the intraocular portion of the surgery. Decisions may need to be made during the treatment to modify or abort certain steps. We make it a point to hold the patient's head and talk them through the surgery. Of course, the status of the suction ring needs to be monitored so that any suction break will be recognized.

The Intraocular Portion of ReLACS

The key difference in the intraocular portion of laser cataract surgery is that the surgeon has to assess and recognize the steps that the laser has done before he begins the manual part of the surgery. In most instances, the laser has done about half of the case. For example, rather than performing the primary incision, the surgeon evaluates the laser incisions and determines whether the placement is correct, if they are complete and if any modifications are called for (see Fig. 13.3).

Incisions and Capsulotomy

Typically, there is no need to recut the main or the stab incisions. I simply verify they are open using a blunt instrument. I go in through the sideport at the first step, put in the SugharCaine and then the viscoelastic agent (Duovisc, Alcon Laboratories), and then open the primary. The surgeon should then carefully inspect the completeness of the capsulotomy and look for any tags. One needs to be careful to make sure that the capsulotomy is complete before removal to avoid any extension of an incomplete capsulorhexis. I use a cystotome or forceps to confirm that the capsulotomy is free. I then use a gentle hydrodissection under the edge of the capsule to detach the nucleus (see Fig. 13.4).

Nucleus

I currently use a four chop radial pattern with circular cuts as well. Divide and conquer works well. I am currently pre-chopping more, and use a new coaxial prechopper to separate the quadrants followed by phacoemulsification with an Ozil 45 Kelman Mini Flare Tip. We are often able to produce segments that do not need to be pre-chopped. Colleagues have asked me how this procedure will impact phacoemulsification. I think that it is the perfect partner for phacoemulsification, because it

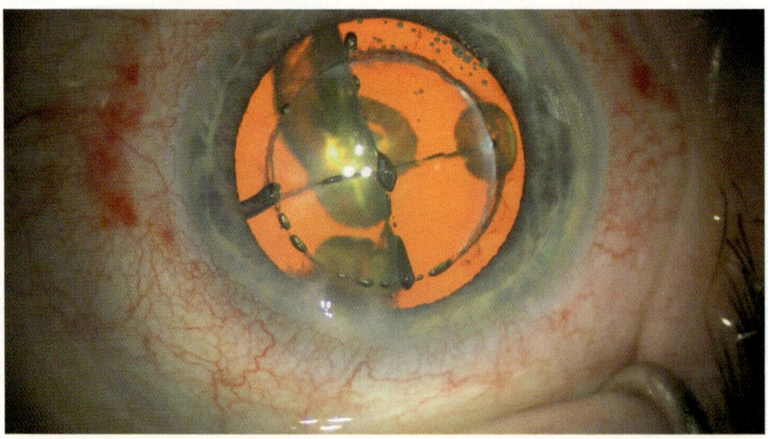

Fig. 13.3 The eye as it presents to the surgeon in the operating room. Corneal incisions have been made as well as the capsulotomy. In this case the cross-shaped nuclear chop pattern is also evident as are gas bubbles behind the posterior aspect of the nucleus and in front of the posterior cortex and capsule

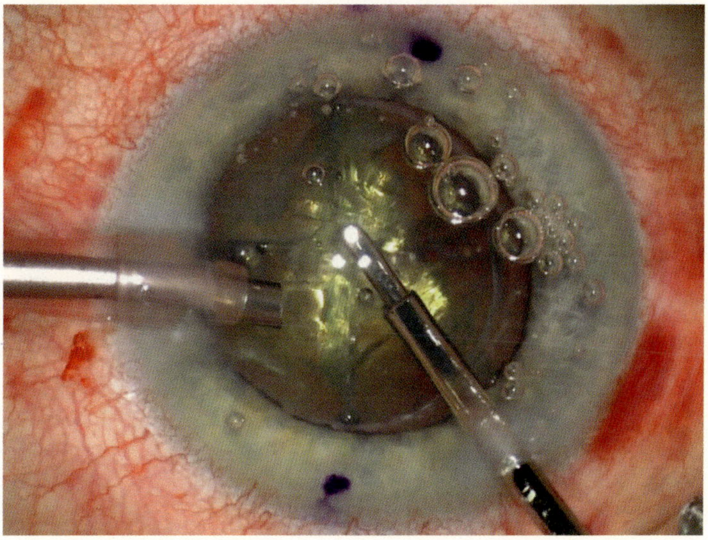

Fig. 13.4 A laser specific Coaxial Prechopper (Storz, ASICO Instruments) performing nuclear cracking

will allow us to optimize our phaco machines and our techniques. We can still use our preferred technique to remove the fragmented nucleus. For now, my staff and I are concentrating on optimizing our cataract surgeries using the INFINITI Vision System, OZil IP torsional ultrasound (Alcon Laboratories, Inc., Fort Worth, TX), with different tips and settings. I am impressed with this system's capacity for adjusting amplitude and flow rates in response to the varieties of nuclei. We are exploring how to adapt these technologies to use them together. For example, for soft nuclei, we can use a series of soft cylinders to liquefy the cataract, pick a specific phaco hand-piece tip and then perform I/A. In the majority of cases, we use the blend of FS laser and phacoemulsification to improve our speed, safety, and outcomes.

Cortex

The epinucleus is typically disengaged from the cortex by the LenSx laser's gas hydrodissection, and is easy to emulsify. Likewise, the cortex has a well-defined edge and aspirates well, often in one piece. The cortex may take longer to remove than the surgeon is used to in some cases, as one doesn't have the tags to grab. Additionally, I think that the gas pressure of the lens chop somehow plasters the cortex against the capsule harder. I try to hydrodissect it from the capsule at the start, or after the nucleus is out, come back, and run fluid or viscoelastic agent under it.

Clinical Results of FS Laser Capsulotomy and Lens Fragmentation: Safety and Outcomes

Safety

Patients want two things from eye surgery: safety and the best possible glasses-free vision as soon after surgery as possible. ReLACS helps to deliver both. I believe that FS lasers offer important advantages over manual cataract surgery in terms of safety:

1. Reduction in ultrasound energy
   My colleagues and I have shown that using that the laser to pre-chop the nucleus decreases phaco time, power, and time in the eye (Fig. 13.5) [5, 6].
2. Corneal and Endothelial Cell Safety
   We have shown, statistically significantly, that using the FS laser to pre-chop the nucleus and perform the capsulorhexis decreases phaco time and power. This leads to less endothelial cell loss. Comparing my laser cases' endothelial cell counts, to published series of post cataract endothelial cell counts, we can show a

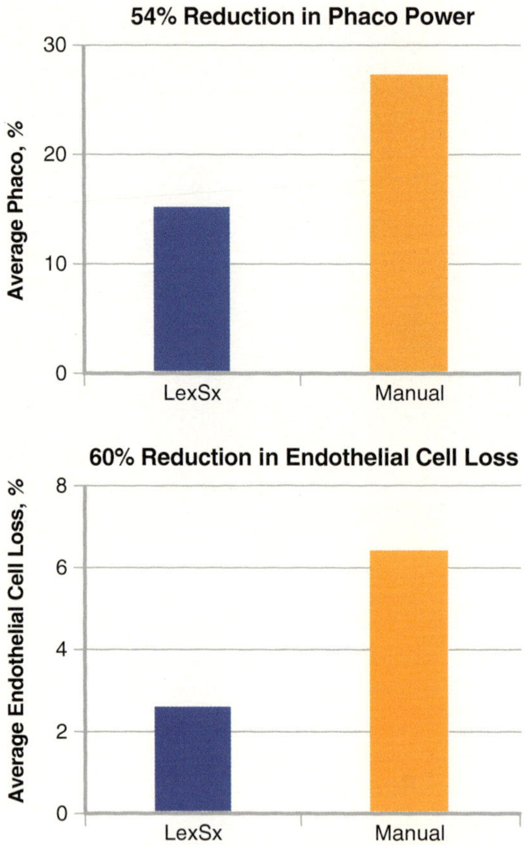

Fig. 13.5 In two separate studies the effect of the laser on phaco time and endothelial cell loss was studied. We found that there was a significant decrease in effective phacoemusification time and power delivered to the eye with the laser. Further, our cases with the laser showed less endothelial cell loss when compared to historical reported values [5, 6]. Image courtesy of Melvin Sarayaba

lower cell loss with the laser (Fig. 13.5). This may mean better results and fewer complications of cloudy corneas leading to PKPs and DSAEKs and the associated complications. Anecdotally, both my partner and I independently have felt that the corneas on day 1 are exceptionally clear, perhaps due to less intraocular maneuvering, less fluid flow in the eye during phacoemulsification and cortex irrigation and manipulation of the corneal tissue.

3. Improved Accuracy
We have shown that controlling and standardizing the size and centration of the capsulorhexis increases the accuracy of the spherical component of the IOL. (Presented Data ASCRS 2011 and in publication) The capsular contraction is more uniform so the IOL effective lens position (ELP) is less variable. If the lens is more accurate, then there may be fewer IOL exchanges and fewer secondary procedures like LASIK or PRK for accuracy, each of which carry their own surgical risks.
4. Reduced manipulation in difficult cases
FS lasers may have advantages for difficult cases as well, including cases of compromised zonules, traumatic cataracts, and pseudo exfoliation. With the laser, we do not have to stress the zonules when making the capsulorhexis or chopping the nucleus, which could mean fewer dislocated lenses and dropped nuclei. The laser also helps with white cataracts, dislocated lenses, and fibrous capsules. We are better able to optimize the dimensions and construction of the cataract incision and do it time after time with the laser [7]. This may lead to fewer wound leaks, improved lens stability and lower infection rates. Better wounds could also actually lower induced astigmatism, resulting in fewer secondary procedures with their associated risks. There are advantages for many of our more difficult cases as well. There is added safety in a "no touch" capsulorhexis in cases of compromised zonules, traumatic cataracts, and psuedoexfoliation.

Efficacy

Refractive Accuracy and IOL Results

Background

Modern cataract surgery with advanced technology IOLs (multifocal or accommodating) has raised patients' expectations as they hope for little-to-no dependence on spectacles or contact lenses postoperatively. Attaining this goal typically requires eliminating astigmatism and achieving a precise postoperative plano-refraction within ±0.25D [8].

The accuracy of predicting the necessary power for an IOL is directly related to the accuracy of several measurements. They include central corneal refractive power (keratometry readings), axial length (biometry), horizontal corneal diameter (horizontal white-to-white), anterior chamber depth, lenticular thickness, preoperative refraction, and the age of the patient [9, 10].

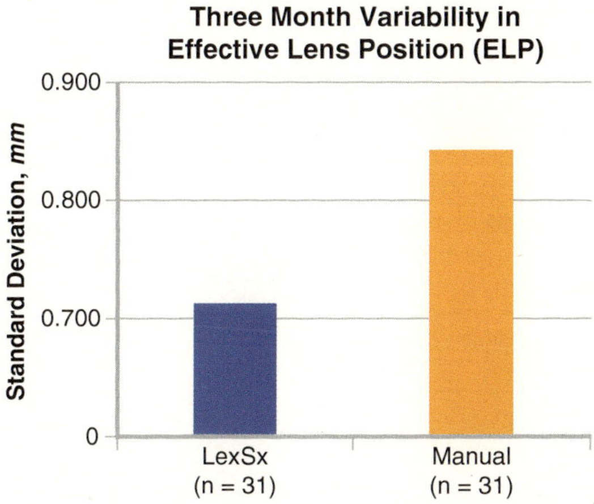

Fig. 13.6 Three-month variability in ELP, Refractive Predictability. The standard deviation (SD) was 0.40D and 0.60D in the study and control group, respectively ($p=0.04$). The laser group was also significantly improved compared to historical data acquired with other Crystalens models (Five-O, HD, and AO) ($p<0.05$) [16] Image courtesy of Melvin Sarayaba

A study done by Norrby showed that one of the largest sources of error in postoperative refraction is the estimation of effective lens position (ELP) [11]. If IOL is 0.5 mm posterior to the assumed plane, a 21D lens will produce only 20D of correction, producing a hyperopic outcome. Conversely, if IOL is 0.5 mm anterior to the assumed plane, a 21D lens will produce 22D of correction, producing a myopic outcome. The key to highly accurate IOL power calculation is being able to correctly predict ELP for any given patient and IOL [12]. The five most commonly used formulas in modern IOL power calculations assume that the IOL position will be at the plane of the lens zonules plus some estimation factor (A Constant or Surgeon Factor). It has been determined that capsulotomy size affects ELP. A 4 mm capsulorhexis results in longer postoperative ELP than does a 6 mm capsulorhexis for the type of IOL used [13–15].To ensure that an IOL's position in the bag matches the anticipated formula used to calculate its power, the capsulorhexis should be round, centered and smaller than the IOL's optic. This encourages consistent refractive outcomes [16].

Our Clinical Results

Study Design

We have specifically compared the predictability of ELP in eyes that had laser vs. manual capsulotomy. We also compared the refractive outcomes between the two groups. Thirty-one consecutive patients were analyzed, being treated with a 5.5 mm laser capsulotomy using the FS laser (LenSx Laser) and implanted with the same Crystalens AO IOL (Bausch and Lomb, Rochester, NY). Subjects were examined preoperatively and at 3 month postoperatively. Warren Hill's formula was used to determine ELP by entering axial length, keratometry, IOL power and refractive outcome to the calculator. To determine the accuracy of capsulotomy diameter, the intended and achieved diameters of the anterior capsulotomy were collected. The achieved capsulotomy diameter was measured by exporting intraoperative photos from 14 eyes to Scion Image (Scion Image, Corp.). Since the cornea magnifies intraocular image by approximately 15%, the measurement scale was set using the IOL optic diameter as reference and the capsulotomy diameter was measured vertically and horizontally. To determine refractive predictability, refractive spherical equivalent (SEQ) outcome was compared to target SEQ outcome. For the control group, the last 31 consecutive Crystalens patients that had manual capsulotomy were identified and analyzed similarly.

Results

Diameter Accuracy

Capsulotomy diameter was highly accurate with the use of the LenSx laser. The mean error between intended and achieved diameter was 0.04 mm (+/– 0.03 mm). There were no cases in which the delta between intended and achieved capsulotomy diameter was greater than 0.10 mm.

Effective Lens Position

The standard deviation of ELP was 0.76 and 0.90 mm for the LenSx and manual group, respectively. There was significant difference in the variability of ELP between the two groups (F test $p<0.05$) (Figs. 13.6, 13.7, and 13.8) [17].

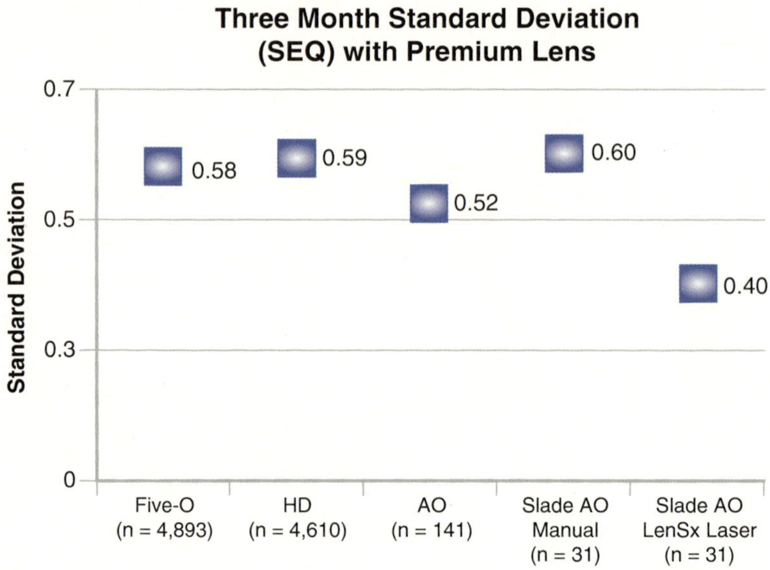

Fig. 13.7 Three-month variability in deviation from target refraction (Target SEQ minus Achieved SEQ). A laser capsulotomy creates accurate and reproducible diameter. Since capsulotomy diameter directly affects the position of the IOL, refractive predictability improvement is expected to follow, also as shown in this study. Assuming normal distribution of refractive outcomes, a variability of 0.60D in the manual group would result in 59% of patients achieving SEQ of ±0.50D. On the other hand, a variability of 0.40D in the laser group would result in 80% of patients achieving SEQ of ±0.50D. Image courtesy of Melvin Sarayaba

Treatment of Astigmatism

Background

Seventy-two percent of the US population has at least 0.5D of astigmatism. This will affect a patient's ability to see well after surgery without glasses if left uncorrected. Since the lens in these patients is being removed, corneal astigmatism is what is of interest and targeted. A literature review of current success rates with both toric IOLs and LRIs (limbal relaxing incisions) was performed. The best-published results we found for LRIs were from a study by Poll et al. [18] and showed an average postoperative residual astigmatism to be 0.42D ($n=77$) after Toric IOL and 0.46D ($n=115$) in the LRI group.

Our Clinical Studies and Results

We designed a study to compare our results with corneal incisions. We decided to put the incision at 9 mm rather than the limbus for efficacy and control with the laser. All incisions were done with the laser with direct image guidance and OCT depth measurement and placement at the desired position. We initially compared results with two groups, a manual LRI group ($N=20$) and a laser arcuate incision group ($n=15$).

In the LRI group, two limbal incisions were performed along the steepest meridian using preset guarded stainless steel knives with preset guards of 550-μm depths. The length of the incision depended on the degree of the astigmatism, and was calculated using a personal monogram. In the laser group, a new nomogram was calculated based on the nomogram created by Eric Donnenfeld (www.lricalculator.com) with his help. Even with this initial nomogram and experience, our results with the laser incisions exceeded that of our own and others' LRI results and were close to the Jed results [18] (Fig. 13.9). We believe that with refinement of the technique and feedback to the nomogram, we will be able to routinely exceed current results with treating astigmatism. We now routinely treat corneal astigmatism with arcuate cuts with the laser at the time of the lens surgery. These have the further advantage of being adjustable postoperatively at the slit lamp if a

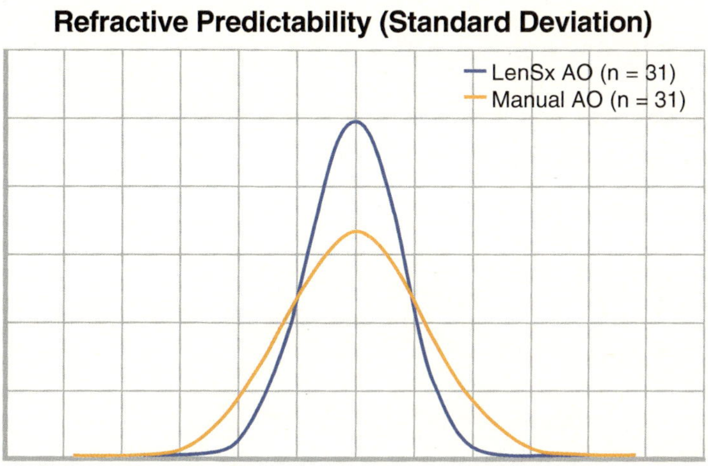

Fig. 13.8 Projected refractive predictability of LenSx vs. manual capsulotomy. The 21% difference is clinically significant as it represents more patients achieving their "promised" outcome. This study showed improved ELP and refractive predictability in eyes that had laser capsulotomy over those that had manual capsulotomy. Image courtesy of Melvin Sarayaba

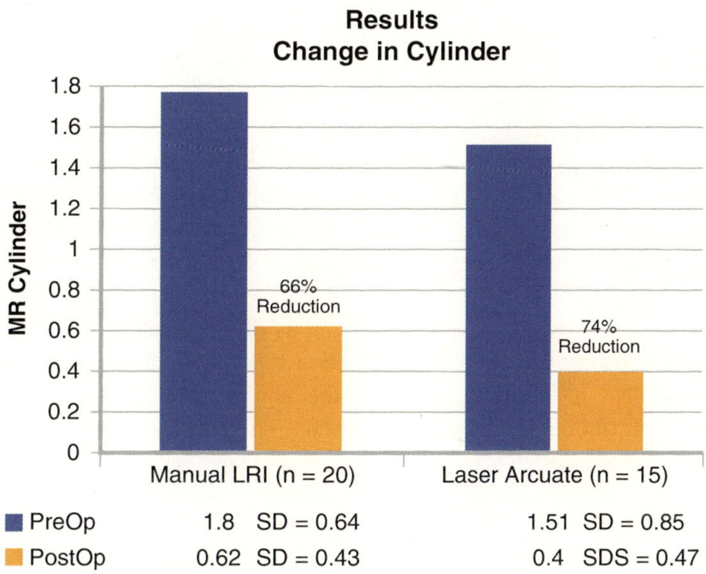

Fig. 13.9 Manual versus FS laser Astigmatic Incisions. The taller bars show the preop in both Manual LRI on the right, and in Laser Arcuate on the left pair while the shorter bars show postoperative astigmatism. Image courtesy of Melvin Sarayaba

portion of the incision is left unopened manually after the surgery.

Where to Locate the Laser in the ASC: OR Versus Outside the OR

We keep the LenSx laser in a separate, environment-controlled area, next to but not in the actual operating room. The OR is typically the most cost intensive area in the clinic or surgery center. We try to limit its use to what it is designed for: intraocular surgery. If the laser is placed inside the OR, the OR cannot be used for intraocular surgery while the laser procedure is being done. If the laser is placed outside of the OR, both the OR and laser area function as they are tasked. A single laser can thus serve multiple ORs. A second surgeon or medical ophthalmologist can perform the laser portion of the cases while and intraocular specialist rotates between the ORs, for maximum efficiency. While the laser adds total time to the patient treatment, the laser can cut the length of the intraocular portion of the cataract procedure in half.

Reimbursement Logistics

Much of the heated debate about ReLACS has not been about the capabilities of the technology, however, but rather its real-world practicality. Will patients seek it out? Is it economical? Who will pay for it? I have a unique perspective here. I have been performing ReLACS commercially in Houston since early 2010 on all of our practice's premium IOL patients and most of our other cataract patients.

Many surgeons I speak with ask me who is going to pay for the procedure. That is an easy one to answer: The patient. Patients have and always will pay for cataract surgery and the technology employed to make it better and safer. They pay for cataract surgery in one of three ways. The first two methods are indirect, where payments are "covered" by Medicare or private insurance. But keep in mind that Medicare is paid for by taxes and insurance by employer or self-funded premiums. The third method, self-pay, has always been the case for RLE-based procedures and more recently for those who choose to select an advanced implant as offered by presbyopia or astigmatic-correcting IOLs. So regardless of how it gets paid, the consumer always ultimately pays for cataract surgery, directly or through taxes.

My cataract candidates both comprehend the benefits of laser-based surgery for astigmatism or a presbyopia correcting IOL and are willing to pay an additional fee to receive them. Within this first year of having the technology, ReLACS has become the primary procedure I perform. The timing is right: Approximately 3.3 million cataract procedures are performed in the USA annually, and this figure will continue to rise as more baby boomers reach the age of 65 every year. In fact, projections show that 10,000 people turn 65 each day in the USA, and that the number of Americans aged 65 years and older will double in 7 years [19]. If the number of ophthalmic residents doubled tomorrow, there would still not be enough ophthalmologists to serve this coming growth.

In my experience, patients easily understand and prefer the use of the "laser" in ReLACS, and they seek it out. Yes, there are added costs. Medicare does not cover this advanced technology for astigmatism, however, but patients can assume these costs if they so choose. In other words, patients can elect to pay for what they decide provides a better postoperative result.

Summary

Patients and physicians alike always seek out better technology. I am excited about the potential of ReLACS and how it will continually improve with the input and experience of more and more surgeons. I am further greatly encouraged by the acceptance of the technology by other surgeons in the USA as more and more lasers are placed. With this larger user base, we are able to confer with one another and compare our results for continual refinement. Indeed, we have greatly accelerated the development of the technology with the synergy of our shared experiences.

The advantages of automating certain surgical steps are precision and reproducibility. Rather than measuring, positioning, and creating the incisions and capsulorhexis, we are now identifying and monitoring these steps. In my experience and that of my colleagues, controlling and standardizing the size and centration of the capsulotomy with a FS laser increases the accuracy of the spherical component of the IOL. The capsular contraction is more uniform, so the IOL's effective lens position is less variable. We have also achieved excellent results when using the laser to treat astigmatism at the time of cataract surgery. Thus, ReLACS contributes to a higher rate of glasses-free postoperative vision sooner after surgery. Of course, if the lens is more accurately positioned, fewer IOLs will require exchange, and fewer secondary procedures like LASIK or PRK will be necessary, which increases safety for the patient.

In conclusion, my initial experience with ReLACS has been extremely positive. In my years as a refractive and cataract surgeon, I have had the good fortune to be deeply involved with the introduction of a number of new technologies including LASIK, accommodating IOLs and the FS laser for corneal flaps. These technologies have profoundly changed what we are able to offer our patients. Yet what have we done in cataract surgery? Think of it. If an ophthalmologist from the 1980s appeared by time travel in our offices today, the phaco might be the only thing he would recognize. All of the diagnostic devices, drugs, excimers lasers, YAG lasers, etc. would be new to him. It is time to change the way we do cataract surgery. With this laser, I believe that we will soon have a cataract surgery technology that may enhance the performance of premium IOLs. We are facing a wave of baby boomers, all with extremely high expectations for their cataract surgery outcome.

Key Points

1. Since the laser does much of the cutting, planning surgery and data entry take on a new level of importance.
2. Coupling the laser to the eye with the docking process is the main technical challenge that is overcome with a learning curve.
3. Each laser has unique technical nuances, so strategies to streamline surgical workflow and optimizing treatment will vary.
4. Once in the OR, it is important to assess the laser's incisions BEFORE entering the eye, especially the completeness of the capsulotomy.
5. Pupil dilation may be difficult to maintain in some cases: use all means possible to maintain pharmacologic mydriasis.
6. ReLACS reduces endothelial cell loss and ultrasound power usage.
7. Early data demonstrates improved refractive outcomes from laser versus manual capsulotomy and LRI techniques for spherical equivalent and astigmatism, respectively.
8. Patients rapidly accept ReLACS, needing less explaining, education and/or counseling that any of the other new incremental technologies offered in refractive and cataract surgery.

References

1. Nagy Z. Use of the femtosecond laser in cataract surgery. Paper presented at the AAO annual meeting, San Francisco, CA, 27 Oct 2009
2. Cumming JS, Colvard DM, Dell SJ, Doane J, Fine IH, Hoffman RS, Packer M, Slade SG. Clinical evaluation of the Crystalens AT-45 accommodating intraocular lens: results of the U.S. Food and Drug Administration clinical trial. J Cataract Refract Surg. 2006;32(5): 812–25.
3. Nagy Z, Takacs A, Filkorn T, Sarayba M. Initial clinical evaluation of an intraocular femtosecond laser in cataract surgery. J Refract Surg. 2009;25(12): 1053–60.
4. Nagy Z. Intraocular femtosecond laser applications in cataract surgery: precise laser incisions may enable surgeons to deliver more reproducible outcomes. Cataract Refract Surg Today. 2009;9(9):29–30.
5. Wong T, Hingorani M, Lee V. Phacoemulsification time and power requirements in phaco chop and divide and conquer nucleofractis techniques. J Cataract Refract Surg. 2000;26(9):1374–8.
6. Storr-Paulsen A, Norregaard JC, Ahmed S, Storr-Paulsen T, Pedersen TH. Endothelial cell damage after cataract surgery: divide-and-conquer versus phaco-chop technique. J Cataract Refract Surg. 2008;34(6): 996–1000.
7. Slade SG, Culbertson WW, Krueger RR. Femtosecond lasers for refractive cataract surgery. Cataract Refract Surg Today. 2010;10(8):67–9.
8. Holladay JT. IOL power calculations for multifocal lenses. J Cataract Refract Surg Today. 2007;7:71–3.
9. Holladay JT, Prager TC, Ruiz RS, Lewis JW. Improving the predictability of intraocular lens calculations. Arch Ophthalmol. 1986;104:539–41.
10. Holladay JT, Prager TC, Chandler TY. A three-part system for refining intraocular lens power calculations. J Cataract Refract Surg. 1988;13:17–24.
11. Norrby S. Sources of error in intraocular lens power calculation. J Cataract Refract Surg. 2008;34(3):368–76.
12. Hill W. Intraocular lens power calculations: are we stuck in the past? Clin Experiment Ophthalmol. 2009; 37:761–2.
13. Aykan U, Bilge AH, Karadayi K. The effect of capsulorhexis size on development of posterior capsule opacification: small (4.5 to 5.0 mm) versus large (6.0 to 7.0 mm). Eur J Ophthalmol. 2003;13:541–5.
14. Hollick EJ, Spalton DJ, Meacock WR. The effect of capsulorhexis size on posterior capsular opacification: one-year results of a randomized prospective trial. Am J Ophthalmol. 1999;128:271–9.
15. Cekiç O, Batman C. The relationship between capsulorhexis size and anterior chamber depth relation. Ophthalmic Surg Lasers. 1999 Mar;30(3):185-90. Erratum in: Ophthalmic Surg Lasers 1999 Nov-Dec;30(9):714.

16. Nagy Z. Use of femtosecond laser system in cataract surgery. Presented at the XXVII Congress of the ESCRS, Barcelona, Spain, 15 Sept 2009
17. Stonecipher KG, Kezirian GM. Wavefront-optimized versus wavefront-guided LASIK for myopic astigmatism with the ALLEGRETTO WAVE: three-month results of a prospective FDA trial. J Refract Surg. 2008;24(4):S424–30.
18. Poll JT, Wang L, Koch DD, Weikert MP. Correction of astigmatism during cataract surgery: toric intraocular lens compared to peripheral corneal relaxing incisions. J Refract Surg. 2011;27(3): 165–71.
19. http://www.census.gov. Accessed Jun 2012

Global Implications of Refractive Laser Assisted Cataract Surgery (ReLACS)

14

Michael A. Lawless and Christopher Hodge,

Introduction/Background

With an estimated 19.5 million cataract procedures to be performed in the world in calendar year 2011, 3.4 million in the United States and 200,000 in Australia, any possible improvement to the safety and accuracy of cataract surgery is to be welcomed.

An operation as common as cataract surgery has implications, not just for the patient and the surgeon but also for a variety of stakeholders, and in this chapter I, [MAL], look at the implications for the following:

1. Patients and their relatives.
2. Ophthalmologists.
3. Government and regulatory authorities.
4. Private hospitals, ambulatory surgery centers, and health insurers.
5. Universities and teaching institutions.
6. Manufacturers.
7. Optometrists.

In addition to taking this global view I review the initial instillation of the laser into our center in Sydney where we began surgery on 6th April 2011. This is a multi-surgeon ambulatory surgery center with ten surgeons trained to use the device. These surgeons range from traditional cataract surgeons with an elderly population base to refractive lens surgeons.

M.A. Lawless, M.B.B.S., F.R.A.N.Z.C.O., (✉)
• C. Hodge, B.App.Sc. (Orth.)
Vision Eye Institute Chatswood, Level 3 270 Victoria Avenue, Chatswood, NSW 2067, Australia
e-mail: Michael.lawless@vgaustralia.com

Societal Implications of Reduced Complication Rates and Improved Outcomes

Capsular Rupture

The incidence of anterior capsular tears is 0.79–3.8% [1, 2] with 0.79% the reported incidence in the hands of one highly experienced surgeon. Of those with an anterior capsular tear in the experienced surgeon study, 40% extended to the posterior capsule and 20% required a vitrectomy. In Australia this would equate to approximately 320 vitrectomies per year (0.16% of the total cataract cases) and in the United States 5,440 vitrectomies annually. This is the best case scenario.

Unal et al. [3] has shown that when residents perform cataract surgery in teaching institutions, the anterior capsular tear rate is 5.3%, the rate of irregular capsulotomy 9.3% and posterior tear with vitreous loss 6.6%. At this figure there would be 13,200 vitrectomies in Australia annually and 224,000 vitrectomies associated with cataract surgery in the United States alone. The reality is somewhere in between the experienced surgeon and training resident rate.

In a retrospective audit Ang et al. [4] reported that 64.4% of patients with a posterior capsule tear required anterior vitrectomy. This led on average

R.R. Krueger et al. (eds.), *Textbook of Refractive Laser Assisted Cataract Surgery (ReLACS)*,
DOI 10.1007/978-1-4614-1010-2_14, © Springer Science+Business Media, LLC 2013

to an additional 3.9 visits over 11.7 weeks. Of these patients 51% suffered additional complications including a rise in intraocular pressure, persistent uveitis, cystoid macular oedema, retinal detachment, and retained soft lens matter requiring removal. Capsular rupture also leads to other problems; Hatch [5] has shown that endophthalmitis rates are significantly higher in cases with capsular rupture. Patients with capsular rupture were 9.56 times more likely to develop infection than uncomplicated cataract surgery patients. Bhagwandien [6] suggests the relationship is higher at just over 16 times more likely to develop infective endophthalmitis if capsular rupture occurs.

If laser-based surgery can produce a reproducibly round, centered, and intact anterior capsule, this alone would improve the safety of cataract surgery in a way that justifies the introduction of the technology.

Endophthalmitis

Endophthalmitis is the most feared complication of cataract surgery. The risk is between 0.06 and 0.39% in longitudinal studies conducted in various developed countries [7–10].

A systemic review of pooled data provided an average rate of 0.128% [11]. This review showed a significant increase in the rate of endophthalmitis after the year 2000, and incision type appeared to significantly influence the risk of endophthalmitis. If we take the pooled average rate of 0.128% then this means in Australia there would 256 cases of endophthalmitis and in the United States 4,352 per year.

Endophthalmitis after cataract surgery negatively impacts on self-perceived vision-related quality of life, resulting in poorer psychological well-being and a decreased ability to maintain a role in daily life compared to uncomplicated controls [12]. As well as the emotional and clinical costs, the additional financial cost of treating endophthalmitis, including hospital stay, has been calculated at €3,688 in a European study [13]. Schmier et al. [14] found that patients with endophthalmitis represented an increase in claims and reimbursements 1.45 greater than controls with each case resulting in approximately an extra $US 3,500 in Medicare billings. These are just the minimal increased costs to society as they do not include loss of productivity for patients and caregivers.

This analysis could be done at every level of the common complications of cataract surgery such as posterior capsule opacification, cystoid macular edema, vitreous loss, and corneal endothelial cell damage as well as other significant vision threatening complications such as retinal detachment, persistent cystoid macular edema, and endophthalmitis.

Refractive Outcomes

ReLACS should have an impact on the accuracy of surgery. Limited data is available on long-term cataract surgical outcomes. Kanthan et al. [15] have looked at the intermediate and longer term visual outcomes after cataract surgery in the Blue Mountains Eye Study. At 10-year follow-up 23% of eyes had presenting visual acuity of less than 20/40. Uncorrected refractive error accounted for 66% of these eyes. Uncorrected refractive error and posterior capsule opacification were the main causes of poor vision long term. In addition, in this study 26% of eyes without astigmatism before cataract surgery developed astigmatism during the early postoperative period, a proportion that increased to 41% during the long term after surgery. If the capsulotomy can be placed with greater precision and the wound can be improved by a laser-based approach, significant refractive errors following surgery should be reduced and there will be consequent improved visual quality and savings for society.

Stakeholders: Who Will Be Interested in This Technology?

ReLACS should enable the surgeon to perform the incisions, capsulotomy and nucleus removal more safely, more reproducibly and with greater precision. The beginning surgeon will be interested, but also the experienced surgeon. Those interested will be the risk averse, those who seek perfection, those who want a form of "insurance" that their surgery will be better than conventional methods, and for those who wish to achieve greater spectacle independence.

In short this means *every* patient, relative and surgeon will be interested in this technology.

Let's look at some of the stakeholders.

Patients and Their Relatives

The patient with a cataract or the person seeking refractive lens surgery would understand that a laser-based approach can add precision and reproducibility. The question they would ask is how this will apply to me as an individual.

1. How much extra benefit will I gain from having this procedure?
   The procedure should raise the bar of accuracy and safety at every level, but how far the bar is raised is not clear. For example, if we quote the anterior capsular tear rate of a middle range of 2%, this can probably either be eliminated or reduced to <0.2% so that patient can be told that the tear rate for them will go from approximately 2 out of a 100 to about 1 in 500. If by a better quality and more secure incision the endophthalmitis rate can be reduced from 0.128% to half this value, this would also resonate with an individual patient.
2. Are there particular eye problems where improved safety may be even greater?
   For example, the patient with pseudoexfoliation or a reduced endothelial cell count can be counselled that the safety impact in their circumstances will be greater than that of the general population because they are more at risk of capsule problems and endothelial cell loss. There are individual patients who will need to be told that they are unsuitable for surgery even though it would be potentially advantageous, such as those with small pupils (small pupil surgery cannot be performed with a laser approach as it is a closed system). For these patients it may be that simply performing the incisions will be appropriate and then the wound opened and the pupil manually increased with OVD or other methods. Those with a narrow palpebral fissure may need to be excluded as well. The current devices lock onto the eye, and as such must have adequate orbital rim clearance. For example, the system I am familiar with, the Alcon LenSx System, uses a curved applanation plate which is a "one size fits all." Our experience is that with smaller hyperopic eyes with steeper corneas it is more difficult to achieve suction and full contact applanation, and some of these patients are unable to be treated until improvements in the applanation mechanism can allow for unusually shaped eyes to be treated. These patients need to decide whether they wish to proceed with conventional surgery or wait until technology catches up with their anatomy.
3. What will this cost me?
   This is front and center in a patient's mind. I can only say what I personally charge in Sydney. My conventional cataract surgical fee is $US 2,400 and to have surgery performed with a laser approach is an extra $US 900, making the cost $US 3,300 per eye, or a 37% increase. In the middle class area in which I practice there has been little or no price resistance to this increase as patients perceive the advantages that it can convey and consider it a value proposition. A patient and their relatives in a regional center will often ask: "this is not available in my center, is it necessary to travel?" In Australia, the distances can be large. Some patients are traveling interstate and from rural areas in order to avail themselves of this technology, but the majority are not. Most are seeking the advice of their current ophthalmologist and are either proceeding with conventional surgery or waiting until it is available in their area.

The Ophthalmic Surgeon

1. What they may think:
   The view of ophthalmologists range from "this is ridiculous: I can perform a capsulotomy with a needle and forceps perfectly well and I am not interested in this technology" to "how can I get

the first one in my region? I need this and want to offer it to my patients." Some of these opinions are based on fear and ignorance, but a skeptical view at this point is not unreasonable.

2. Where is the proof?

   A surgeon can reasonably ask: where is the proof for the claims of improved safety and efficacy? Nagy [16] demonstrated that in a porcine eye the capsulotomy diameter was more precise and rounder than with a manual technique, and the chance of achieving a capsulotomy diameter within 0.25% of intended was 100% in the capsulotomy group and 10% in the manual group. Palanker et al. [17] demonstrated a mean circularity of 0.942 in 29 lasered eyes compared with 0.774 in 30 manual eyes with a 12 fold improvement in the precision of the capsulotomy diameter. More recently Friedman [18] and authors have showed the deviation from the intended diameter was 29 μm ± 26 (SD) for the laser technique and 337 ± 258 μm for the manual technique with a mean deviation from circularity was 6 and 20%, respectively.

   Both Nagy and Friedman [16, 18] also show that the capsule strength is as good, or greater, than a manual capsulorrhexis and the smoothness of the capsulotomy edge is similar to that of a manual capsulotomy. These benefits coexist with an approximately 50% reduction in both average phaco power and effective phaco time. These studies represent small patient cohorts, and a surgeon could reasonably say "well show me more data over a larger cohort." Some surgeons and patients will wish to wait for confirmation of the initial clinical data, and this is their choice.

3. Will the transition be difficult?

   My personal view is that the surgical transition to ReLACS should be easier for those who are already accustomed to femtosecond (FS) LASIK given that the application of a suction device and manipulation of data during the procedure are second nature to a FS LASIK surgeon and unfamiliar to a general cataract surgeon. Our practice of ten visiting surgeons has shown that this has been the case. Over the initial 200 cases there was a statistically significant difference in terms of intraoperative issues between FS LASIK surgeons and general cataract surgeons (data submitted for publication). With well-trained technical staff though, the transition to laser-based cataract surgery will be made easier for the general cataract surgeons.

4. Will my surgical volume increase or decrease?

   The simple answer is that if the surgery is safer and more accurate, more patients will avail themselves of the surgery over time with an overall increase in volume. My personal view is that not all surgeons will share in this increase. Some will increase and some will decrease. If a surgeon decides to access the technology, they have to decide if it will be in their own ambulatory center or if a local hospital will purchase the technology. As a general rule, an institution, whether it is an ambulatory surgical center, a private hospital, or a public hospital, would need to be doing a minimum of 1,000 cataract procedures per year to justify the instillation of this technology under current terms. As the technology evolves and more competition enters the market, the cost structure may be applicable to smaller centers, but my personal feeling is that FS laser technology will lead to the closure of small centers doing only 200–300 cases per year with the consolidation of surgery into centers performing more surgery. I believe this trend will increase, which will be a dilemma for regional centers, as it may be that both surgeons and patients will need to travel to avail themselves of this technology.

5. What are the technology choices and how will surgical workflow be affected?

   One could not make a choice in 2011 on the basis of technology differences as the current systems all appear to be well thought out. As such, choices will be based more on availability, technical support, and price. Once a laser system is installed, the surgeon will have to decide, can he or she delegate part of the procedure, and in particular can the laser portion of the procedure be delegated to either other ophthalmologists or other staff (MD or paraprofessional) to allow for an increase in volume and flow? Having just been through an instillation and being involved with ten surgeons now training on the device, it is absolutely clear that none of this can be delegated in its current form. A few years from now, the situation may be different. Right now, FS laser technology makes a relatively easy operation more difficult for the surgeon requiring more concentration and manual skill, and leads to an overall increase in operating time. For the patient, ReLACS technology leads to clear benefits. For the surgeon, it is at the present time a more difficult way to perform what was for them a relatively routine and comfortable operation. To delegate any part of the procedure at this stage seems imprudent. To those surgeons who feel that their role as a surgeon is under threat, I would say relax and appreciate the introduction of this technology for the improved satisfaction it can bring to you as a professional and the improved safety and efficacy it can bring to your patients as a benefit.

Government and Regulatory Authorities

Governments are in the business of rationing goods and services because they cannot provide everything society wants. They will need to look at the finances involved, and it will take some years of accurate data accumulation to make a decision at a government level as to whether this technology translates into a benefit for society in a way that requires it to be subsidized at a federal level? If one were to extrapolate the situation that has evolved at our surgical center, adding $US 900 to the cost of a procedure with 200,000 procedures performed in Australia in any given year would add $US 180,000,000 to the cost of performing cataract surgery. This will be borne by the patient and the patient's relatives. Should the government contribute? Governments will make their own decisions based on data, pressure from relevant groups (manufacturers, the providers of ambulatory surgery centers, and private hospitals), and in particular from an aging voting demographic that feels it could benefit from this surgery and would like the technology to be subsidized. At this stage, there is no government in the world that appears interested in underwriting the additional costs of this procedure in either the public or private sector, but it is only barely on their radar in 2011.

Private Hospitals, Ambulatory Surgery Centers, Health Insurers

Private hospitals and ambulatory surgery centers will, as a general rule, be confident they are able to perform approximately 1,000 procedures per year to make ReLACS technology economically feasible. These devices are difficult and expensive to manufacture, and will not be able to be rolled out quickly. Once installed, they require intensive technical support and surgeon training. Private hospitals and ambulatory surgery centers will have to decide whether they will take a loss-leader position and whether they can link the FS laser to other products from the manufacturer to offset the initial capital cost (i.e., whether it can be linked to IOL supply and custom and pick packs). There are many issues to deal with, but the underlying premise is an understanding that this technology will dominate cataract surgery in the developed world within the next 5 years, and that the concentration of surgery within a smaller number of larger facilities is also likely to occur, with the consequence that smaller facilities will be likely to move their focus away from ophthalmology.

Universities and Training Facilities

Those responsible for training resident ophthalmologists have to work out how they place these systems in what are generally public facilities in most parts of the world, and have to convince their government or private backers that this is an appropriate technology for a training institution. They therefore must decide if they are adding ReLACS for safety or for safety and accuracy. Safety can be easily measured over time, with consequent benefits for the individual patient and society. Accuracy is a different matter. If teaching hospitals are adding FS laser technology partly to improve the accuracy of procedures, they must have an intraocular lens supply that will allow benefit to be gained from a more accurate procedure. Many public facilities do not offer a range of toric, multifocal, or accommodative lenses to make best use of the perceived increased accuracy of ReLACS. In addition to the supply of a new range of IOL's, such hospitals would need to have a mindset that incorporates the goal of surgical accuracy into clinical decision making. This is generally done well outside the training milieu and in the private sector where patients are undergoing surgery with a refractive emphasis foremost (as the safety profile has already been optimized), as opposed to a public or training facility where they are having the procedure on therapeutic grounds and where the emphasis on safety may be foremost.

Those responsible for training will also be concerned that a laser-based cataract surgery rollout may devalue other surgical skills. The short answer is that yes, it will, just as phacoemulsification decreased the ability of residents to master suturing techniques, and in my view decreased their ability to handle penetrating trauma. This is the fate and reality of improvements on the one hand causing collateral damage on the other, and those responsible for training need to think of innovative ways to help trainees master some of these technical skills.

Industry

Manufacturers wish to have a return on their investment, and that investment has been considerable. Their dilemma is, are FS lasers for premium refractive cataract surgery or regular cataract surgery as well? In many markets, local conditions will determine how industry positions FS laser technology. However, in the end, despite the distortions imposed by reimbursement, government regulators and historical norms, a procedure that is safer and more accurate will resonate with patients and society. If the safety and accuracy bar can be raised, this combination will mean that the technology becomes widespread.

At present (mid-2011), manufacturers are facing the dilemma of a rollout which is slower than they (and surgeons) would like. Our experience in Australia has shown that the slow rollout has some advantage, because if FS lasers were quickly available at a many sites there is just not enough technical support to take the surgeons through the learning curve. Although the slow rollout will be aggravating for many surgeons, it is inevitable and probably to their benefit as experience is gained and modifications and improvements are made to technique, hardware and software. Many of the manufacturers have an interest in other products such as custom packs and intraocular lenses, and companies without that capability may need to offer better technology and/or greater flexibility.

Optometrists

Optometrists are naturally interested in this technology. At a basic level they give advice to patients on a daily basis and are trusted advisers. They must have an understanding of ReLACS technology and what it can offer, and for those patients for whom it may have a greater initial safety impact. Education is needed to give appropriate advice, although increased awareness of FS laser technology may impact traditional referral patterns whereby the optometrist would generally refer to a local ophthalmologist who may or may not have access to the technology.

Personal Experience with ReLACS: Lessons Learned

We performed our first surgeries with the Alcon LenSx system in Sydney on 6th April 2011. Previously, I had had the privilege of visiting Professor Zoltan Nagy in Budapest and perform surgery on his system.

Our facility is a group private multispecialty practice with its own ambulatory day surgery center and refractive laser facility located in suburban Sydney, 15 min from the Central Business District in a middle class locality.

We have located the laser in a dedicated room adjacent to the entrance of the ambulatory day

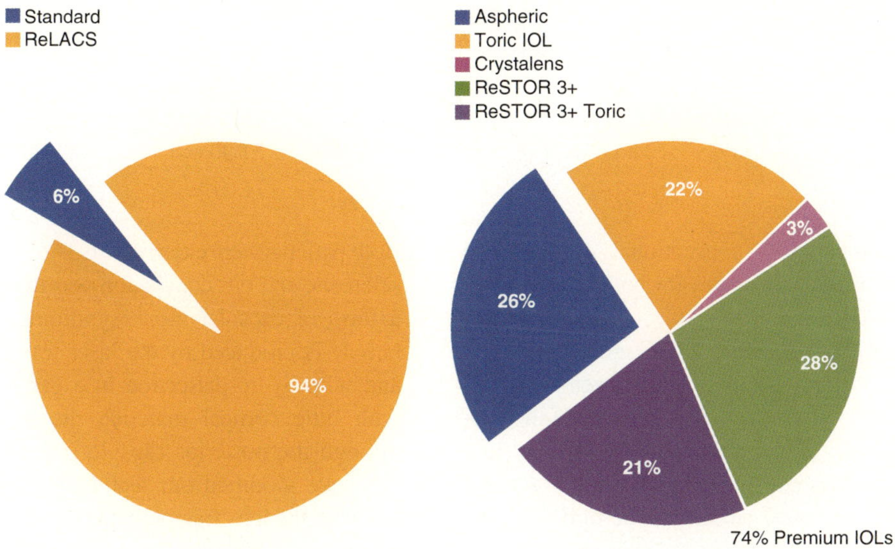

Fig. 14.1 Percentage of standard cataract procedures compared to ReLACS following the introduction of FS technology

surgery center. The patient walks with assistance into the laser room and is placed on a stretcher, where the procedure is performed under topical anesthesia. The patient is then escorted and walks approximately 3 m to the ambulatory surgery facility where they are then given intravenous sedation and the lens removal and IOL implantation performed under topical anesthesia with intravenous sedation.

The lessons we have learnt in the first 2 months are as follows:

1. Patient and surgeon acceptance of the approximately 30% increase in the surgical fee has been very easy.

   Both patients and surgeons perceive the value of ReLACS to be real and significant, so there has been almost no reluctance to proceed. The surgeons have introduced the technology to their patients in a variety of ways. All of my patients who are technically suitable (i.e., those who have large enough pupils and an appropriate palpebral fissure and orbit), receive ReLACS. Some surgeons have been more circumspect, but this is very quickly moving to a level where it is the preferred mechanism for all patients who are technically suitable. Figure 14.1 shows the breakdown of my patients undergoing standard cataract surgery compared to ReLACS since the introduction of the LenSx unit. A breakdown of the IOLs implanted over this time period is also provided.
2. The process is quite comfortable for patients; however, technical difficulty for surgeons has increased.

   To aid patients we use oral Temazepam 45 min prior to the laser procedure. The docking applanation and procedure is rated as easy from a patient perspective. From a surgeon's perspective, however, docking is quite difficult. Mastery of docking entails a stressful learning curve with more technical demands and increases the length of time for the cataract procedure as a whole. In addition OR time is also increased during early cases. In my initial 50 eyes, the average time spent in the operating theater was 19 min with a range of 15–23 min. To be clear, this time is the time spent in the ambulatory surgery center once the LenSx procedure has been performed, and represents an average increase of approximately 4 min per case compared to conventional surgery. The revised operational flow has also had an impact on the overall time a patient will spend at the center. The overall average length of stay for the patients is approximately 1 h and 10 min longer for patients undergoing the LenSx proce-

Table 14.1 Comparison of surgery times between conventional phacoemulsification and ReLACS

	Standard cataract		ReLACS (Alcon LenSx)	
	Average time	Range	Average time	Range
Time spent in Ambulatory Center	15.66 min	11–19 min	19.83 min	15–23 min
Total length of stay	2 h 27 min	2 h 10 min to 3 h 15 min	3 h 40 min	3 h to 4 h 30 min

dure compared to conventional surgery. The average times and ranges for both surgeries are provided in Table 14.1.

3. Suction is not possible in all patients.
   In a minority of patients I have been unable to achieve good suction. This is because the current curved applanation under relatively low pressure does not sit well in those with a small palpebral fissure, smaller hyperopic eyes or steep corneas. There is also a learning curve in this regard, and both the ability to obtain suction and the centration of the applanation has improved as I have gained more experience.
4. The capsulotomy is beautiful to behold as are the corneal incisions. Adjustments to the procedure were initially necessary, though.
   The precision of the surgery makes my conventional capsulotomies and incisions appear crude in comparison. In the beginning we had problems with pupils constricting during the laser capsulotomy. This is because the Z-axis offset above and below the capsulotomy was too generous resulting in a greater length of time and energy being dissipated. Decreasing these Z axis offsets has resolved the issue and pupil constriction during laser capsulotomy is no longer a problem. The initial anterior and posterior offsets were set at 300 μm eventually reducing to 150 μm.

   In our facility one of the surgeons has had two separate incidences of capsular block syndrome after laser treatment. In both cases the laser ablation was performed without incident by standard practice of capsulotomy, followed by phacofragmentation and then corneal incisions. In the operating room the wound was opened, OVD injected and the anterior chamber deepened normally. The capsulotomy was completed without incident. Gas bubbles were noted posterior to the lens fragmentation pattern. During hydro-dissection a posterior capsule rupture occurred. In both cases the cataract was then removed via a vitreoretinal approach. Both patients were elderly with 3+ to 4+ nuclear sclerosis, and our conclusion was that this was a form of capsular block syndrome. The gas bubble is produced by the laser fragmentation and with hydro-dissection in a dense nucleus with little cortical material, the gas pushed through the posterior capsule (see Fig. 14.2). We have modified our technique moving the offset of the lens fragmentation from the initial settings of 800 μm to a minimum 1,200 μm from the posterior capsule; we decompress the eye prior to hydro-dissection and are more cautious about the use of hydro-dissection. These two cases were adverse events reported to both the Australian TGA (Therapeutic Goods Administration) and the American FDA.

   With ReLACS, cortical removal is different from a standard cataract operation, as there are fewer tags or strands of cortical material. The cortical material needs to be removed in a more painstaking and piecemeal fashion.
5. Subconjunctival hemorrhages.
   Subconjunctival hemorrhages are common and the patients are informed of these prior to discharge.

Postscript

Now at mid September 2011 our unit at Chatswood has performed 620 fs laser cataract procedures. Of these I have performed 199. The only problems I have personally encountered are two suction breaks during the procedure which meant that the incisions had to be completed manually, five cases of pupillary constriction after the laser capsulotomy and three small anterior capsular tags. All these occurred in the first 50 cases and none in the subsequent 149. None were visually threatening or led to any detrimental effect for patients. In particular I have not experienced anterior capsular tears nor capsular block syndrome.

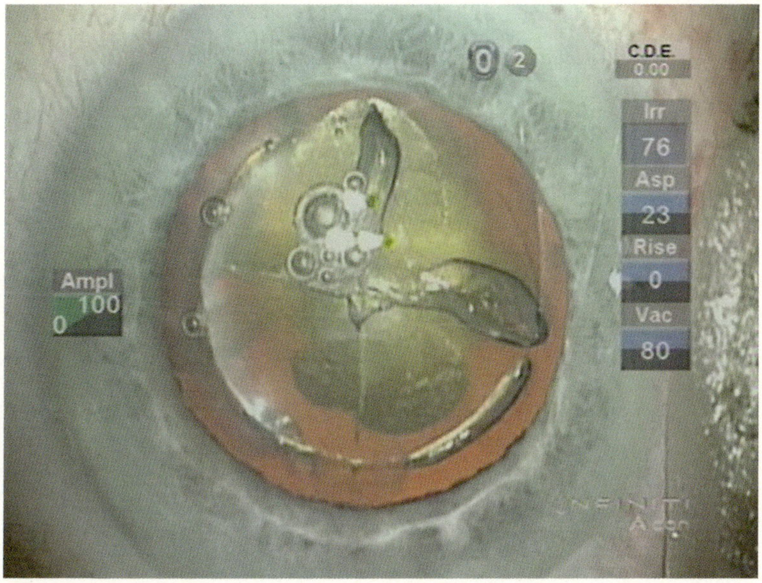

Fig. 14.2 Image immediately following FS laser delivery in ReLACS

With changes in software, technique and pharmacological manipulation, in experienced hands the complication rate would seem to be very close to zero. The technique and technology is evolving. We have had a new laser installed after 4 months and a number of software changes, and with this the incision has moved from a standard incision to a reverse trapezoidal three plane incision 1.8 mm in length. Most capsulotomies are now free, without adhesive tags, and this in combination with improvements in nucleus division have enabled me to modify how I approach these cases. For example, one improvement has been moving to a technique recently described by Dr. Steve Slade which involves minimal intraocular manipulation (personal communication, 2011). OVD is injected and then the phaco handpiece is used to remove the anterior capsule and nucleus without the need for hydro-dissection or nucleus chopping.

With an aspheric intraocular lens, my mean absolute difference from intended spherical equivalent is 0.24 dioptres (±0.15 D), which is better than I was able to achieve with a manual technique. An analysis of the initial cases completed with the assistance of the LenSx FS laser has shown a reduction in terms of both mean absolute mean prediction error and the standard deviation compared to a small cohort of patients undertaking routine surgery. The comparative group was assessed retrospectively; however, the cases represent consecutive surgeries undertaken immediately prior to the installation of the laser unit.

Table 14.2 Results of LenSx group vs. routine group

	LenSx group ($N=21$)	Routine group ($N=16$)
Pre-op sphere	−0.08 ± 4.51 D	0.91 ± 2.21 D
Pre-op cylinder	−0.71 ± 0.38 D	−0.53 ± 0.35 D
Pre-op SE	−0.43 ± 0.45 D	0.64 ± 2.28 D
Post-op sphere	−0.31 ± 0.79 D	0.23 ± 0.77 D
Post-op cylinder	−0.43 ± 0.30 D	−0.56 ± 0.50 D
Post-op SE	−0.52 ± 0.82 D	−0.05 ± 0.61 D

Mann-Whitney comparison was used to ensure that the two groups were statistically similar preoperatively ($P=0.368$). The difference in mean absolute error from the intended correction suggests an improvement for the delivery in ReLACS cohort although this did not reach statistical significance ($P=0.068$). The results are listed in Tables 14.2 and 14.3.

The observation that it will take some years and a large volume of cases to show improved safety and efficacy with ReLACS vs. manual techniques, will, I think, prove to be incorrect.

As we have moved beyond the first 2 months of the learning curve, we now feel much more

Table 14.3 Difference in mean absolute error from intended correction

	LenSx group	Routine group
Absolute mean prediction error	0.27±0.16 D	0.45±0.38 D
Minimum	0.01 D	0.00 D
Maximum	0.54 D	1.63 D

confident as a team of surgeons that this is the right technology for patients. Laser surgery turns cataract and refractive lensectomy surgery from a relatively easy quick procedure into a more technically demanding and lengthy procedure for the surgeon. Despite this, the benefits to patients are obvious to those surgeons who have experienced the technology, and patients are comfortable that they are receiving the best possible care and keen to avail themselves of ReLACS technology.

Key Points

1. Improvements in capsulotomy alone justify the introduction of ReLACS technology.
2. While easy for patients, the addition of ReLACS turns cataract and refractive lensectomy surgery from a relatively quick procedure into a more technically demanding and lengthy procedure for the surgeon.
3. Surgeons with experience performing FS LASIK surgery may find the transition easier.
4. Initial cases will require more time in the operating room as well as at the laser.
5. Patient acceptance of increased costs has been rapid due to perceived increased safety.
6. Once established, ReLACS technology will lead to the closure of small centers doing 200–300 cases per year with the amalgamation and concentration of surgery into centers performing more surgery.

References

1. Marques FF, Marques DM, Osher RH, Osher JM. Phakic anterior capsular tears during cataract surgery. J Cataract Refract Surg. 2005;32(10):1638–42.
2. Ng DT, Rowe NA, Francis IC, et al. Intraoperative complications of 1,000 phacoemulsification procedures: a prospective study. J Cataract Refract Surg. 1998;24(10):1390–5.
3. Unal M, Yucel I, Sarici A, et al. Phacoemulsification with topical anaesthesia: resident experience. J Cataract Refract Surg. 2006;32:1361–5.
4. Ang GS, Whyte IF. Effect and outcomes of posterior capsule rupture in a district general hospital setting. J Cataract Refract Surg. 2006;32(4):623–7.
5. Hatch WV, Cernat G, Wong D, et al. Risk factors for acute endophthalmitis after cataract surgery: a population based study. Ophthalmology. 2009;116(3): 425–30.
6. Bhagwandien AC, Cheng YY, Wolfs RC, et al. Relationship between retinal detachment and biometry in 4,262 cataractous eyes. Ophthalmology. 2006; 113(4):643–9.
7. Endophthalmitis Study Group, ESCRS. Prophylaxis of post-operative endophthalmitis following cataract surgery: results of the ESCRS multicenter study and identification of risk factors. J Cataract Refract Surg. 2007;33(6):978–88.
8. Patwardhan A, Rao GP, Saha K, Craig EA. Incidents and outcomes evaluation of endophthalmitis management after phacoemulsification and three-piece silicone intraocular lens implantation over six years in a single eye unit. J Cataract Refract Surg. 2006;32(6): 1018–21.
9. Haapala TT, Nelimarkka L, Saari JM, et al. Endophthalmitis following cataract surgery in South-West Finland from 1987 to 2000. Graefes Arch Clin Exp Opthalmol. 2005;243(100):1010–7.
10. Montan P, Lundstrom M, Stenevi U, Thorburn W. Endophthalmitis following cataract surgery in Sweden: The 1998 National Prospective Survey. Acta Ophthalmol Scand. 2001;80(3):258–61.
11. Taban M, Behrens A, Newcomb RL, et al. Acute endophthalmitis following cataract surgery: a systematic review of the literature. Arch Ophthalmol. 2005;123(5):613–20.
12. Clark A, Ng JQ, Morlet N, et al. Quality of life after post-operative endophthalmitis. Clin Exp Ophthalmol. 2008;36(6):526–31.
13. Colin X, Berdeaux G, Lafuma A, et al. Inpatient costs of endophthalmitis evaluated for the whole of France. Appl Econ Health Policy 8(1):53–60.
14. Schmier JK, Halpern MT, Covert DW, et al. Evaluation of Medicare costs of endophthalmitis among patients after cataract surgery. Ophthalmology. 2007; 114(6):1094–9.
15. Kanthan GL, Mitchel P, Burlutsky G, Wang JJ. Intermediate and longer term visual outcomes after cataract surgery: The Blue Mountains Eye Study. Clin Exp Ophthalmol. 2011;39:201–6.
16. Nagy Z, Takacs A, Filkorn T, Sarayba M. Initial clinical evaluation of an intraocular femtosecond laser in cataract surgery. J Refract Surg. 2009;25:1053–60.
17. Palanker DV, Blumenkranz MS, Andersen D, et al. Femtosecond laser assisted cataract surgery with integrated optical coherence tomography. Sci Transl Med. 2010;2:58ra85.
18. Friedman NJ, Palanker DV, Schuele G, Andersen D, et al. Femtosecond laser capsulotomy. J Cataract Refract Surg. 2011;37(7):1189–98.

Commercially Available Systems: Alcon/LenSx

15

Zoltan Z. Nagy

Background and Motivation

The development of femtosecond (FS) lasers in ophthalmology has been reviewed elsewhere (Chaps. 3 and 4). Their widespread application in corneal refractive surgery is one of the factors that led to an overall improvement in the clinical results of LASIK during the decade from 1995 to 2005, when rates of postoperative 20/20 UCVA increased from approximately 50–60% to nearly 90%. Similar to early stage corneal refractive surgery, rates of postoperative 20/20 UCVA in refractive cataract surgery currently stand at around 50–60%, affecting both distance and near corrections [1–3].

Beginning around 2007, several factors critical for commercial innovation came together to support the development of FS lasers for refractive cataract surgery. These included (1) an unmet clinical need for better uncorrected visual acuity outcomes, (2) strong evidence for clinical and technical feasibility, and (3) a business model that benefited major stakeholders (providers, patients, and industry). These same factors strongly influenced product requirements for the Alcon LenSx® Laser, which was designed specifically to provide integrated planning, positioning and creation of precise corneal and lenticular laser incisions to enhance refractive cataract surgery outcomes.

Z.Z. Nagy, M.D., Ph.D., D.Sc. (✉)
Department of Ophthalmology, Semmelweis University, Maria u. 39, Budapest H-1085, Hungary
e-mail: zoltan.nagy100@gmail.com; nz@szem1.sote.hu

Technical Aspects

Laser System and Delivery

The Alcon LenSx® Laser System (Fig. 15.1) includes a proprietary solid-state laser source that produces thousands of FS pulses per second, which are then delivered to the eye via a sophisticated beam delivery system. The beam delivery system includes an articulated arm to allow flexible positioning, as well as a series of lenses, scanners, and monitors that deliver a series of precisely focused spots within the three-dimensional surgical field. In contrast to corneal FS lasers, which only need to be focused in the corneal stroma, the LenSx Laser delivery system optics utilizes a variable numerical aperture for optimal performance in both the cornea and lens. This feature, as well as other proprietary scanning techniques, allows the LenSx System to minmize the effects of small aberrations at the corneal plane, such as corneal wrinkles, that can impact performance with optical systems that were designed primarily for only corneal or lens applications.

Docking Sytem and Coupling to the Eye

The surgeon couples the patient's eye to the distal end of the focusing objective using a sterile disposable patient interface (PI) that consists of a curved contact lens integrated with a limbal suction ring. Tubing connects to an onboard vacuum system that

R.R. Krueger et al. (eds.), *Textbook of Refractive Laser Assisted Cataract Surgery (ReLACS)*,
DOI 10.1007/978-1-4614-1010-2_15, © Springer Science+Business Media, LLC 2013

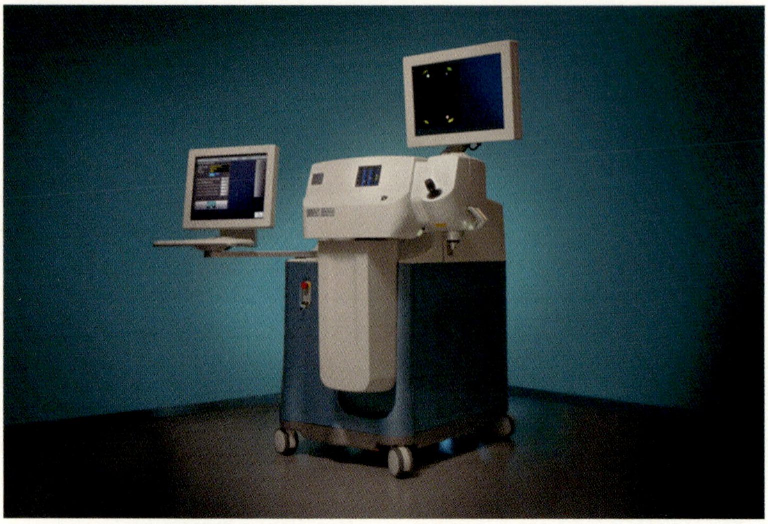

Fig. 15.1 Alcon LenSx® Laser System

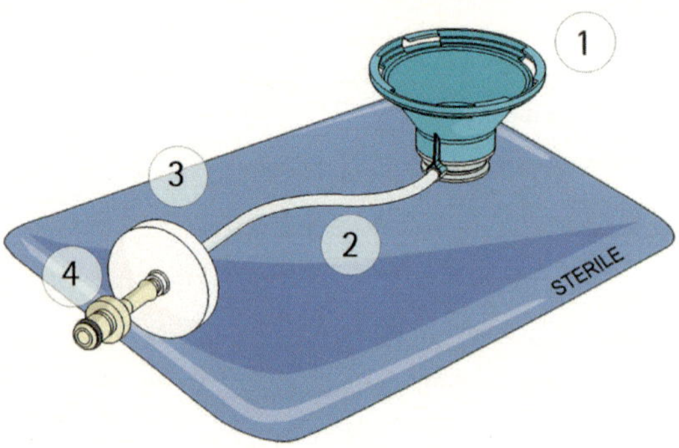

Fig. 15.2 Alcon LenSx® Laser PI—(1) interface cone and gripper, (2) tubing, (3) filter, and (4) vacuum port

allows for straightforward fixation of the eye (see Fig. 15.2). At <20 mm in maximal outer diameter, the LenSx PI is the smallest of any FS laser. While fitting easily into almost any eye, the system also delivers the largest viewing and surgical diameter range. The LenSx PI is easy to apply and maintain sterility, both of which have yet to be demonstrated with more complicated docking systems.

As with all FS laser systems that deliver laser pulses with micron level accuracy, the eye must be fixated prior to imaging and laser application. Since this process can take approximately 1–2 min, consideration of ocular perfusion is appropriate. In the supine position, mean ocular perfusion pressure, defined as the difference between mean arterial pressure and IOP, averages about 60 mmHg in a population typical of that undergoing cataract surgery [4, 5]. Since the LenSx Laser PI elevates IOP by approximately 30 mmHg during the procedure, ocular perfusion and visual perception is maintained. As with retrobulbar blocks, any IOP increase may be contraindicated in patients with a history of low arterial blood pressure, glaucoma or high IOP [6]. Importantly, the secure fixation of the LenSx PI does not require any specialized bed or head restraints, allowing patients to remain on the same surgical bed during laser treatment and in the operating room, thereby providing maximal flexibility for patient flow.

Imaging and Pattern Programming

The LenSx Laser uses live video and optical coherence tomography (OCT) imaging to guide both docking of the PI onto the eye as well as subsequent surgical pattern localization. Since application of the suction ring used in all FS laser systems can alter the position of target tissues, pattern positioning is performed after docking. The LenSx OCT utilizes the same optical path as the laser pulse and so is fully integrated and cross calibrated. Importantly, the range of the LenSx OCT covers the entire anterior segment of the eye (see Fig. 15.3) and does not rely on multiple scans that must be stitched together

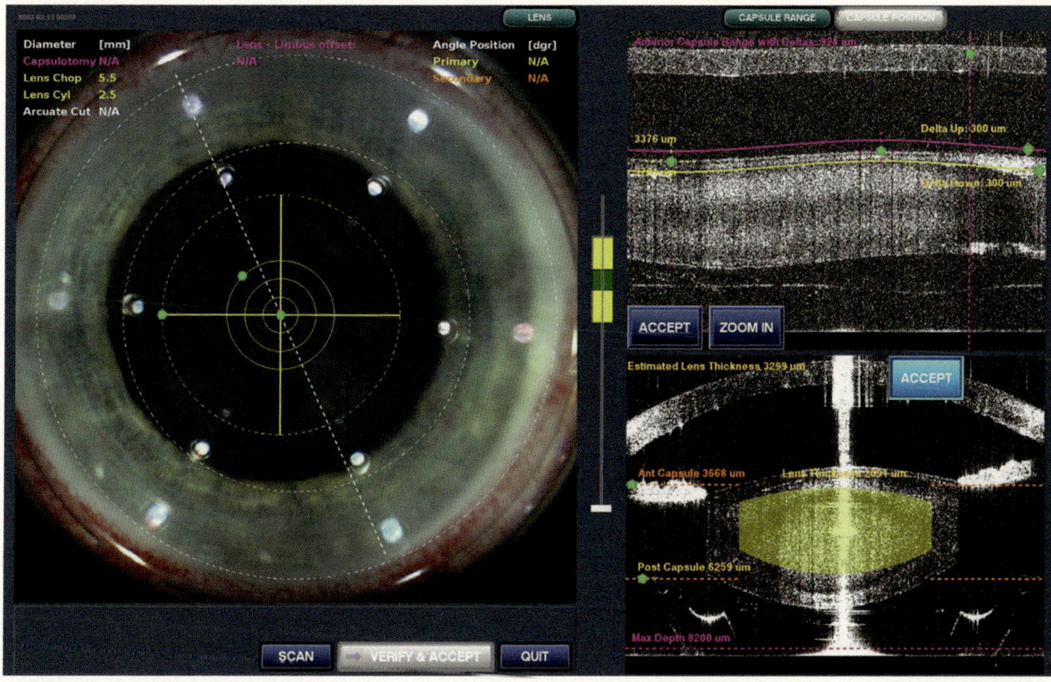

Fig. 15.3 Alcon LenSx® Laser System video microscope and OCT user interface

(which necessitates additional calibration steps). Automatic pre-positioning of the surgical patterns is also performed, with only quick adjustments by the surgeon used to finalize position of all corneal and lenticular incisions. The combination of circular and linear OCT scans efficiently provides both depth and tilt information, the latter which is used to fix the limits of laser placement. While FS laser pulses produce shock waves that propogate <100 μm, a 500 μm safety zone from posterior capsule is recommended for all laser systems.

Early Technical Obstacles and How They Were Overcome

The primary technical challenges for ReLACS include the requirements for laser pulse delivery over an extended volume, an integrated imaging system, and a high average power laser source. These challenges, and their solutions, are summarized in Chap. 4.

Equally challenging has been the recognition of clinical situations that are not commonly seen in conventional cataract surgery, as well as the development of surgical techniques that take best advantage of the precise execution of laser incisions. To address these challenges, the clinical experience of initial users has been collected and discussed in various forums to facilitiate consensus strategies, both with respect to laser and manual surgical technique. This process no doubt will continue during the next several years via scientific meetings, presentations, and publications. A brief summary of some of the major findings to date is provided below.

Subconjunctival Hemorrhage: Mild to moderate subconjunctival hemorrhage was noted initially, but procedure time reduction and improvements in the PI design have significantly reduced their frequency and severity.

Pupillary Constriction: Pupil dilation is required for both laser and operative procedures, increasing duration requirements for mydriatic agents. Shock waves from laser pulses delivered close to the iris can also lead to miosis. Though easily addressed in the OR with intracameral mydriatics, programming the capsulotomy at a diameter that is smaller than the dilated pupil is advised.

Capsular Block Syndrome: Intraoperative capsular block syndrome following ReLACS was first reported by Roberts et al. [7]. The authors describe posterior capsular rupture in two patients during hydrodissection following uncomplicated laser procedures. Potential etiologies include the following: (1) the uniform capsulotomy created with the FS laser that may increase the potential for blockage of fluid egress by the elevated nucleus following hydrodissection; (2) the presence of intracapsular gas may represent an additional factor that could impede the flow of injected fluid around the lens nucleus. Modifications to surgical technique to avoid capsular block syndrome include slow, titrated injection of fluid during hydrodissection and/or splitting of the laser cut lens nucleus prior to hydrodissection to allow release of fluid and/or gas.

Corneal Incision Sizing and Positioning: Laser created corneal entry incision widths may appear narrower than those created with manual blades, possibly due to lateral extension inherent with manual incisions. Adjustment of programmed incision width eliminates this issue and ensures that stretching of the wound will not impact its self-sealing properties. Positioning of incisions at the limbus is enabled to a diameter of 12.5 mm.

Clinical Capabilities and Parameters for Cataract Surgery

Indications for Use

The Alcon LenSx® Laser is indicated for use in patients undergoing cataract surgery for removal of the crystalline lens. Intended uses in cataract surgery include anterior capsulotomy, laser phacofragmentation, and the creation of single plane and multi-plane arc cuts/incisions in the cornea, each of which may be performed either individually or consecutively during the same procedure. Surgeons can select from a range of parameters for each of the surgical procedure patterns to customize the procedure to the individual eye.

Currently, lens fragmentation can be accomplished using one of three patterns, with additional patterns planned. In the most common fragmentation pattern used currently, a central core is outlined with a cylinder pattern, while the peripheral nucleus is segmented into quarters. This allows easy removal of the central nucleus, which then gives ideal access to the residual quadrants for removal with reduced phaco time and power as compared to completely ultrasonic techniques, using stop and chop or mechanical chopping [8, 9]. These observations may account for reduced corneal edema and better one day visual acuity noted by many surgeons with laser cases. While no reports of cystoid macular edema after ReLACS have yet appeared, a relative reduction in retinal thickness after ReLACS has been noted, presumabely due to less applied ultrasound power compared to standard procedures [10]. Additional benefits include reduced movement and manipulation in the eye enabled by the pre-fragmented lens nucleus. Laser lens fragmentation has been performed on all grades of cataract, including brunescent lenses.

The capsulotomy can be sized and positioned over a wide range, allowing additional customization, and delivering unparalleled accuracy and reproducibility [11]. Small residual attachments can be easily separated using standard capsulorhexis techniques to continue the circumferential cut. A number of cases have been performed on white cataracts and those with weak zonules, further demonstrating the flexibility of the device.

Similarly, a wide range of single and multiple plane corneal incisions can be sized and positioned to optimize postoperative uncorrected visual acuity. Corneal incisions can be full or partial thickness, giving the surgeon extensive flexiblity in how such incisions are performed and opened. Many surgeons choose to place, but not open, partial thickness arcuate incisions until guided by postoperative refractive measurements.

Ergonomic Simplicity of Operation

Device Logistics

The Alcon LenSx® Laser fits well into a variety of surgical venues, with a footprint of 60 in. in width and 72 in. in length. Minimum suggested room dimensions are 11 ft. × 14 ft. The system, which is self-calibrating, can be repositioned by the user before and after surgery. The system is compatible with a variety of patient beds and use of a universal power supply (UPS) is recommended.

Device Operation

The planned series of procedures (lens fragmentation, capsulotomy, and corneal incisions) is selected and the PI connected to the system.

The LenSx Laser features a fully integrated OCT imaging system, focus tracking, and automated pattern pre-positioning which greatly streamlines docking and treatment planning. The PI was designed for maximum patient comfort utilizing low suction while maintaining contact with the corneal surface. The LenSx Laser's delivery system was designed specifically for this small, universal PI, which has been validated in thousands of procedures to date. Using the gantry joystick and visualization via the video microscope, the surgeon is guided to the corneal surface for placement of the PI. Suction is activated, and the system quickly scans the entire anterior segment to provide the surgeon with 3 dimensional cross-sectional images extending from the corneal epithelium to beyond the posterior capsule. Software allows the surgeon to quickly confirm all pre-positioned incision and fragmentation parameters which are represented as overlays on the video microscope. Adjustments are easily made, if required, and when accepted by the surgeon the entire procedure is initiated by pressing the footswitch. The procedure may be stopped at any time by releasing the footswitch. When the procedure is completed, suction is released and the focusing objective is lifted, removing the applanation lens from the surface of the eye.

Perceived Benefits of the Alcon LenSx® Laser

A number of factors establish the LenSx® Laser in the field of ReLACS:

1. The LenSx Laser was the first FS laser cleared by the US FDA for clinical applications in cataract surgery (2009) [12].
2. Commercialized in 2010, the LenSx Laser has a global user base and a rapidly growing body of clinical data.
3. Validated and published in peer reviewed literature, the LenSx Laser is a precise surgical instrument that has demonstrated precision and predictability for the key steps of ReLACS.
4. Alcon has a mature customer support infrastructure, including global clinical trainers and field service.
5. Alcon has the industry leading development team dedicated to further technical and clinical advances.
6. The LenSx Laser's design, mobility, and size give flexibility for surgical venue and patient flow optimization.

Ten Compelling Reasons Why a Customer Should Buy the Alcon LenSx® Laser

1. The Alcon LenSx Laser was designed to bring the precision of a FS laser to refractive cataract surgery. This precision, which has been demonstrated clinically and published in peer reviewed literature, contributes to the efficacy of refractive IOLs by addressing critical factors such as effective lens position variability and centration [10–13]. Arcuate incisions may also be performed at the time of lens replacement surgery to meet the refractive goals of the patient.
2. The Alcon LenSx Laser technology adds to the complement of Alcon products and services for the patient who requests that refractive error be addressed at the time of lens replacement surgery.

3. As the first system commercialized for ReLACS, and with the largest global installed base, LenSx technology has already demonstrated the ability to meet patient expectations in a private pay environment.
4. The world leader in ophthalmic surgery innovation chose to invest early during development of the category, and selected LenSx technology as the most robust and predictable platform to complement their existing and future product portfolio.
5. Based on early clinical validation, the Alcon LenSx Laser gives surgeons the ability to offer patients the comfort and confidence of a laser procedure for lens replacement surgery.
6. The Alcon LenSx Laser enables the surgeon and staff to deliver a truly premium surgical experience for the patient, and to more predictably meet surgical goals and expectations.
7. With over 1 year of global commercial experience, the LenSx Laser has established patient acceptance and willingness to pay ReLACS.
8. The Alcon LenSx Laser was the first to market and rapidly advance the technology based upon actual commercial clinical feedback. All components are proprietary and designed in-house which facilitates rapid innovation.
9. The Alcon LenSx Laser is the product of the most successful team in FS laser technology. The experience and expertise of the LenSx team to scale and globally commercialize FS laser technology and field support is well established.
10. The Alcon legacy of product innovation, commitment to excellence, and exceptional customer support enable surgeons to consistently deliver the most compelling surgical advancements to patients worldwide.

Future Developments and Upgradability

The Alcon LenSx® Laser is designed for rapid innovation that will no doubt occur as the category of ReLACS develops. Alcon is committed to maintaining its leadership position and continues to invest heavily in the LenSx platform. As the technology is currently in its infancy, surgeons should expect additional clinical applications and surgical innovations by Alcon and the LenSx Laser technology team.

Principle Contact Information

Eric Weinberg
Vice-President, Alcon LenSx, Inc.
33 Journey, Aliso Viejo, CA 92656
949-360-6010

References

1. Gale RP, Saldana M, Johnston RL, et al. Benchmark standards for refractive outcomes after NHS cataract surgery. Eye. 2009;23(1):149–52.
2. Eleftheriadis H. IOLMaster biometry: refractive results of 100 consecutive cases. Br J Ophthalmol. 2003;87(8):960–3.
3. Murphy C, Tufy SJ, Minassian DC. Refractive error and visual outcome after cataract extraction. J Cataract Refract Surg. 2002;28:62–6.
4. Yip JL, Broadway DC, Luben R, Garway-Heath DF, Hayat S, Dalzell N, Lee PS, Bhaniani A, Wareham NJ, Khaw KT, Foster PJ. Physical activity and ocular perfusion pressure: the EPIC-Norfolk Eye Study. Invest Ophthalmol Vis Sci. 2011;52(11):8186–92.
5. Caprioli J, Coleman A. Blood pressure, perfusion pressure, and glaucoma. Am J Ophthalmol. 2010;149(5):704–12.
6. O'Donoghue E, Batterbury M, Lavy T. Effect on intraocular pressure of local anaesthesia in eyes undergoing intraocular surgery. Br J Ophthalmol. 1994;78(8):605–7.
7. Roberts T, Sutton G, Lawless M, Jindal-Bali S. Capsular block syndrome associated with femtosecond laser-assisted cataract surgery. J Cataract Refract Surg. 2011;37:2068–70.
8. Knorz M, Thompson V, Cionni R. Reduction in mean Cumulative Dissipated Energy (CDE) following lens fragmentation with an intraocular femtosecond laser. ESCRS 2011, Abstract FP-5420.
9. Nagy Z, Miháltz K, Kránitz K, Takacs A. Comparison of conventional and femtosecond laser assisted phacoemulsification on dense nuclear cataracts. AAO 2011, PA008.
10. Ecsedy M, Mihāltz K, Kovács I, Takács A, Filkorn T, Nagy ZZ. Effect of femtosecond laser cataract surgery on the macula. J Refract Surg. 2011;31:1–6.
11. Kránitz K, Takacs A, Mihāltz K, Kovács I, Knorz MC, Nagy ZZ. Femtosecond laser capsulotomy and manual continuous curvilinear capsulorrhexis parameters and their effects on intraocular lens centration. J Refract Surg. 2011;27(8):558–63.

12. Nagy Z, Takacs A, Filkorn T, Sarayba M. Initial clinical evaluation of an intraocular femtosecond laser in cataract surgery. J Refract Surg. 2009;25(12):1053–60.
13. Nagy ZZ, Kránitz K, Takacs AI, Miháltz K, Kovács I, Knorz MC. Comparison of intraocular lens decentration parameters after femtosecond and manual capsulotomies. J Refract Surg. 2011;27(8):564–9.

Commercially Available Systems: LensAR Laser System

16

Harvey S. Uy, Ronald R. Krueger, Keith H. Edwards, Randy Frey, and Simone Schneider

Historical Background and Beginning in Femto-lasers and Femto-cataract Surgery

LensAR Inc. was founded by Randy Frey in 2004. Prior to this time, he had been founder, CEO, and Chairman of Autonomous Technologies which had roots in the Star Wars program and later converted into a medical laser company. Autonomous developed the LADAR system which was the first laser radar system that enabled pupil tracking and enhanced the effectiveness of LASIK treatment. After the merger with Summit Technologies and the subsequent sale to Alcon, Randy Frey founded Lasersoft Vision with the idea of treating presbyopia by using a laser to soften the natural crystalline lens in situ to restore accommodation. These were ideas that were previously investigated and patented by Ray Myers, O.D. and Ronald Krueger, M.D., and they joined forces as cofounders of the new company. Randy also brought in some of his previous partners at Autonomous and was able to interest investors in his idea.

H.S. Uy, M.D. (✉)
Pacific Eye and Laser Institute, Makati City, Manila, The Philippines
e-mail: harveyuy@yahoo.com

R.R. Krueger, M.D., M.S.E.
Cole Eye Institute, Department of Refractive Surgery, Cleveland Clinic Lerner College of Medicine, Cleveland, OH 44106, USA

K.H. Edwards, F.C.Optom., Dip.C.L.P.
Clinical & Regulatory Affairs, LensAR Inc., 2800 Discovery Drive, Orlando, FL 32826, USA

R. Frey
LensAR Inc., 2800 Discovery Drive, Orlando, FL 32826, USA

S. Schneider, Ph.D., M.Sc.
Clinical Department, Clinical & Regulatory Affairs, LensAR Inc., 2800 Discovery Drive, Orlando, FL 32826, USA

Motivating Concept for What ReLACS Would Do for the Worldwide Market and Surgical Outcomes

During the course of studying the laser techniques for presbyopia on eye models and monkeys, some Lasersoft Vision medical advisors suggested that the technology could facilitate removal of lenticular material during the cataract procedure. In particular, laser lens fragmentation could simplify the breaking up and removal of higher grade cataracts with which surgeons experience the most difficulties. Initial work was conducted on animal and cadaver eyes which verified proof of concept that laser lens fragmentation improved nuclear disassembly by making lenticular extraction faster, less

R.R. Krueger et al. (eds.), *Textbook of Refractive Laser Assisted Cataract Surgery (ReLACS)*,
DOI 10.1007/978-1-4614-1010-2_16,

traumatic and more efficient in terms of required ultrasound energy. The latter, in particular, has been associated with endothelial cell loss and anterior segment trauma.

After successful animal trials and upgrades to the system software, the company changed its name in 2007 from Lasersoft Vision to LensAR, which stood for "Lens Accommodation Restoration," being the primary focus of the company at its inception. Meanwhile, venture capital was acquired, and it was decided to shift the company's main focus to cataract surgery, since accommodation restoration was scientifically more challenging, and would later benefit from the experience, technology and resources gained from laser cataract surgery.

The aim was to develop and design a highly integrated and automated measurement technology using a 3D scanning laser system with confocal, structured illumination for enhanced viewing of the most and least reflective structures in the anterior segment of the eye. This computer generated image, referred to as "Augmented Reality", is nicely highlighted in the company name, LensAR, (previously Lens Accommodation Restoration, but now Lens Augmented Reality). After previous 510 (k) approval for capsulotomy and fragmentation using the LensAR laser prototype, LensAR then received 510 (k) clearance for lens fragmentation with or without capulotomy for their commercial device in June 2012.

Technical Requirements for Adequate Nucleus Fragmentation

Laser System and Delivery

The LensAR Laser System incorporates a unique laser specifically designed for the application, and operates in the infrared range. The parameters of the laser were generated specifically for optimal photodisruption in the lens, reflecting the initial presbyopia application that also enhances the phaco-fragmentation potential of the system. The selection of wavelength, pulse width, and energy for each application was made after extensive laboratory and clinical research, and although it remains proprietary information, can be characterized as having a similar infrared laser wavelength, a whole order of magnitude greater pulse energy, and higher pulse widths than the refractive and corneal femtosecond (FS) lasers. The patterns used were investigated during a clinical study in the Philippines and compared both the reduction in ultrasound energy as well as surgeon subjective feedback—see Figs. 16.1 and 16.2. As a result a "pie" algorithm was selected as being the most effective across the complete range of cataract densities. In the FDA submission cohort, reductions in CDE using the Alcon Infiniti system with the Ozil handpiece ranged between 38.8 and 100% depending on cataract grade (see Table 16.1).

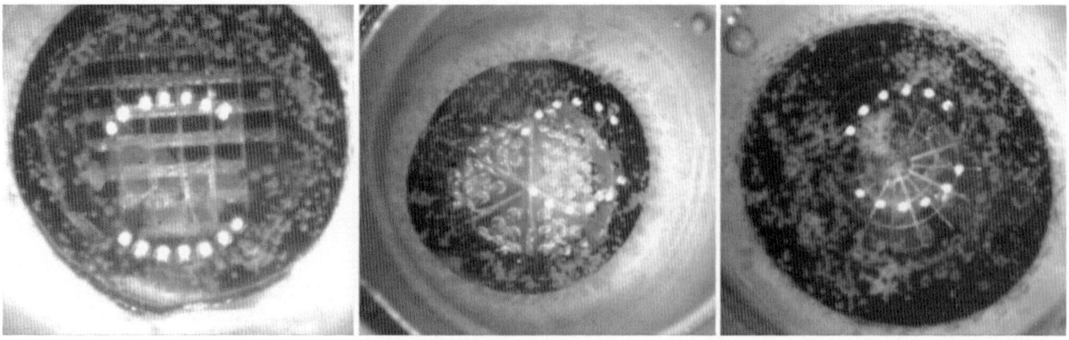

Fig. 16.1 Examples of the fragmentation patterns cut in the lens; "*Cubes*" at *left*, "*Spheres*" *center*, and "*Pies*" at *right*

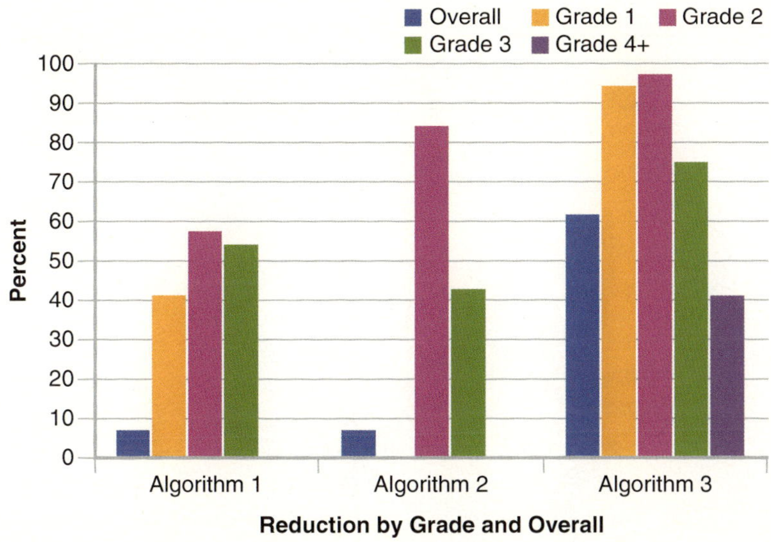

Fig. 16.2 Results from the assessment of different patterns and algorithms showing the reduction in ultrasound energy compared to conventional phacoemulsification. Algorithm 3 was the "Pies" algorithm showing effectiveness across all cataract grades and subsequently used in the clinical studies

Table 1A: Reduction in ultrasound energy (CDE) following laser phaco-fragmentation in ReLACS

Table. Analysis of mean (SD) CDE as a function of preoperative nuclear cataract grade

Treatment groups	For Grade 0[1]	For Grade 1	For Grade 2	For Grade 3	For Grade 4+[2]
	Mean (SD)	Mean (SD)	Mean (SD)	Mean (SD)	Mean (SD)
	N	*N*	*N*	*N*	*N*
Laser treatments	1.9 (3.2)	0.0 (0.0)	3.0 (4.0)	9.3 (9.4)	24.0 (18.8)
	3	4	29	25	27
Control group	7.8 (–)	4.4 (2.4)	8.2 (6.1)	15.2 (13.0)	41.2 (24.7)
	1	7	24	15	7
% Difference control versus combined laser cohorts	–75.6	–100.0	–63.4	–38.8	–41.7

[1]No nuclear cataract (cortical and/or subcapsular only)
[2]Grade 4+ includes all higher graded cataracts

Table 1B: Significant reduction in Cumulative Dissipated Energy following laser phaco fragmentation in ReLACS for Grades 1, 2 and 4 at 95% level of significance

Grade ≤1		Grade 1		Grade 2		Grade 3		Grade 4	
Laser	Phaco	Laser	Phaco	Laser	Phaco	Laser	Phaco	Laser	Phaco
$N=7$	$N=8$	$N=4$	$N=7$	$N=29$	$N=24$	$N=25$	$N=15$	$N=27$	$N=7$
$p=0.006$		$p=0.006$		$p<0.001$		$p=0.069$		$p=0.052$	

While the prototype laser utilized pulse energies in the picosecond range, as inferred in the characterization above, the commercial system has been validated, tested and fully approved for equivalency in the femtosecond range in order to optimize the laser delivery for lens fragmentation and capsulotomy. This refinement was not only made to improve the lens based applications, but also to optimize the corneal incisional applications, which await imminent FDA approval.

Docking System and Coupling to the Eye

The original docking system incorporated an applanating patient interface (PI). However, this was found to distort the cornea and induce striae which interfered with the imaging of the more posterior ocular structures. Over time this was changed to a curved interface, and then the current design which incorporates a corneal no touch, fluid-filled interface (see Fig. 16.3). The latter

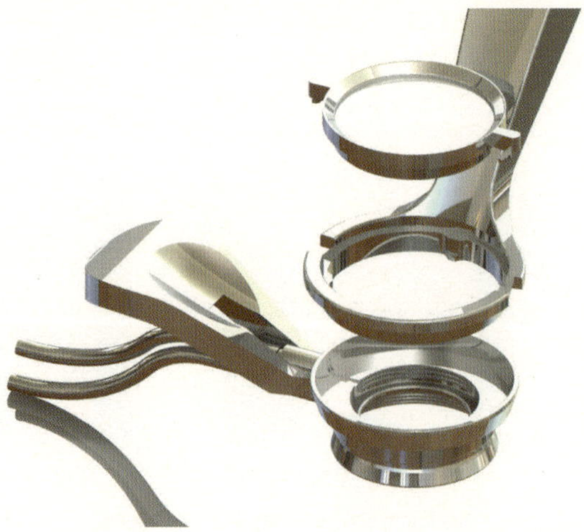

Fig. 16.3 PI device comprising a suction ring, PI arm, and reference glass. All these pieces together provide a non-corneal contact docking procedure

approach ensures no corneal distortion which can affect the imaging of deeper structures (Fig. 16.4) as well as impacting the ability to make accurate corneal cuts for surgical incisions and peripheral incisions to manage astigmatism. The PI incorporates a low-pressure suction device that is attached to the eye and then filled with a balanced salt solution. All controls for suction and saline flow are incorporated into the foot pedal. Once the suction ring is in place and filled with saline, the laser is docked to the interface via a servo-controlled docking head and a PI arm. The software images through the interface arm, automatically calibrating the system via identification of key elements within the interface window. Once fully docked, imaging and treatment proceeds.

The PI comprises both disposable and reusable elements. The PI arm is reusable after autoclave sterilization, while the PI device, interface window, and small saline bag are all single-use items (see Fig. 16.3).

Imaging System

The LensAR Laser System incorporates the proprietary 3D-CSI imaging and biometry system.

The LensAR Laser System incorporates the proprietary "Augmented Reality" imaging and biometry system. The "Augmented Reality" system is based on 3D confocal, structured illumination (3D CSI), as featured below:

- A scanning, diagnostic laser that can scan at varying rates for different ocular structures within the anterior segment. This ensures that the image has optimum contrast for both highly reflecting surfaces, such as the anterior corneal surface, as well as lower reflecting surfaces, such as the posterior lens capsule. At the same time, image background noise is minimized, thus permitting accurate imaging and measurement through all densities of nuclei. Since the images are of high quality, the software can automatically detect the key interfaces including anterior and posterior corneal surfaces and anterior and posterior capsules.
- Confocal alignment of the imaging and laser delivery systems that ensures an identical optical pathway, once the eye is docked. In this way, there is no systematic error between imaging and treatment, ensuring the ability to direct laser pulses exactly to where the imaging system detects the target structures.
- Multiple images that can be used to generate an accurate three-dimensional model using

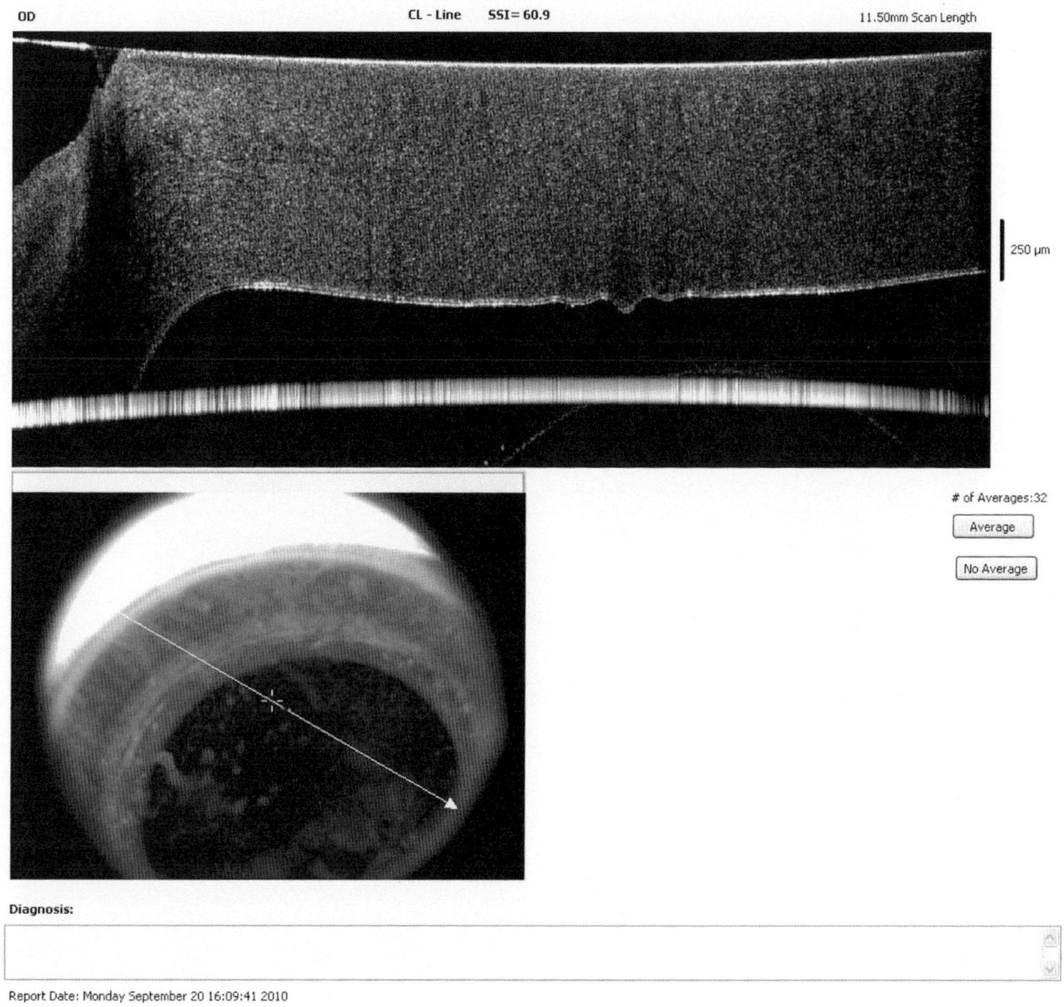

Fig. 16.4 OCT of an applanated cornea showing striae in the posterior cornea, as well as endothelial artifacts, which can affect the diagnostic imaging and therapeutic laser pulse delivery to anterior segment structures

optical ray tracing. A minimum of three individual images is required and a maximum of eight can be captured.

- Enhanced depth of field of ocular structures through incorporation of the Scheimpflug imaging principle. This permits an in-focus image from the anterior cornea to the posterior lens capsule in a single video frame. There is no need to stitch adjacent images together.

The 3D-CSI system collects biometric data including anterior and posterior corneal radius of curvature, corneal thickness, anterior chamber depth, anterior and posterior lens radius of curvature and lens thickness. Since the system detects the anterior and posterior apices of the lens it can determine lens tilt from the optical axis of the lens. This has the advantage of allowing the surgeon to center the anterior capsulotomy over the optical axis of the crystalline lens prior to removal. Provided that the IOL is centered under the capsulotomy this should ensure that there is no change in overall optical axis of the eye's components after the surgery. As an alternative, the surgeon can elect to center the capsulotomy over the pupil center or the anterior lens apex. Figure 16.5 shows the auto-surface detection on an individual image while Fig. 16.6 shows the 3D reconstruction process together with the biometric data derived from the images.

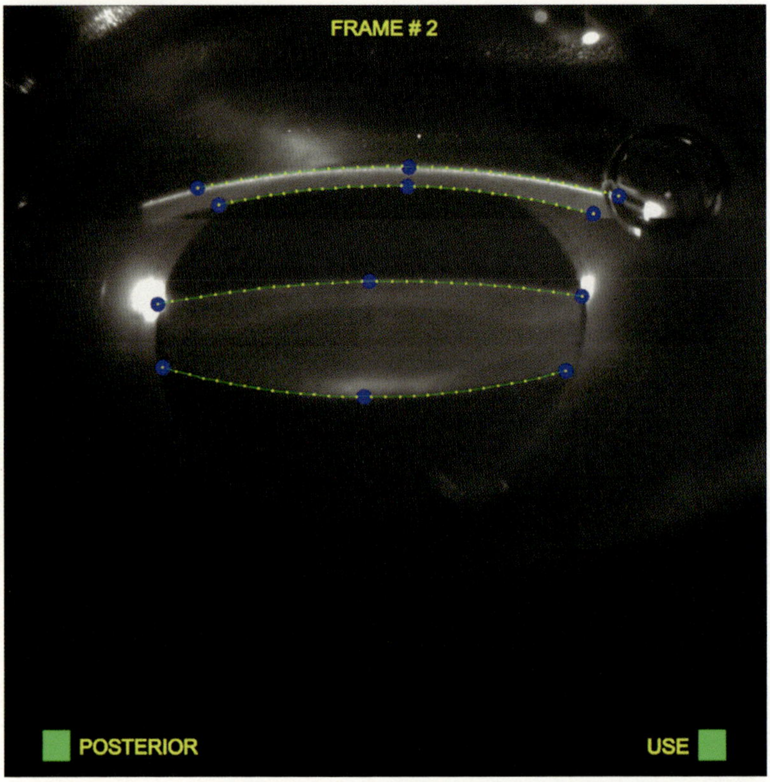

Fig. 16.5 Software screen showing automated surface detection of key ocular surfaces

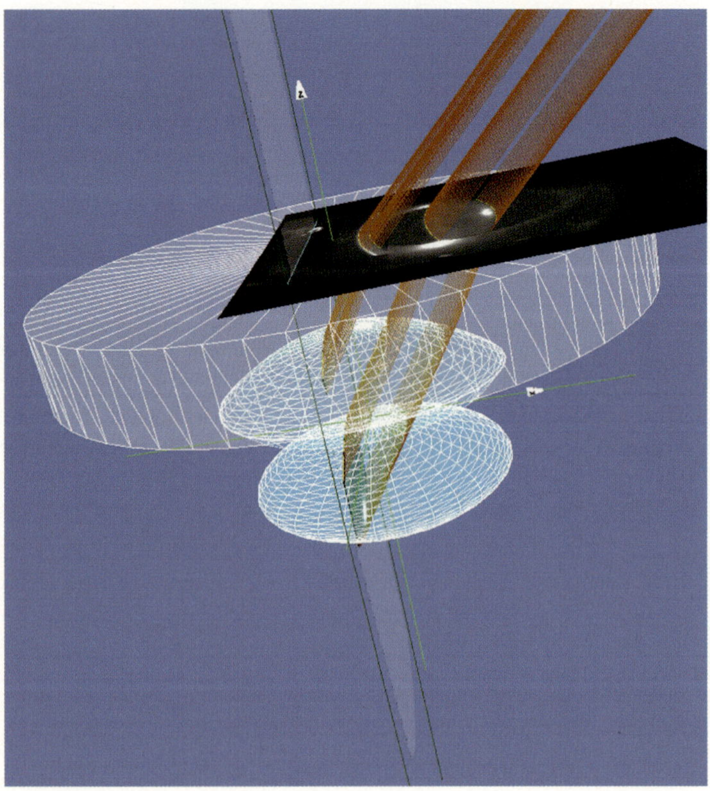

Fig. 16.6 Graphic representation of 3D reconstruction from individual images. Biometric data are shown on the *lower right part* of the screen

At all stages the surgeon can elect to accept or modify the software analysis of the surface prior to the final 3D reconstruction, allowing an additional safety margin.

Once the 3D reconstruction is complete, the software creates patient specific parameters for capsulotomy and lens fragmentation (Fig. 16.7). This is based on surgeon preferences that are preprogrammed taking into account the IOL to be implanted and the preferred fragmentation parameters, etc. The software takes into account any lens tilt and the required capsular clearance of 500 μm to maintain a safe margin from the capsule. This safety clearance may be increased if necessary, as when dealing with hard nuclei where an increased posterior epinuclear layer may protect the posterior capsule from the hard nuclear particles circulating during nuclear disassembly. In this case, one may consider a safety clearance of 750 μm or more.

Clinical Capabilities and Parameters for Cataract Surgery

Nucleus Fragmentation

In the original feasibility series a number of cutting patterns were assessed including "spheres," "cubes" and "pies." Figure 16.1 shows examples of the patterns assessed. The pies algorithm was found to be the most effective across the whole range of cataract grades (Fig. 16.2).

The LensAR system has been used to fragment nuclei with a wide range of nuclear opalescence grades (LOCS II, 0–4 and LOCS III, 0.1–6.9), including brown and some white cataracts. In the case of white (opaque) cataract the ability to fragment the lens below the surface is limited. This is because the infrared laser light is highly absorbed and poorly transmitted through the white, opaque lens. Work continues to refine the algorithms for denser nuclei. Table 16.1 shows the overall reduction in CDE when using laser phaco-fragmentation compared to conventional phacoemulsification in 142 eyes analyzed in the Philippines [1]. In each grade of nucleus density, laser fragmentation was associated with a statistically significant reduction in cumulative dispersed energy (CDE) in comparison to phacoemulsification alone. Finally, no significant changes in intraocular pressure and corneal endothelial cell count were observed in a series of 60 eyes that underwent laser anterior capsulotomy and fragmentation in Mexico [2].

Capsulotomy

Anterior capsulotomy size and shape was assessed in a clinical study in Mexico [3]. Capsular buttons were retrieved and compared in size to the target, as well as for regularity of shape. Compared to manual capsulorrhexis, the laser capsulotomy was found to be closer to the target diameter and with less variation. The mean deviation ± SD from target was 0.16 ± 0.17 mm for the laser capsulotomy compared to 0.42 ± 0.54 mm for the manual capsulorrhexis ($p = 0.03$). Mean absolute deviation from the intended diameter was 0.20 ± 0.12 for the laser compared with 0.49 ± 0.47 for the manual method. The mean of the average squared residuals (a measure of regularity of shape) was 0.01 ± 0.03 for the laser and 0.02 ± 0.04 for the manual ($p = 0.09$).

An assessment of capsular strength was undertaken using porcine eyes which revealed that laser capsulotomies were more robust than those made with a manual capsulorrhexis technique [4]. The research showed that the mean force necessary to rupture the capsular edge was significantly greater at 177 ± 53 mN with the laser versus 125 ± 43 mN with CCC ($p < 0.05$). The mean capsular edge distention prior to capsular rupture was significantly greater with the laser at 7.45 ± 0.47 mm than that following CCC at 4.68 ± 1.01 mm ($p < 0.001$).

A review of post operative refractive outcomes in patients undergoing laser capsulotomy compared to manual capsulorrhexis, reveals a 6-month mean deviation of MRSE from predicted target of −0.21 ± 0.39 D for the laser capsulotomy ($n = 249$ eyes) compared with +0.55 ± 0.41 D for manual capsulorrhexis ($n = 123$ eyes), ($p = 0.001$). The absolute deviation in MRSE was less (laser, 0.42 ± 0.39 D; manual, −.59 ± 0.35 D) but still

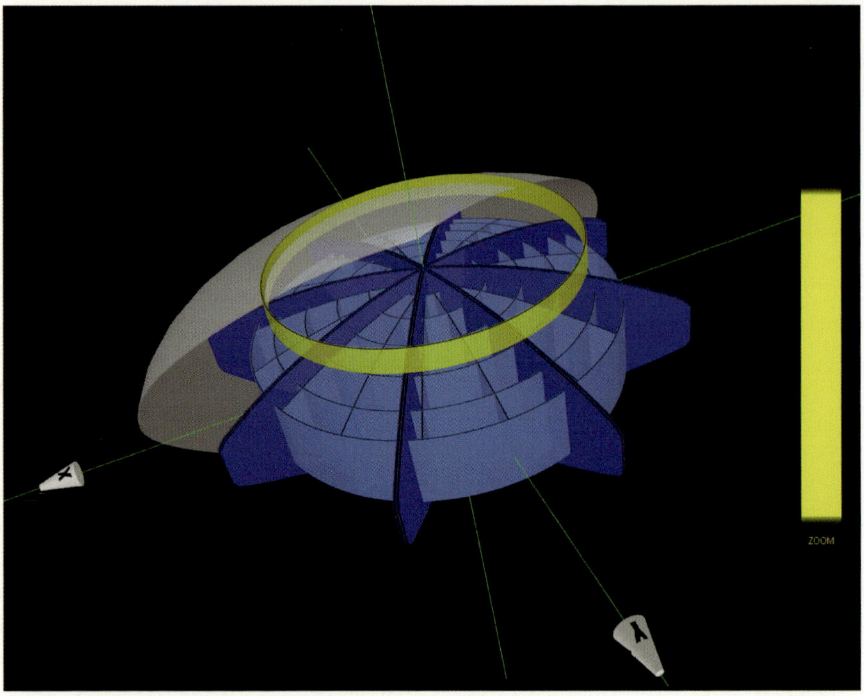

Fig. 16.7 Software generated treatment algorithm for capsulotomy (*lighter shade top circle*) and phaco-fragmentation (*darker shade central pattern with multiple rings*). The capsular bag is represented by the outer shell

statistically significant, demonstrating better predictability in the laser group. According to frequency of cases within a certain range of target MRSE, 47% of the laser group were within 0.25 D of target MRSE versus 22% of the manual group ($p=0.003$); 79% of the laser group were within 0.5 D of target MRSE versus 53% of manually treated eyes ($p=0.003$). These results show improved predictability of refractive outcomes for eyes that underwent laser anterior capsulotomy compared to manual capsulorrhexis [5].

Corneal Incisions

Treatment parameters for creation of transcorneal entry incisions and limbal relaxing incisions were a particular challenge for the no touch, fluid filled interface, since small microsaccadic movements of the eye could effect the precise placement of these incisions. Consequently, LensAR designed a real-time, dynamic adjustment for motion, based on feedback from its Augmented Reality Imaging system. The incision site is first imaged at 3 cross-sectional angles and referenced based on location markers on its 3D reconstructed model. The specific location of the first and each subsequent laser pulse is then imaged and adjusted for by computing the real-time error (within milliseconds) at each location. The laser incision is therefore modified as it is created, and the entire process is automated according to the surgeon's treatment plan.

The corneal, no touch, fluid filled interface allows for no compression or distortion of the corneal architecture. In the same way that immersion ultrasound is better than contact ultrasound for biometry, the fluid filled interface is the better than a contact interface for imaging and laser treatment of corneal and deeper anterior segment structures. It is this technology with therapeutic laser delivery in the femtosecond range that is supporting the ongoing development of the LensAR laser system for transcorneal entry incisions and peripheral corneal relaxing incisions.

Ergonomics

The LensAR Laser System was designed after extensive input from surgeons and operating room staff. It is designed to work within a perioperative

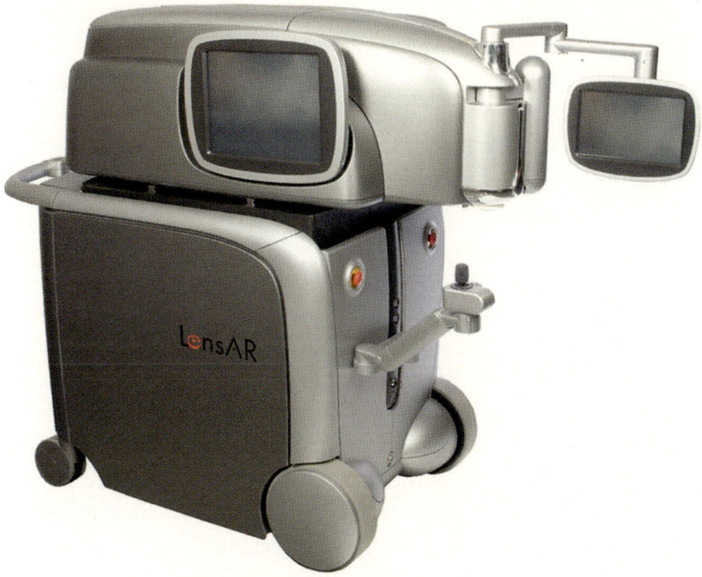

Fig. 16.8 The LensAR Laser System. Compact with several ergonomic features (see text)

treatment room or within the operating room itself. The device has a small footprint and several space-saving features (see Fig. 16.8). The laser head is on an extending arm that can be deployed to a neutral position once the patient is in the room. After the PI device is placed on the eye, the laser head is docked to the interface via the PI arm. The laser head is under servo control and maintains a predetermined force on the eye at all times. Control of the docking is by a joystick and progress is monitored via the surgeon's monitor. There are two further screens that give access to the software for a circulating nurse or technician. The system is designed to allow for any patient orientation for either eye so that the surgeon's preferences for seating relative to the operative eye can be maintained. Once the imaging and treatment are complete, the head can be retracted to the parked position, which is out of the way of the surgeon and allows an operating microscope to be brought in should the procedure have been carried out in the O.R. Once the laser pretreatment is complete, cataract surgery can begin. To allow an even greater working distance than what currently exists, the system can be preprogrammed to automatically move back an additional 18–24 in. to give even more unrestricted access to the patient.

Control of the essential elements of the procedure is conducted from the foot pedal (vacuum for suction, saline fill of the interface and firing of the laser) or joystick (docking/undocking) while progress is seen on the surgeon's monitor.

The graphic user interface allows the surgeon to customize the treatment beyond the software recommended parameters. Capsulotomy size can be programmed according to the IOL to be implanted and can be centered over the pupil, over the anterior lens apex or over the optical axis of the lens. The width of the fragmentation pattern can be extended or reduced within the pupil diameter subject to a preprogrammed safety margin. The depth of the pattern can also be reduced if a larger epinuclear plate is required. The LensAR system is fully automated while providing the surgeon opportunities at each step to override the system-recommended settings.

Ten Compelling Reasons Why a Customer Would Buy the LensAR System

1. The LensAR Laser System has been designed to be compact and ergonomically flexible in order to work either within a standard operating room or in a separate treatment room. It has a PI arm that can be moved into the operative area for docking and treatment, and then retracted away when the laser treatment is

completed. This allows maximum flexibility to the surgeon and/or surgery center.
2. The low-pressure suction ring allows immobilization of the eye without dramatic rises in IOP while the fluid filled interface allows the cornea to remain uncompressed, avoiding corneal striae and the resulting imaging artifacts. In the same way that immersion ultrasound is better for biometry than contact ultrasound, the fluid filled interface is better than the contact interface for both corneal imaging and laser delivery.
3. The Augmented Reality imaging and biometry system allows high quality images to be obtained without the need for image processing and/or OCT image stitching. This provides an in-focus image from anterior cornea to posterior capsule in a single image while retaining the detail within the imaged structures. The fact that the imaging and treatment systems have a parallel optical pathway ensures precise alignment of laser pulses with the detected surfaces.
4. The Augmented Reality imaging system increases the rate of laser scanning for deeper, low reflecting lens structures, such as the posterior capsule, so that it can be visualized even in dense nuclei, where failure to image the posterior capsule, as with some OCT imaging systems, would prevent the implementation of lens fragmentation.
5. The automation of the surface detection and the fact that the capsulotomy is cut before the fragmentation means that surgeon or technician manipulation of the images prior to treatment is minimized or eliminated.
6. The LensAR system has compensating software that measures and adjusts for lens tilt, which is frequently seen after suction and docking. This feature ensures proper centration of the capsulotomy and treats the lens nucleus as if it was perpendicularly aligned, eliminating the risk of posterior capsule rupture at the site of anterior tilting.
7. The LensAR system was the first system to receive FDA clearance with FDA labeling of specific ultrasound energy reductions across a full range of cataract grades, including dense brunescent cataracts.
8. To compensate for microsaccadic movement of the eye with a fluid filled interface, a real-time, dynamic adjustment for motion is implemented through closed loop feedback from the Augmented Reality Imaging system, so that each subsequent laser pulse is positionally modified to follow the imaged location of the previous pulse base on the surgeons treatment plan
9. The LensAR system is the only laser system that is being investigated for the treatment of presbyopia by laser induced accommodation restoration, and while still in early feasibility trials, has shown safety in preventing progressive cataracts with central sparing treatment algorithms.
10. Since the treatment patterns and algorithms for both cataract and accommodation restoration procedures are controlled by the software, future developments can easily be accommodated through software upgrades.

Future Developments and Upgradability

The future of LensAR and its capabilities will naturally be subject to the successes of the present, and hence it is difficult to fully project where this technology will go. However, there are a number of ideas and initiatives that are under development, and these are mentioned here for consideration.

Accommodation Restoration

The company name LensAR was conceptualized and designed to stand for "Lens Accommodation Restoration." Hence, the original focus of LensAR was to surgically treat the lens with laser in order to facilitate a greater flexibility and sliding of the protein fibers within the lens that are compacted, making a lens nucleus harder with age. Two of the company founders, Ronald Krueger, M.D. and Raymond Myers, O.D. had proposed this concept and published on it years earlier [6], and subsequent experimental studies demonstrated its potential efficacy ex vivo with cadaver eyes

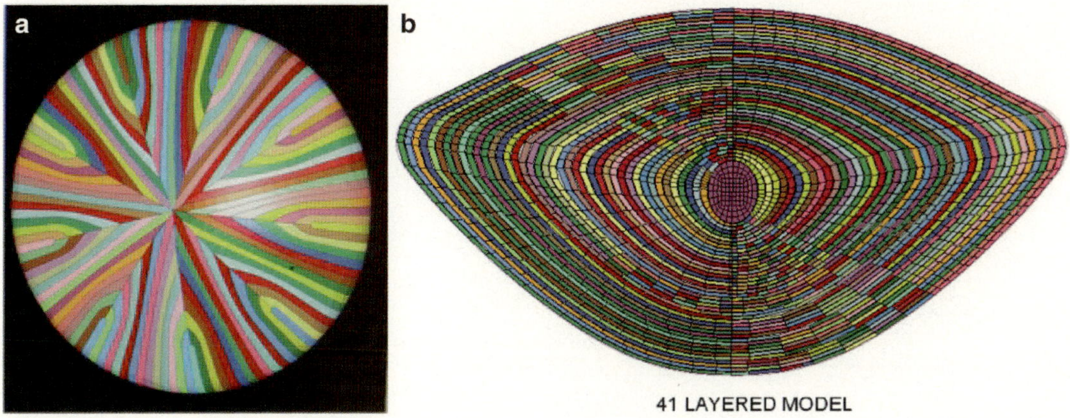

Fig. 16.9 Complex, multilayered, finite element model (FEM) of the human crystalline lens, showing the curved orientation of fibers that overlap at the lens sutures in the coronal view (**a**) and the multitude of sliding layers of lens fibers that extend from anterior to posterior in the sagittal view (**b**)

[7] and safety in vivo with rabbit eye morphology, light scattering and healing studies [8].

One of the first things LensAR did when it was founded in 2004, was to design a complex finite element model of the crystalline lens that could be used to test out their hypothesis mathematically, and help determine the best patterns for intralenticular laser treatment. They enlisted the expert consultation of Adrian Glasser, Ph.D. on the mechanisms of accommodation and presbyopia and Jer Kuszak, Ph.D. on the embryology and microanatomy of the crystalline lens to design a complex multilayered model of the human crystalline lens (Fig. 16.9a, b).

Following extensive laboratory studies and refinement in their laser development, LensAR conducted preclinical studies in nonhuman primate eyes at the University of Wisconsin under the direction of Paul Kaufman, M.D., demonstrating effective delivery of the laser into specific pattern in the lens and safety by avoiding the formation of cataracts up to 4+ years after the treatment. Figure 16.10 shows the appearance of the treated lens after 3 years with only a few microtranslucencies and a clear view to the retina (left) in comparison to the contralateral nontreated monkey eye (right). The early follow-up on these nonhuman primate eyes spurred on the early clinical work in this area.

The first clinical treatments for lens accommodation restoration were performed in 2007 in Mexico City by Dr. Ramon Naranjo Tachman. These demonstrated that a laser pattern with a central clear zone might be preferable in order minimize unwanted dysphotopsias and photic side effects from the most centrally placed laser spots. The model for this investigation was based on a recruitment of eyes with only low grade cataracts for refractive lens exchange, that were enlisted to participation in laser treatment and follow-up for 1 month prior to lens extraction. From these early experiences, further clinical investigation with the same model progressed in Makati City, Manila in the Philippines under the direction of Dr. Harvey Uy. To date, over 80 eyes have undergone this investigational treatment with various patterns of laser application. These have validated the visual safety of the treatment, when sparing the center of the lens, demonstrating no progressive cataract formation (Fig. 16.11a, b). They have also shown a variable margin of efficacy with 50% of subjects reporting some subjective accommodation with the push up test, 1/3 revealing some objective accommodation with the Grand Seiko autorefractor, and 40% reading better with an improved best distance corrected near visual acuity (BDCNVA) during the first month of follow-up. Ongoing clinical investigation with new patterns are underway in an attempt to improve the degree and magnitude of efficacy.

Lens Densitometry Guided Surgery

The clinical application of Scheimpflug tomography has not only been useful in measuring the thickness and curvature of the cornea, but has been

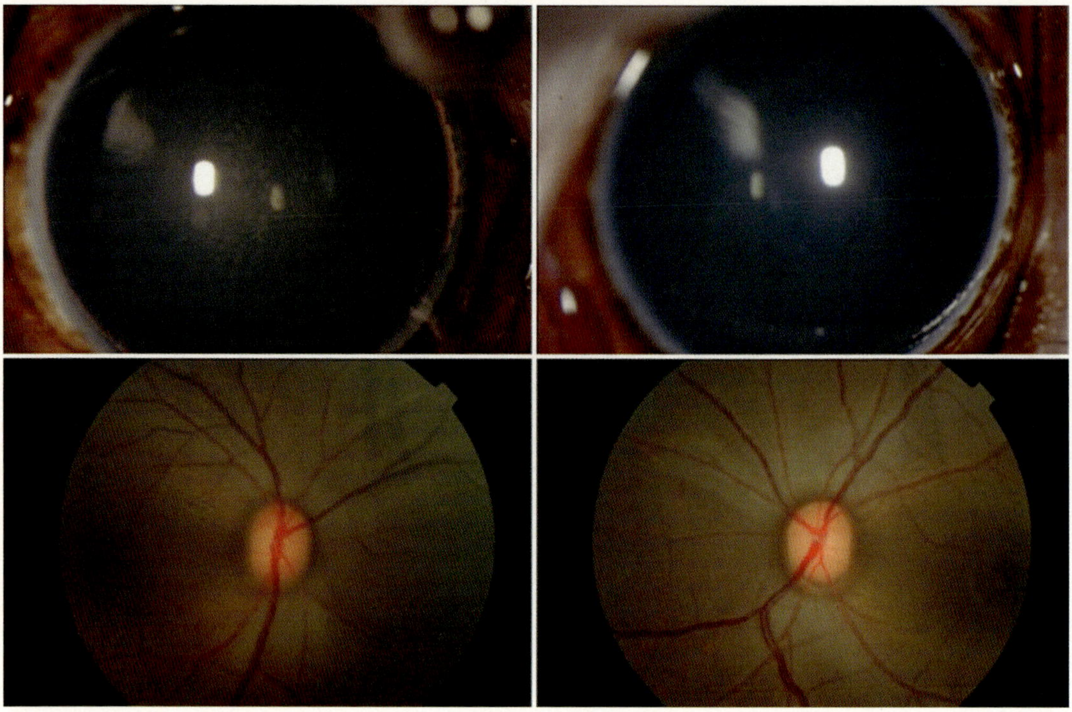

Fig. 16.10 Rhesus monkey eyes, revealing (**a**) faint microtranslucencies of the crystalline lens and clear visualization of the retina 3 years after picosecond laser lens treatment with over ten million pulses of 25 μJ pulse energy and (**b**) clear crystalline lens and similar clear visualization of the retina in the untreated, contralateral, control eye

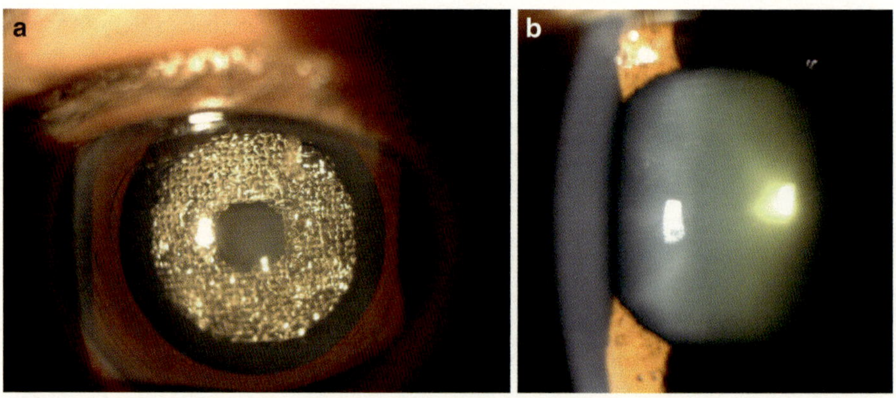

Fig. 16.11 Slit lamp photograph of crystalline lens, showing the fragmentation ("waffle") pattern for accommodative restoration performed using the LensAR system. Note (**a**) the numerous, intralenticular, gas bubbles, but clear central zone immediately post-treatment and (**b**) the faint superior, pinpoint opacities, clear visual axis, the absence of residual gas bubbles and no progressive cataract formation at 1 month post-treatment

is particularly useful in qualitatively and quantitatively assessing the density and level of opacity of ocular structures, especially the crystalline lens. This is known as lens densitometry, and it can also be implemented, to an even greater degree, with the advanced imaging system of LensAR.

The 3D-confocal structured illumination (3D-CSI) technology utilizes a confocal laser (superluminescent diode) imaging technique that is optically captured at a Scheimpflug angle and is optically enhanced with a form of structured illumination, that scans less reflective structures (posterior capsule) more than highly reflective structures (anterior corneal surface). Lens densitometry is also possible with this technology, similar to and exceeding that experienced with Scheimpflug tomography (see Fig. 19.4 of Chap. 19). Although not currently utilized, lens densitometry could quantitatively access the level of hardness and adjust the laser energy to match this density as a future improvement to this technology. If this titratable energy delivery could improve the efficiency of lens fragmentation and disassembly, then it would be preferable in enhancing safety, as well (less energy, less risk). Beyond the measurement and manual adjustment of therapeutic laser energy for fragmentation, a closed loop system could also be designed in the future to assess the lens density and then automatically adjust the laser energy for optimal fragmentation. Since the densitometry dependent adjustment of laser energy is not currently being performed, it still has not been shown whether this would improve outcomes, and hence is still only a speculative future development.

Upgradability

The future developments of accommodation restoration and lens densitometry guided surgery are only still speculative as their full proof of concept remains to be demonstrated. However, the modular nature of the LensAR Laser System will make it easily upgradable for these developments, should they mature into clinical use, and for any further refinement and development in ReLACS techniques and technology.

Company Details

Nicholas Curtis
Chief Executive Officer
Chief Commercial Officer
LensAR Inc.
2800 Discovery Drive
Orlando FL 32826
USA
Email: nick.curtis@lensar.com

References

1. Edwards K, Uy HS, Schneider S. The effect of laser lens fragmentation on use of ultrasound energy in cataract surgery. Association for research in vision and ophthalmology annual meeting. Poster #D768, 4 May 2011. Fort Lauderdale, FL.
2. Edwards KH, Frey RW, Tackman RN, et al. Clinical outcomes following laser cataract surgery. Invest Ophthalmol Vis Sci 2010;51 [E-Abstract 5394].
3. Naranjo Tackman R, Villar Kuri J, Nichamin LD, Edwards K. Anterior capsulotomy with an ultrashort-pulse laser. J Cataract Refract Surg. 2011;37:819–24.
4. Frey RW, Teuma EV, O'Suilleabhain D, Elliot D, Downes GR Jr, Downes GR III, Bielitzki J. Evaluation of the mechanical properties of the crystalline lens capsule following photodisruption capsulotomy and continuous curvilinear capsulorrhexis. Invest Ophthalmol Vis Sci 2009;50 [E-Abstract 1141].
5. Uy H, Hill WE, Edwards K. Refractive results after laser anterior capsulotomy. Invest Ophthalmol Vis Sci 2011;52 [E-abstract 5695].
6. Myers RI, Krueger RR. Novel approaches to correction of presbyopia with laser modification of the crystalline lens. J Refract Surg. 1998;14:136–9.
7. Krueger RR, Sun XK, Stroh J, Myers R. Experimental increase in accommodative potential after neodymium: yttrium-aluminum-garnet laser photodisruption of paired cadaver lenses. Ophthalmology. 2001; 108(11):2122–9.
8. Krueger RR, Kuszak J, Lubatschowski H, Myers RI, Ripken T, Heisterkamp A. First safety study of femtosecond laser photodisruption in animal lenses: tissue morphology and cataractogenesis. J Cataract Refract Surg. 2005;31:2386–94.

Commercially Available Systems: OptiMedica's Catalys Precision Laser System

17

William W. Culbertson

Introduction By Mark Forchette: OptiMedica and Pattern Scanning Lasers

OptiMedica was founded in Silicon Valley in 2004 to deliver innovative ophthalmic technologies and transform existing standards of care in retina, glaucoma and cataract. Our breakthrough technologies include the PASCAL® (Pattern SCAnning Laser) family of photocoagulators for the treatment of retinal disease and glaucoma and the Catalys™ Precision Laser System for the treatment of cataract [1–4].

While we have been focused on both technologies from the very beginning, OptiMedica achieved its first commercial success with PASCAL. Launched worldwide in 2006, PASCAL was designed to dramatically improve the precision, efficiency and comfort of panretinal photocoagulation (PRP) procedures [1–4]. While a PRP treatment can require up to 2,000 laser spots, traditional single spot green laser photocoagulators required ophthalmologists to deliver them one at a time with a pulse duration of 100 ms. With the PASCAL pattern scanning technique, ophthalmologists could for the first time deliver up to 56 laser spots in half a second with a pulse duration of just 10 ms. This marked advancement brought significant benefits to ophthalmologists and patients, as treatments that previously required retrobulbar anesthetic blocks and multiple office visits could be completed in one visit with no block and with much less collateral tissue damage (see Fig. 17.1a–c).

The benefits of our PASCAL technology led to rapid and broad adoption by ophthalmologists worldwide. By mid-2010, OptiMedica manufactured and shipped more than 600 PASCAL units in more than 40 markets around the world, with more than 750,000 patients treated and more than 30 million patterns delivered. This clinical and commercial success drew great interest from a number of other companies in the ophthalmic device industry, including Topcon Corp. Topcon added PASCAL to its product portfolio in 2008 and ultimately chose to acquire the technology in August 2010. The transaction, which represented the largest acquisition in the history of Topcon Corp.'s medical device business, delivered to Topcon Corp. a significant therapeutic product portfolio and a pipeline of retina innovation. At the same time, it was a strategic move for OptiMedica that gave us significant funding and the ability to apply undiluted focus to the development of our Catalys Precision Laser System.

Cataract procedures are in the midst of a revolutionary change, and we strongly believe that

W.W. Culbertson, M.D. (✉)
Department of Ophthalmology, Bascom Palmer Eye Institute, University of Miami Miller School of Medicine, 900 N.W. 17th St., Miami, FL 33136, USA
e-mail: wculbertson@med.miami.edu

R.R. Krueger et al. (eds.), *Textbook of Refractive Laser Assisted Cataract Surgery (ReLACS)*,
DOI 10.1007/978-1-4614-1010-2_17, © Springer Science+Business Media, LLC 2013

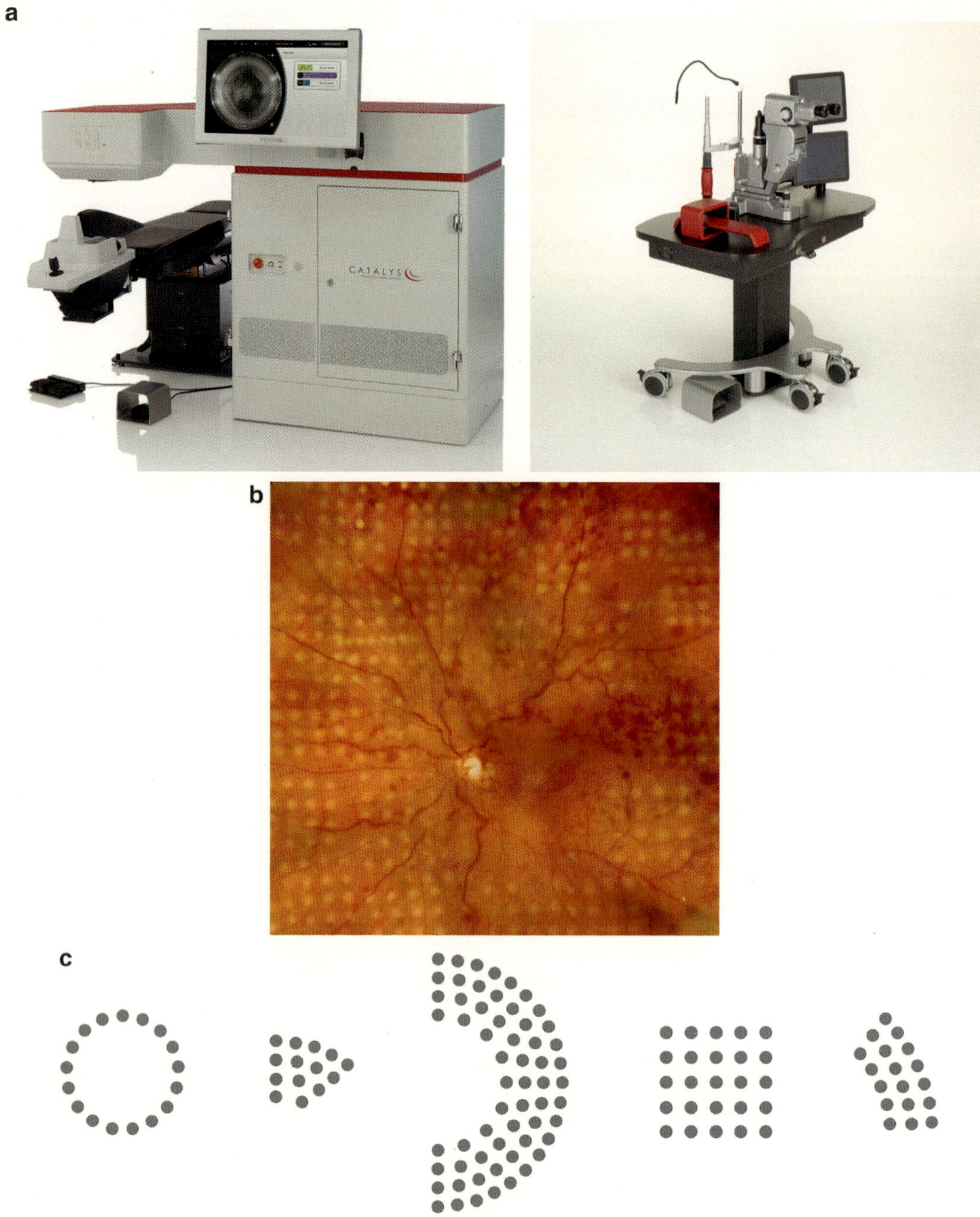

Fig. 17.1 (**a**) PASCAL photocoagulator. (**b** and **c**) Patterns from the PASCAL Streamline photocoagulator, the retinal photocoagulation product line developed by OptiMedica (image courtesy of OptiMedica Corporation, Sunnyvale, CA) https://optimedica.box.com/s/k7etsumdy08o2ms90do7

OptiMedica is poised to provide leadership in the technology that satisfies the high expectations of surgeons and their patients. As evidenced by our success with PASCAL, OptiMedica has a deep knowledge of laser–tissue interaction and the delivery of laser with high-speed scanning. Our research, development, and manufacturing teams excel in high quality optical design, integration of complex control systems, system ergonomics, and intuitive graphic user interface (GUI) design.

We have a deep history of partnerships and personal relationships within the ophthalmic community, and our reputation for excellent customer service and support is second to none.

The Catalys™ Precision Laser System received CE Mark approval in Europe and FDA clearance in 2011 and 2012 for anterior capsulotomy, lens fragmentation, arcuate incisions and multiplanar primary and sideport cataract incisions. There are over 25 laser systems in operation in the USA and around the world at the time of this writing.

Motivating Concept: The Potential Impact of ReLACS on the Worldwide Market and Surgical Outcomes

From its founding in 2004, OptiMedica has been committed to delivering on the tremendous potential of ReLACS to ophthalmic surgeons and their patients. Together with Stanford University Chairman of Ophthalmology, Mark S. Blumenkranz, M.D., and Stanford research scientist, Daniel Palanker, Ph.D., the OptiMedica team began developing an OCT-guided FS laser with the idea that it could enhance cataract surgery by creating new levels of precision. Soon after the company's inception, the initial patent for FS laser cataract surgery was filed.

In 2005, at the beginning of the ReLACS, development process, William Culbertson, I began working with OptiMedica after having spent 3 years using the Intralase FS laser in making flaps for LASIK at the Bascom Palmer Eye Institute. The fundamental precision of the Intralase instrument was immediately apparent, and we found that we could program the instrument to create LASIK flaps with diameters, shapes, thicknesses, and positions within 20 μm of what we intended to achieve. For the first time, we were able to customize the flap dimensions to the patient's eye and to the intended type of correction. These results were far superior to what we could achieve using a microkeratome. Although the microkeratome usually made smooth interfaces, the inconsistencies of diameter, thickness, shape, and position made us largely abandon it for flap making.

I also found that the Intralase FS laser was a useful tool in performing other types of corneal surgery with dependability and accuracy that far exceeded what could be achieved with traditional manual techniques. Along with others, I created channels for INTACS rings, performed anterior lamellar keratoplasty with a perfect fit between donor and host [5], corneal incisions using preprogrammed dimensions and shapes, including arcuate incisions for correction of astigmatism [6], special shaped cataract incisions that seal better than manually created ones [7]. The software was even expanded to allow for custom shaped penetrating keratoplasty and deep anterior lamellar keratoplasty ("zig-zag," "mushroom," and "tophat" shapes).

In developing the Catalys Precision Laser System, our goal was to deliver the precision and safety benefits of FS laser technology to the practice of cataract surgery. Once we were able to demonstrate the feasibility of this concept in our initial bench laboratory work, we performed safety studies, and energy and scanning parameters were developed. A prototype FS laser with integral OCT imaging specifically designed for cataract surgery was constructed, initially employing a fixed curved single lens contact interface.

Following investigational review board (IRB) approval, human studies began in the Dominican Republic at the Clinica Centro Laser of Juan Batlle, M.D., in Santo Domingo in June 2009. Results from the very first cases confirmed our initial assumptions regarding the safety and accuracy of the laser, and we proceeded to develop a refined commercial instrument, which OptiMedica named "Catalys."

The global market opportunity for FS lasers that perform cataract surgery is substantial. As the world's population ages, surgical volumes are growing and cataract surgery patients are increasingly demanding the best visual outcomes made possible by new IOL technologies. Leading refractive cataract surgeons have recognized this trend and are dedicated to delivering the refractive outcomes that these patients expect. By creating consistent, reproducible cuts and pretreating the cornea and lens, Catalys has the potential to help cataract surgeons achieve the patient's refractive goals.

Technical Aspects of the Commercial System

Laser System and Delivery

The Catalys FS laser engine is a diode-pumped solid state laser with a pulse duration <600 fs and near infrared wavelength of approximately 1,032 nm. A large focal depth of greater than 8 mm is required to fragment and soften cataractous tissue deep in the crystalline lens. The laser-focusing system needed to support this larger range of focal depth has special requirements, namely, a reduced numerical aperture and increased focal beam diameter. Therefore, as laser physics dictate, a higher threshold energy is needed for photodisruption of ocular tissues than with corneal FS laser surgery.

OptiMedica conducted preclinical and clinical studies to determine the operating parameter ranges for both safety and efficacy. The primary safety concerns of pulsed lasers at high repetition rates are heating of the retina (as described by the American National Standards Institute ocular laser safety standards) and of thermo-mechanical damage to retinal pigment epithelial cells. As a result of the safety studies, the repetition rate of the laser engine was modulated in application to maintain an average power based on pulse energy. To determine operating parameter ranges for efficacy, both preclinical and clinical studies were completed. With freshly enucleated porcine eyes and then 100 samples of enucleated human eyes, the team determined the threshold energy and pattern spot density (in both the lateral and axial dimensions) needed to make a continuous cut in the capsule and to segment the lens. Pulse energy ranged from 3 to 10 μJ with repetition rates between 12 and 80 kHz. Scanning parameters for pattern spot density were 5 μm in the lateral plane of the capsulotomy circle, 10 μm in its cylindrical depth and twice those values for lens fragmentation [8]. Operating parameters were further validated in the IRB-approved prospective clinical study in the Dominican Republic.

Docking System and Coupling to the Eye

The Catalys system includes an advanced Liquid Optics™ Interface, a disposable multi-piece patient–laser interface that serves as the final critical optic for the video and OCT imaging and laser delivery. Liquid Optics was the product of considerable innovative thinking and development. While the initial clinical study with Catalys used a curved applanating patient interface (PI), the surgical

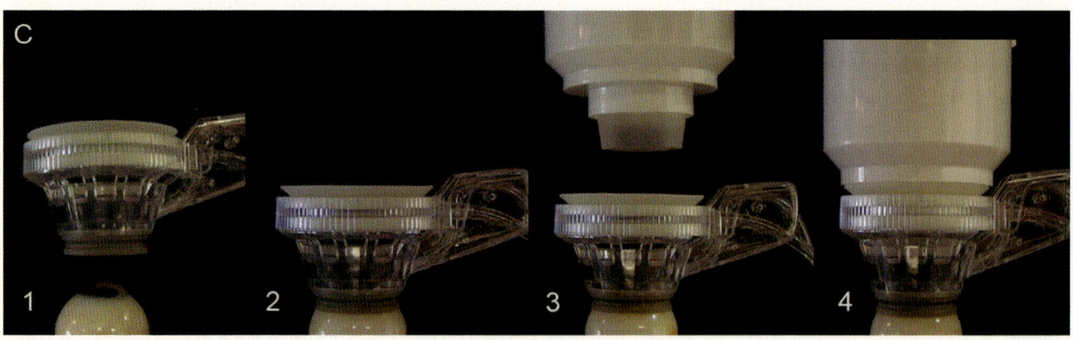

Fig. 17.2 Liquid Optics Interface. Liquid Optics Interface docking system demonstrating the progression of placing the suction ring on the eye and raising the suction ring to engage with the disposable lens (image courtesy of OptiMedica Corporation, Sunnyvale, CA)

team and engineers saw an opportunity to improve the design to eliminate corneal folds, improve incision quality, reduce intraocular pressure (IOP) rise during docking, and reduce the unsightly subconjunctival hemorrhages that persisted for 2–3 weeks post-surgery. The team knew that surgeons and patients would be expecting a comfortable experience for the patient and a predictable refractive outcome that the initial curved lens PI configuration would not deliver to a satisfactory degree. Rather than speeding to market with a suboptimal design, the team committed to an alternative design that addressed all opportunities for improvement. The reengineered interface resulted in a novel, fluid-filled interface which does not distort the cornea and provides a clear optical path for precise OCT, video imaging and laser delivery. Moreover, when compared to the earlier interface, the Liquid Optics Interface has delivered a five-time reduction in IOP rise and has resulted in significantly less eye redness post-surgery [9] (see Fig. 17.2). Please see Chap. 6 for more information on details concerning the fluid-filled PI.

Imaging System

The Catalys system uses a proprietary long-range spectral domain OCT to accurately locate the ocular surfaces in three dimensions. The OCT is integrated with the FS laser optics and applied through the same focusing objective and Liquid Optics Interface as the FS laser. The axial resolution, which is based on the coherence length of the light source, is <15 μm. The lateral resolution, which is based on the optical design, is <40 μm. The image is acquired after the globe is secured to and stabilized by the PI. The accompanying live video system operates at a wavelength nearly coincident with the FS laser, with a field of view that is 17 mm in diameter. Signal processing algorithms use the raw OCT and video data to automatically identify the surfaces of the anterior cornea, posterior cornea, iris, anterior capsule, and posterior capsule.

While anterior segment OCT is broadly used in clinical practices today, as a diagnostic tool, not all OCT systems are designed with equal quality and

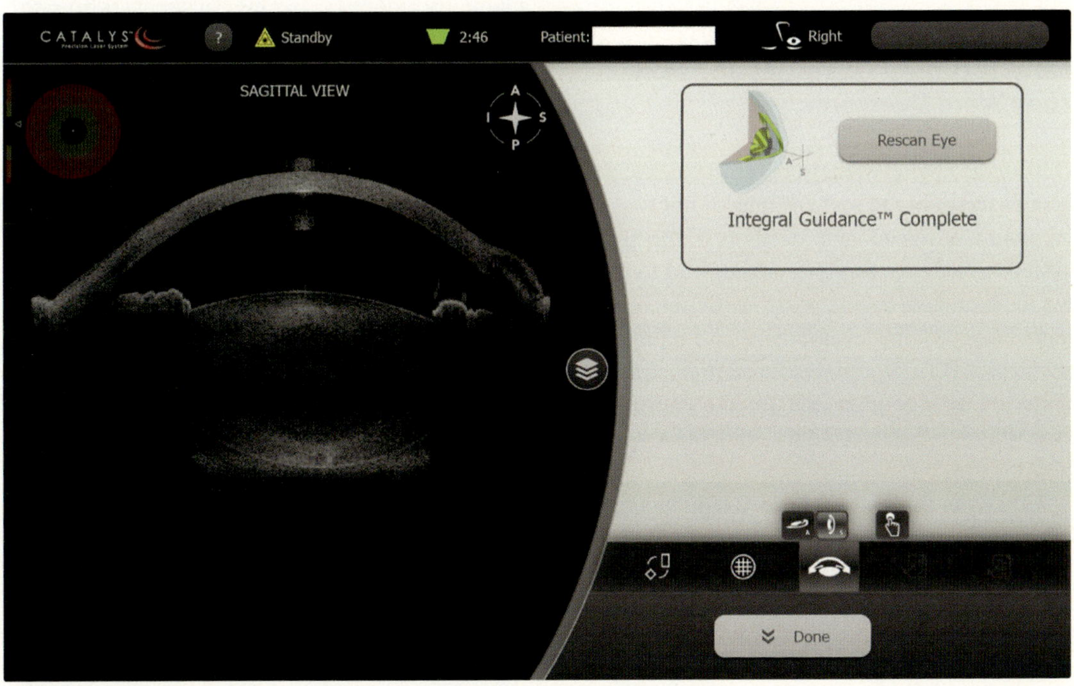

Fig. 17.3 Catalys OCT. A cross-sectional view of the three-dimensional high-resolution spectral domain optical coherence tomography (OCT) from the Catalys graphical user interface (image courtesy of OptiMedica Corporation, Sunnyvale, CA)

technical specifications. For ReLACS, signal processing of 3D OCT images is needed to turn the diagnostic data into a controlled guidance system. OptiMedica's Catalys addresses this requirement with Integral Guidance™, a proprietary image-guidance system that identifies ocular surfaces, creates and maintains exclusion (i.e., safety) zones where the laser cannot fire, helps the surgeon accurately and repeatedly adjust patterns, and ensures that the FS laser pulses are delivered precisely to the intended location.

Integral Guidance removes inverted OCT images (such as seeing a double iris) and other imaging artifacts, so the posterior capsule can be accurately identified. Ocular structures and laser exclusion zones can be created even when the eye is tilted relative to the laser path from docking, or in the case of a tilted crystalline lens with zonular dehiscence. Additionally, ocular surfaces such as the anterior and posterior capsule are identified, so the fragmentation depth can be maximized to safely deliver laser energy deep into the lens in order to make lens disassembly as easy as possible (see Fig. 17.3).

Early Technical Obstacles and How They Were Overcome

OptiMedica believes the success of ReLACS will be measured on the scale of tens of microns. The company designed and developed the Catalys system to leave nothing to chance and to deliver the most precise results possible. Of the four systems currently in development and equipped to perform ReLACS, Catalys has demonstrated the highest levels of precision for the capsulotomy (according to published data available at the time of printing).

Getting to this level of precision did not happen overnight, and it did not happen alone. The multiple years-long development process for Catalys was highly collaborative, bringing together OptiMedica's executive, engineering and development teams and a group of esteemed cataract surgeons from around the world. These surgeons participated closely at every point in the development process, weighing in on everything from clinical considerations and technical requirements to practice integration issues. They also treated hundreds of preclinical eyes, and many participated in IRB-approved clinical studies. In addition, OptiMedica worked closely with a Medical Staff Advisory Board comprised of technicians, nurses and practice administrators, each of whom lent unique perspective to the technology's integration into clinical practice. Together, this extended team was able to develop unique and innovative solutions to address various obstacles during the Catalys system's development.

For example, the Liquid Optics Interface was just one of many subsystems the OptiMedica team refined over time in order to get maximal precision, patient comfort and streamlined workflow. The template-based planning software and automatic surface detection are features that streamline workflow. Planning occurs prior to patient docking and can be completed by someone other than the treating physician. The automatic and highly accurate surface detection algorithms, which are the cornerstone of the Catalys system's Integral Guidance™ process, eliminate the need for the surgeon to manually identify ocular surfaces while the patient is under dock. While it took OptiMedica several years to refine planning and surface detection, the resulting subsystems enhance the accuracy of the procedure and minimize the amount of time that a patient is under dock. This last point is especially critical, as elderly patients may have ocular comorbidities like glaucoma and vascular diseases, so time under dock and intraocular pressure rise should be minimized. Currently we have reduced docked time to approximately 3 min with the expectation that this will decrease with engineering refinements. Since the IOP is only nominally increased during dockage with the Liquid Optics Interface (see Chap. 6), it is unlikely that this period of suction attachment will have any clinical significance.

The supreme measure of the quality of a system is the performance it delivers. Throughout the development process, OptiMedica and its team of advisors prioritized precision, accuracy, safety, and ergonomics as the most important elements to deliver patient benefit with the Catalys system.

Clinical Capabilities and Parameters for Cataract Surgery

The Catalys Precision Laser System is designed to perform the anterior capsulotomy, laser phacofragmentation, corneal arcuate incisions and transcorneal cataract incisions with paracenteses. The capsulotomy is performed first, followed by lens fragmentation and corneal incisions. For each cut, the laser pulses are applied posterior to anterior in order to avoid cavitation and gas bubbles that may be created by treatment posterior to the laser.

Laser Anterior Capsulotomy

Laser Ablation Pattern and Energies/Spacing

OptiMedica conducted extensive preclinical trials with freshly enucleated porcine eyes to determine the laser parameters that enable precise and complete capsulotomies with minimal collateral damage. The experimental design involved extracting the lens, placing it in balanced salt solution (BSS), and vertically directing the laser energy to the anterior capsule through a cover slip. The pattern spot density needed to create a continuous cut with a pulse duration of <600 fs and wavelength of 1,032 nm, was a focal spot size <10 μm, lateral spot spacing of 5 μm and axial spacing of 10 μm [8]. The threshold pulse energy to induce cavitation was approximately 3 μJ. Similar operating parameters were used in clinical trials; the exact values were proprietary at the time of this textbook's publishing.

Vertical Extent of Laser Treatment

Using Integral Guidance, Catalys registers the 3D curvature of the anterior capsule and automatically adjusts the incisional depth so that the depth is consistent along the entire circumference of the capsulotomy. If the lens is tilted relative to the laser pathway, Catalys tilts the laser treatment plane to correspond to the lens tilt. This results in a consistent cut that is simultaneously applied over the 360° of the capsulotomy. For this reason, the system is able to optimize the capsulotomy parameters to ensure a complete cut while minimizing energy applied to the eye.

	Endpoint Measured	Manual Results (Mean ± SD)	Laser Results (Mean ± SD)
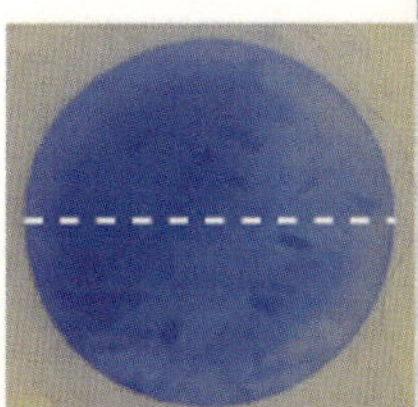	Capsulotomy size (Deviation from intended diameter)	339µm ± 248µm	27µm ± 25µm ($p<0.001$)
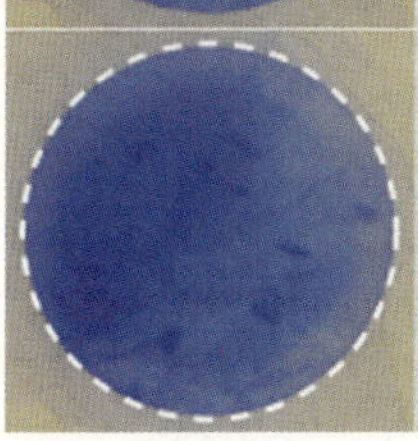	Capsulotomy circularity (1=perfect circle)	0.765 ± 0.148	0.942 ± 0.040 ($p<0.001$)

Fig. 17.4 Capsule size and shape. Laser capsulotomy from the Catalys Precision Laser System stained with trypan blue demonstrating an order of magnitude more precision in size and shape (image courtesy of OptiMedica Corporation, Sunnyvale, CA) https://optimedica.box.com/s/ikmbky7b8p2xvry9gwek

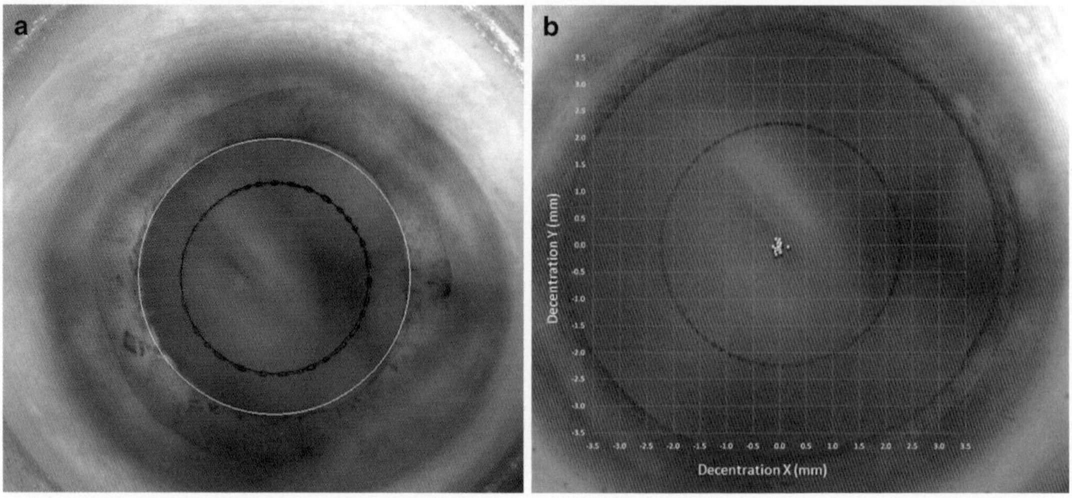

Fig. 17.5 Centration image. (**a**) Laser capsulotomy centration. Still frame from Catalys video system during capsulotomy centration. (**b**) Overlay of *X*/*Y* scatter plot with average root mean square distance of capsulotomy center and dilated pupil center (image courtesy of OptiMedica Corporation, Sunnyvale, CA)

Strength of Cuts

Capsulotomy strength was tested by distending empty porcine capsules and registering the force at rupture. The break force for 3 μJ laser capsulotomy was 152 ± 21 mN compared with 65 ± 21 mN for manual CCC ($p < 0.05$) [10].

Accuracy of Cuts

In a randomized, prospective IRB-approved study, 29 eyes received the Catalys laser procedure and 30 eyes received manual cataract surgery. For all eyes, the anterior capsular disks were removed prior to phacoemulsification so that shape and circularity of the CCC or capsulotomy could be measured.

Size: Size accuracy was calculated as the deviation between intended diameter and observed diameter. The mean deviation for manual capsulorhexis was −0.282 ± 0.305 mm, whereas the mean deviation for laser capsulotomy was just 0.027 ± 0.025 mm ($p < 0.001$). This represented a more than tenfold decrease in deviation from intended diameter. Moreover, the size variability from case to case was much reduced (see Fig. 17.2), demonstrating a much more predictable and repeatable capsulotomy construction with the laser (see Fig. 17.4).

Shape: Circularity was measured as a function of disk size and area. A perfect circle has a circularity value of 1.00. The manual capsulorhexis had a mean circularity of 0.77 ± 0.15 ($n = 22$), while the laser capsulotomy had a mean circularity of 0.95 ± 0.04 ($n = 29$) ($p < 0.001$) [8, 10] (see Fig. 17.4).

Centration: Following laser delivery, centration of the laser capsulotomy was analyzed using still frames from the Catalys video system. Centration accuracy was measured relative to the intended capsulotomy center. The average root mean squared distance from the center of capsulotomy to the intended center was just 0.077 ± 0.047 mm [10]. The manual capsulorhexis was centered by the surgeon's view and could not be measured with micron level accuracy for comparison purposes (see Fig. 17.5a, b).

Postoperative Consistency of Effect

The size and shape of capsule aperture changes over time [11, 12]. Size and shape changes in OptiMedica laser capsulotomy eyes and manual CCC eyes were analyzed at time of surgery and 1 week and 4 weeks postoperatively. The diameter of the laser apertures deviated just 0.1 mm, on average, whereas the manual CCC apertures decreased in size by over half a millimeter.

The laser aperture shape was also more consistent over time [10].

Unique Benefits

The accuracy and precision of capsulotomy size, shape, and centration achieved with Catalys is unmatched by any system, according to published data available at the time of print. Moreover, the surgeon can select the method for centering the capsulotomy preoperatively, such as on the center of the dilated pupil or scanned capsule center as determined by OCT. After the patient is docked to the system, Integral Guidance can automatically adjust the planned capsulotomy according to the chosen target for the patient.

Limitations Overcome

In ReLACS, the cornea is part of the optical system. To enable precise imaging and laser delivery it is critical that both the anterior and posterior surfaces of the cornea are undistorted. In OptiMedica's first approach, the curved lens interface applanated the cornea and induced folds in nearly 75% of cases. These folds reduced the ability of the laser to focus to a point below a fold. The clinical impact was striking, as skips or tags in the capsulotomy were visualized directly posterior to corneal folds [9].

Lens Fragmentation

Geometric Patterns

OptiMedica studied a wide range of patterns in years of preclinical studies and only went to clinical trials with those patterns expected to be successful. The commercial system is equipped with a variety of nuclear fragmentation patterns for segmenting and softening the crystalline lens. Segmentation patterns include a cross design, a sextant pattern and an octant pattern. Softening patterns deliver laser energy to the regions in between the incision lines created by the segmentation patterns (see Fig. 17.6).

Definition of fragmentation, segmentation, softening

- Fragmentation is a general term that refers to both segmentation and softening.
- Segmentation is the breaking up of the lens into several large segments.

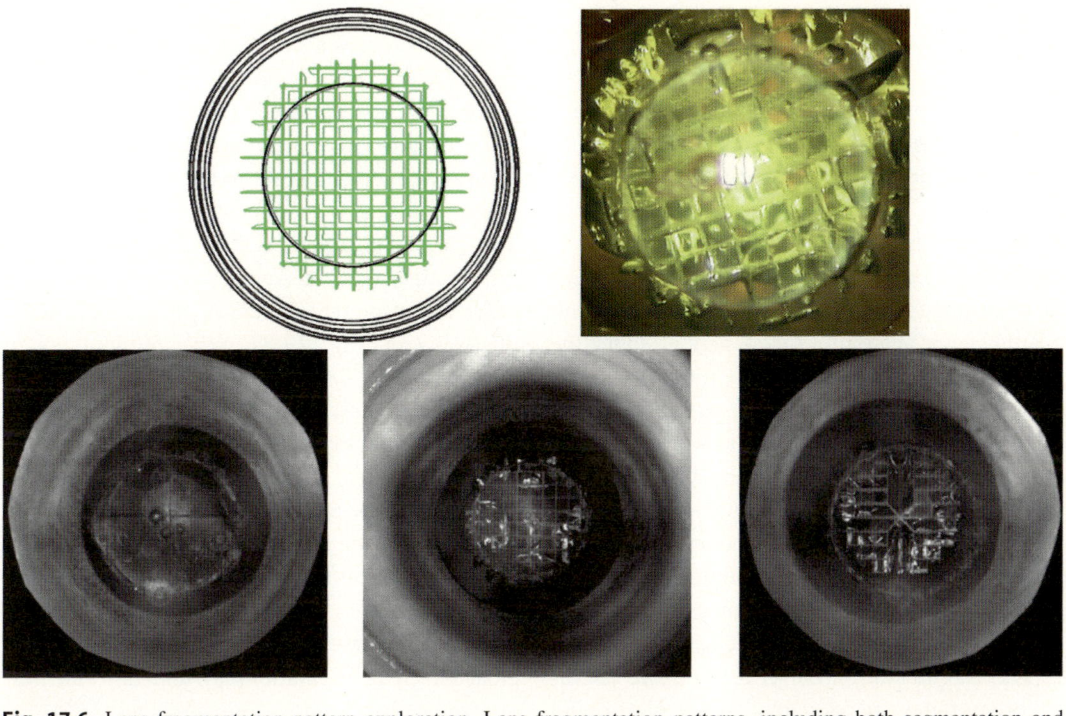

Fig. 17.6 Lens fragmentation pattern exploration. Lens fragmentation patterns, including both segmentation and softening, from the Catalys Precision Laser System (image courtesy of OptiMedica Corporation, Sunnyvale, CA)

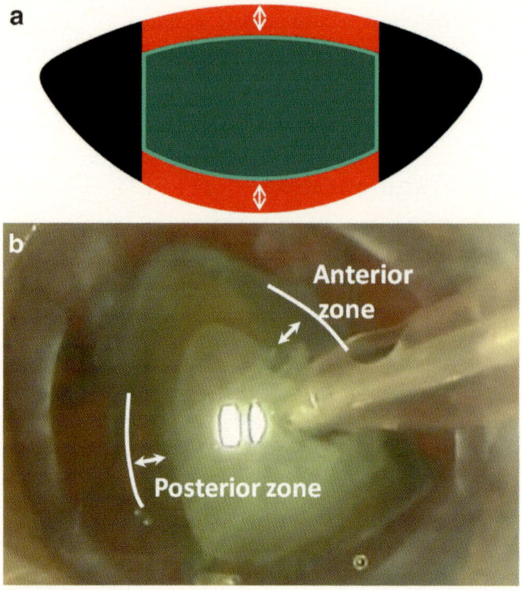

Fig. 17.7 Laser exclusion zones. (**a**) Schematic of anterior and posterior lens safety margins (highlighted with white arrows) and lens fragmentation zone (in the middle) created with Integral Guidance. Safety margins are defined regions where the laser cannot fire. (**b**) Video frame of phaco tip grabbing a lens quadrant following laser lens fragmentation. Anterior and posterior lens safety zones created with Integral Guidance are maintained through laser lens fragmentation and visible during lens removal (image courtesy of OptiMedica Corporation, Sunnyvale, CA)

- Softening is the breaking up of large sections of the lens using a laser pulse pattern with close proximity between cuts.

Fragmentation Dimensions

In a Catalys procedure, the fragmentation dimensions (width and depth) are matched precisely to the 3D ocular anatomy of each patient. Once the patient is under dock, Integral Guidance detects the iris boundaries and posterior capsule and sets exclusion zones to delineate areas where the laser cannot fire. The volume of the lens fragmentation zone is safely maximized in two ways:

1. The fragmentation width is bounded by an iris margin instead of the capsulotomy diameter Catalys is able to fragment more peripherally while still safely avoiding the iris.
2. The fragmentation depth follows the curvature of the posterior capsule instead of being guided by one (or several) manually selected marker(s). This approach allows the lens to be fragmented at a consistent, safe and minimal distance from the posterior capsule. In the IRB-approved study ($n=30$ laser; $n=29$ manual), the fragmentation depth varied from 2.7 to 4.9 mm, as dictated by the thickness of the crystalline lens [13] (see Fig. 17.7a, b).

Effectiveness of Laser Lens Pre-softening

Study Design

Cataracts were graded preoperatively on the LOCSIII scale for density. Most of the patients had advanced cataracts, with almost three-quarters of enrolled patients registering a LOCS grade 3 or 4 cataract. For each patient, one eye was randomized to manual cataract surgery while the other eye received the Catalys laser procedure followed by ultrasound phaco-assisted lens extraction and IOL implantation. After each phacoemulsification procedure, the cumulative dissipated energy (CDE) registered on the Alcon Infiniti system was recorded.

Study Result

Overall, there was approximately a 40% reduction in CDE for the laser pretreated lenses as compared to the non-pretreated lenses ($p=0.028$) [13]. According to anecdotal evidence, laser pretreatment of the lens makes a grade 4 lens feel like a grade 2 during ultrasound phacoemulsification. The CDE data supports this claim, with grade 4 pretreated lenses registering a CDE of 19.5 and grade 2 non-pretreated lenses registering a CDE of 18.2 (see Fig. 17.8). With refinements in patterns and phaco equipment, Professor HB Dick, Chairman of the University Eye Hospital, Bochum Germany, has found a 96% reduction across all grades.

In a follow-up study, surgical video was reviewed and the number of active phaco manipulations (movement of phaco tip in conjunction with use of phaco power) was recorded. The laser pretreated lenses required 45% fewer active surgical phaco manipulations to segment into four quadrants than did non-pretreated lenses [14].

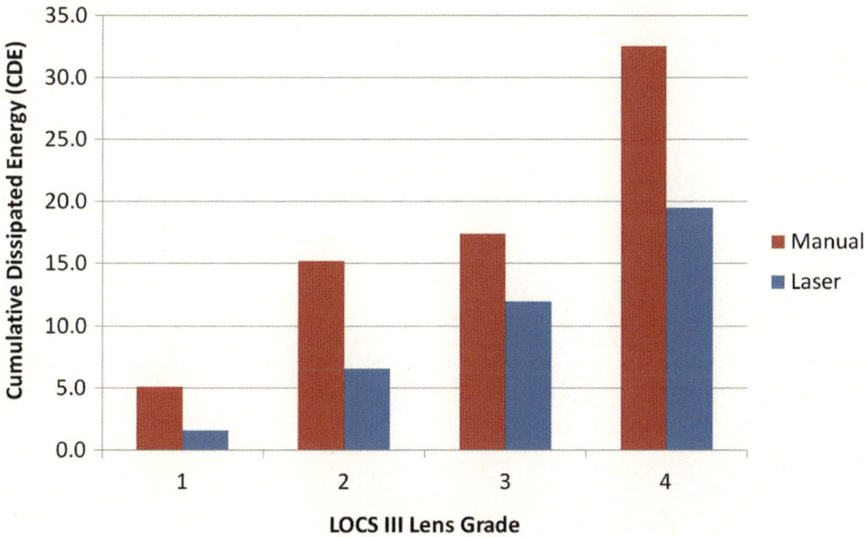

Fig. 17.8 CDE chart by LOCS grade. Comparison of cumulative dissipated energy (CDE) used per case with and without lens segmentation and softening performed with Catalys. Results are grouped by preoperative nuclear color and opalescence based on the Lens Opacities Classification System III (image courtesy of OptiMedica Corporation, Sunnyvale, CA)

Limitations Overcome

Results of OptiMedica's clinical studies demonstrated a progressive decline in phaco energy usage as the surgeons became accustomed to working with laser-segmented and softened lenses.

Unique Benefits

Catalys lens fragmentation is optimized for accuracy, effectiveness, safety and speed. The accuracy is enabled by the system's clear imaging pathway and precise surface detection algorithms. Fragmentation is highly effective, with a near [96] CDE reduction across all cataract grades. Automated exclusion zone registration makes lens treatment safe by ensuring that lasers are delivered a consistent distance from posterior capsule and iris. Lastly, speed is optimized because surface detection does not require manual delineation of ocular surfaces by the surgeon.

Corneal Incisions

Clear Corneal Incisions

The architecture and dimensions of Catalys corneal incisions are customizable for self-sealing architectures. Given the wide inner diameter of the suction ring (14.5 mm), these incisions can be created with high precision at the limbal edge, if desired, without decentering the suction ring. The incision can be configured as fully penetrating or not, as dictated by sterility requirements. Since the system in OptiMedica's Dominican Republic study was located outside of the operating room, the corneal incisions were non-penetrating (see Fig. 17.9a–d).

Corneal Arcuate Incisions

Compared to manual incisions, the laser has the ability to create more consistent, predictable incisions in arc length, depth, angulation, and shape. While the patient is under dock, Integral Guidance registers the corneal thickness at the location of planned arcuate incision. The depth of the incision can be programmed during treatment planning as a set micron value (e.g., 600 μm) or as a percentage of corneal thickness at the treatment location.

Improved consistency in the incision should lead to a more consistent outcome. Given the difference in tissue reaction to laser photocavitation as compared to a blade, large-scale studies will need to be conducted to determine an

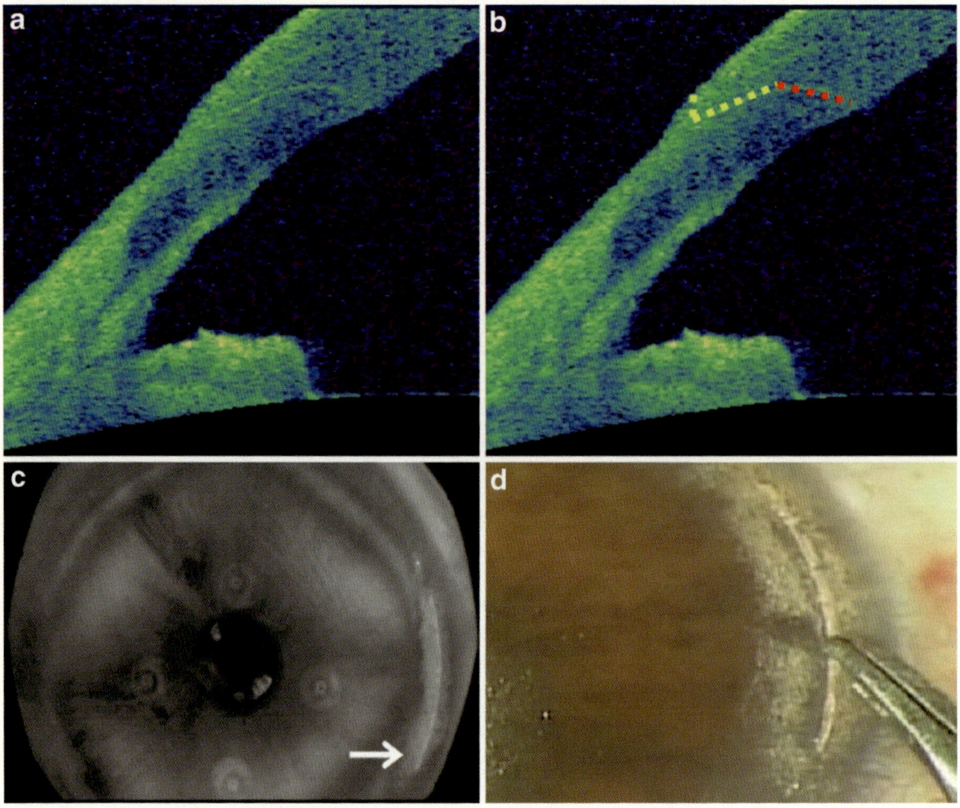

Fig. 17.9 Catalys corneal incisions. (**a** and **b**) Architecture of clear cornea incision initiated with Catalys Precision Laser System. The laser incision (*yellow*) and diamond knife incision (*red*) are highlighted on the post-op OCT image. Laser incision was not fully penetrating so as to maintain sterility of the procedure (image courtesy of OptiMedica Corporation, Sunnyvale, CA). (**c** and **d**) Still frame from video from Catalys Precision Laser video system during creation of arcuate incision (image courtesy of OptiMedica Corporation, Sunnyvale, CA) https://optimedica.box.com/s/nd4bc98nwfpzl6hh1au3

appropriate nomogram for laser corneal arcuate incisions.

Ergonomic Simplicity of Operation

Catalys was designed with superior ergonomics to ensure surgeon ease-of-use and a comfortable patient experience.

Graphical User Interface

The Catalys system's intuitive and elegant touch-screen graphical user interface was designed to simplify the planning process and minimize the time that the patient is under dock. The system is equipped with a high definition 24-in. monitor that can be positioned for comfortable use and visibility from a standing or seated position (see Fig. 17.10).

Mobility of Device

Precision in ReLACS involves more than just controlling the directionality of a laser. It is also critical to control the target. When designing Catalys, safety and precision were OptiMedica's top design objectives. Since success in the procedure is measured in tens of microns, OptiMedica equipped Catalys with an integrated Dexta bed with custom headrest that was explicitly designed to maximize the head stability of elderly cataract patients.

Footprint

Catalys is designed for comfortable use in a 10×10 square foot area; this area includes the system footprint, an integrated patient chair, surgeon chair and service access. For installation, Catalys can fit through a 34-in. doorway.

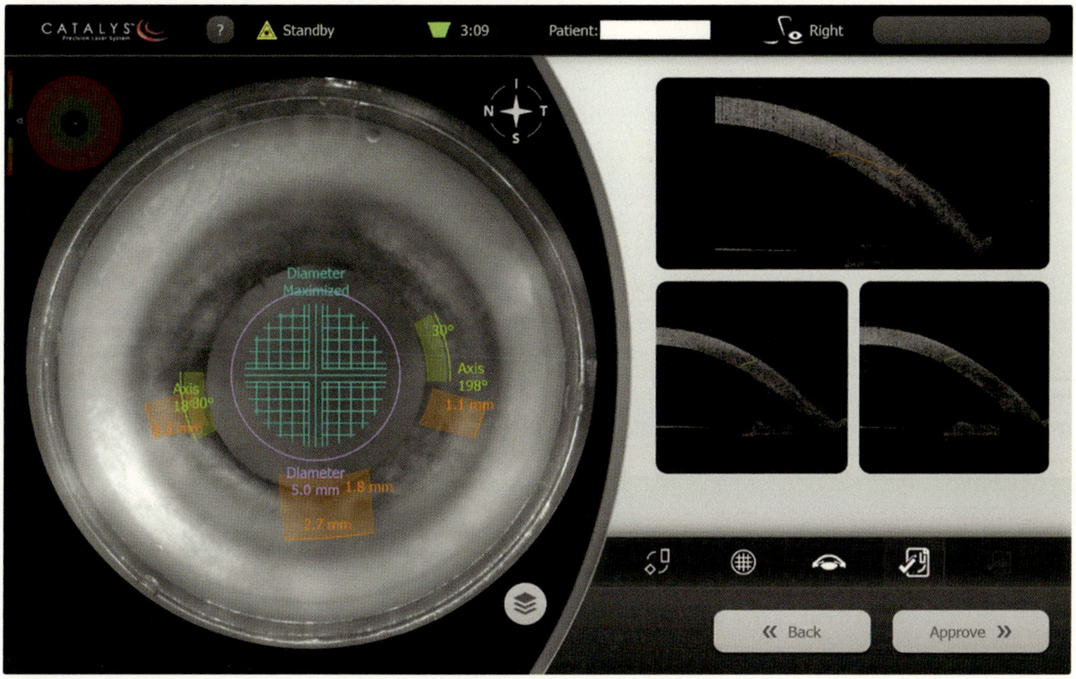

Fig. 17.10 Catalys graphical user interface. Sample Catalys Precision Laser System treatment page as seen on graphical user interface (image courtesy of OptiMedica Corporation, Sunnyvale, CA)

Procedural Workflow

Treatment planning: Planning a treatment on the Catalys system is quick, intuitive and template-based. Templates for each incision can be configured for commonly used treatment parameters. The surgeon or a member of the technical staff can enter the treatment plan for a particular patient in advance of the procedure. The process takes less than one minute.

Patient docking: The Liquid Optics suction ring is placed on the sclera and the connection is stabilized by system-controlled vacuum. The surgeon then fills the ring with balanced saline solution (BSS) and swings the patient bed under the system. Using the joystick on the patient chair, the surgeon maneuvers the chair to mate the suction ring to the disposable lens attached to the system. This connection is stabilized by another vacuum and a mechanical lock.

Treatment customization: Once the patient is under dock, Integral Guidance quickly and accurately customizes the treatment plan to fit the ocular anatomy of the patient. The surgeon simply needs to confirm the customized plan (adjusted if necessary) and then initiate treatment. The system workflow was designed to minimize patient time under dock. Minimizing dock time is relevant to procedure precision because patient stability is critical to accurate laser delivery. In addition, minimizing the amount and duration of IOP rise is a safety standard for elderly patients.

Treatment delivery: The capsulotomy takes 2 s; and the full set of laser incisions takes approximately 40–60 s to complete, depending on the cuts included and the parameters.

Ten Compelling Reasons Why a Customer Should Buy the Catalys Precision Laser System

1. Catalys delivers unsurpassed clinical outcomes, stemming from its superior technology.
2. Catalys offers surgeons the unique benefits of an advanced, proprietary Liquid Optics

Interface™. Designed to be a crucial element in the optical path, the Liquid Optics Interface eliminates corneal folds and results in lower IOP rise and less petechiae after the procedure.
3. Catalys delivers unparalleled precision and safety with Integral Guidance™, which combines proprietary 3D Spectral Domain OCT and signal processing to automatically detect and map the ocular surfaces and automatically create exclusion zones. Integral Guidance customizes the surgeon's treatment plan to the anatomy and the orientation of the patient's eye relative to the laser.
4. Catalys features an easy-to-use and elegant graphical user interface designed to simplify the planning process and minimize the time that the patient is under dock.
5. As evidenced by the features and benefits above, Catalys is the product of a development process based on the deep involvement of physicians and staff, resulting in a detailed understanding of the requirements and workflow.
6. OptiMedica is dedicated to developing superior technology and demonstrating clinical results through rigorous scientific studies.
7. OptiMedica has a history of technology innovation in ophthalmology, including the development of the family of PASCAL photocoagulators. Through that effort, the company developed and brought to market revolutionary technology and sold more than 600 systems worldwide before the business was acquired by Topcon Corp.
8. OptiMedica has an unwavering dedication to supporting ophthalmologists and their staffs in the application of the technology and to creating true partnerships to ensure the successful integration of ReLACS into the practice.
9. OptiMedica has strong financial backing from top investors, including Kleiner Perkins, Caufield & Byers, Alloy Ventures, DAG Ventures, BlackRock, and Bio*One Capital.
10. OptiMedica's management team is a group of industry veterans that brings collective knowledge from ophthalmology and from the broader medical device community. The company's executives have held leadership positions at Alcon, AMO, Intralase, Wavelight, Coherent, Intuitive Surgical, Boston Scientific, Medtronic, and Guidant.

Future Developments and Upgradability

OptiMedica has a strong and highly innovative research and development organization that is working on a range of enhancements to the Catalys Precision Laser System as well as next generation products.

References

1. Bol'shunov AV. The first experience in clinically using a PASCAL laser photocoagulator (OptiMedica, USA). Vestn Oftalmol. 2009;125(4):37–8.
2. Sanghvi C, McLauchlan R, Delgado C, et al. Initial experience with the Pascal photocoagulator: a pilot study of 75 procedures. Br J Ophthalmol. 2008;92(8): 1061–4 [Epub 2008 Jun 27].
3. Modi D, Chiranand P, Akduman L. Efficacy of patterned scan laser in treatment of macular edema and retinal neovascularization. Clin Ophthalmol. 2009;3:465–70 [Epub 2009 Aug 20].
4. Bolz M, Kriechbaum K, Simader C, Diabetic Retinopathy Research Group Vienna, et al. In vivo retinal morphology after grid laser treatment in diabetic macular edema. Ophthalmology. 2010;3:538–44 [Epub 2010 Jan 4].
5. Yoo SH, Kymionis GD, Koreishi A, Ide T, Goldman D, Karp CL, O'Brien TP, Culbertson WW, Alfonso EC. Femtosecond laser-assisted sutureless anterior lamellar keratoplasty. Ophthalmology. 2008;115:1303–7.
6. Kymionis GD, Yoo SH, Ide T, Culbertson WW. Femtosecond-assisted astigmatic keratotomy for post-keratoplasty irregular astigmatism. J Cataract Refract Surg. 2009;35:11–3.
7. Culbertson WW. Presented at the Intralase Users Meeting AAO 11/2006 AAO was in Las Vegas, USA.
8. Palanker DV, Blumenkranz MS, Andersen D, Wiltberger M, Marcellino G, et al. Femtosecond laser-assisted cataract surgery with integrated optical coherence tomography. Sci Transl Med. 2010;2:58ra85.
9. Talamo JH. Optical interface characteristics for laser cataract surgery. In: Proceedings of the American Society of Cataract and Refractive Surgery (ASCRS) 2011 annual meeting, femtosecond laser cataract surgery, session 1-E, 26 March 2011, San Diego, CA. p. 134.

10. Friedman NJ, Palanker DV, Schuele G, et al. Femtosecond laser capsulotomy. J Cataract Refract Surg. 2011;37:1189–98.
11. Park TK, Chung SK, Baek NH. Changes in the area of the anterior capsule opening after intraocular lens implantation. J Cataract Refract Surg. 2002;28:1613–7.
12. Hayashi K, Hayashi H. Intraocular lens factors that may affect anterior capsule contraction. Ophthalmology. 2005;112:286–92.
13. Culbertson WW, Batlle JF, Feliz R, Koch D, et al. Facilitation of nuclear cataract removal by femtosecond laser pretreatment. In: Proceedings of the American Society of Cataract and Refractive Surgery (ASCRS) 2011 annual meeting, femtosecond laser cataract surgery, session 1-E, 26 March 2011, San Diego, CA. p. 134.
14. Koch DD, Culbertson WW, Batlle JF. The use of OCT guided femtosecond laser to facilitate cataract uclear disassembly and aspiration. In: Proceedings of the European Society of Cataract and Refractive Surgery (ESCRS) 2010 annual meeting, Free paper session, Paris, France.

Commercially Available Systems: The TECHNOLAS Femto-Cataract Approach

18

Prasad Kasu Reddy and Kristian Hohla

The Femto-Cataract procedure is an extension of the femtosecond (FS) laser technology offered by Technolas Perfect Vision (Munich, Germany), the TECHNOLAS FS Laser Workstation. In this chapter, we describe how this procedure became reality, the technology, as well as early clinical experience and results and the benefits of this system.

Background

Technolas Perfect Vision (TPV) is a joint venture created in 2009 from the refractive unit of Bausch+Lomb (Rochester, NY) and 20/10 Perfect Vision, a company based in Heidelberg, Germany that had developed the Femtec FS laser, as well as the WaveScan wavefront aberrometry system. Founded in 1999, 20/10 Perfect Vision was the second company to begin the commercial development of an FS laser for corneal surgery, after Intralase. TPV was the first company to develop a curved patient interface (PI) for this purpose, which maintains near-natural curvature of the cornea during the laser procedure, as compared to the IntraLase Laser (AMO, Irvine, CA) which uses a PI that flattens the corneal surface.

P.K. Reddy, M.D. (✉)
Maxivision Eye Care Centres, 6-3-903-/A/1/1 Lane
Beside Yashoda Hospital, Hyderabad 500 082, India
e-mail: drkasuprasad@maxivision.co.in

K. Hohla, Ph.D.
Technolas Perfect Vision GmbH, 1-3 Messerschmittstr.,
Munich, Bavaria 80992, Germany

The initial applications for 20/10 Perfect Vision's FS laser were focused on corneal surgery, including creation of tunnels for implantation of corneal rings, corneal transplantations, and the creation of corneal flaps for laser in situ keratomileusis (LASIK). The company went on to develop INTRACOR, the first noninvasive intra-stromal refractive procedure for the treatment of presbyopia using the company's FS laser, of which the TECHNOLAS Femtosecond Workstation 520F is the successor (with CE Mark approval and US-FDA 510(k) clearance).

From this point, the path to the development of the Femto-Cataract module for the laser was a relatively quick one, with the company announcing the new cataract treatment option in September 2010.

Dr. Reddy was among the first surgeons in the world to begin performing the Femto-Cataract procedure with the Technolas FS laser, beginning in November 2010 at the Maxivision Eye Hospital in Hyderabad, India. He has performed more than 500 cataract surgeries with the system to date.

Technical Features

Laser System

The TECHNOLAS Femtosecond Workstation is a diode-pumped, solid-state laser (DPSSL) with a pulse duration of about 500 fs and a wavelength around 1 μm [1] (see Fig. 18.1). The laser has a pulse repetition rate which can go above 300 kHz and uses a variable pulse energy from sub-microjoules

R.R. Krueger et al. (eds.), *Textbook of Refractive Laser Assisted Cataract Surgery (ReLACS)*,
DOI 10.1007/978-1-4614-1010-2_18, © Springer Science+Business Media, LLC 2013

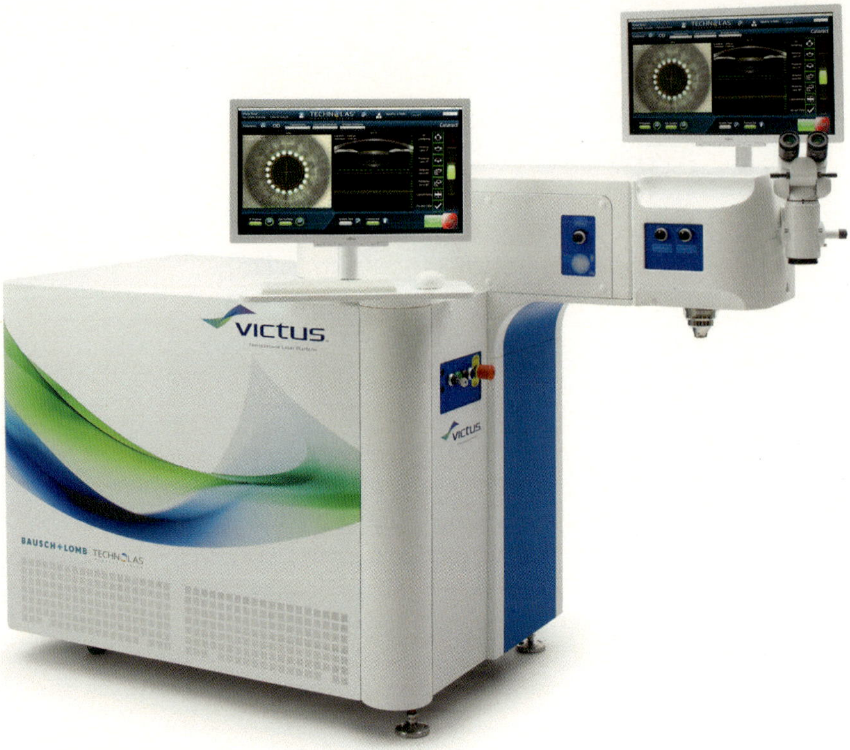

Fig. 18.1 The TECHNOLAS Femtosecond Laser Platform

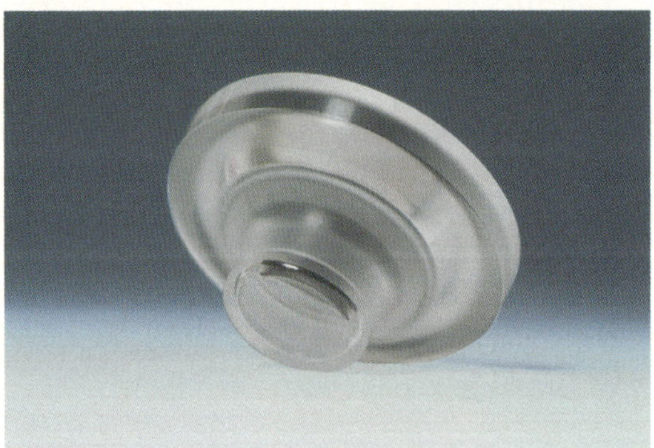

Fig. 18.2 TPV curved PI

to more than 10 μJ, depending on the type of procedure being performed. The system can penetrate the complete volume of the lens, allowing treatment close to the posterior capsule. In addition to the Femto-Cataract procedure, the laser can be programmed to perform a number of corneal procedures:

- LASIK flaps
- Arcuate cuts for Astigmatic Keratotomy (AK)
- Penetrating keratoplasty (PKP) and lamellar keratoplasty (LKP)
- Femtosecond Laser assisted Endothelial Keratoplasty (FLEK)
- Tunnels for Intrastromal Ring Segments (ICRS)
- Pockets for Corneal Cross-Linking procedures (CXL)
- Intrastromal treatment for presbyopia (INTRACOR)

This laser system uses a unique and proprietary curved PI approach for all procedures. The curved PI is a two-piece device. During fixation on the cornea, the system uses a proprietary approach with sensitive sensors (Intelligent Pressure Control) in three dimensions to monitor the pressure (see Fig. 18.2) [1]. The suction ring interacts with the sclera. No gels or other fluids are being used with the PI. TPV's proprietary Intelligent Pressure Control ensures that contact pressures are being used such that corneal

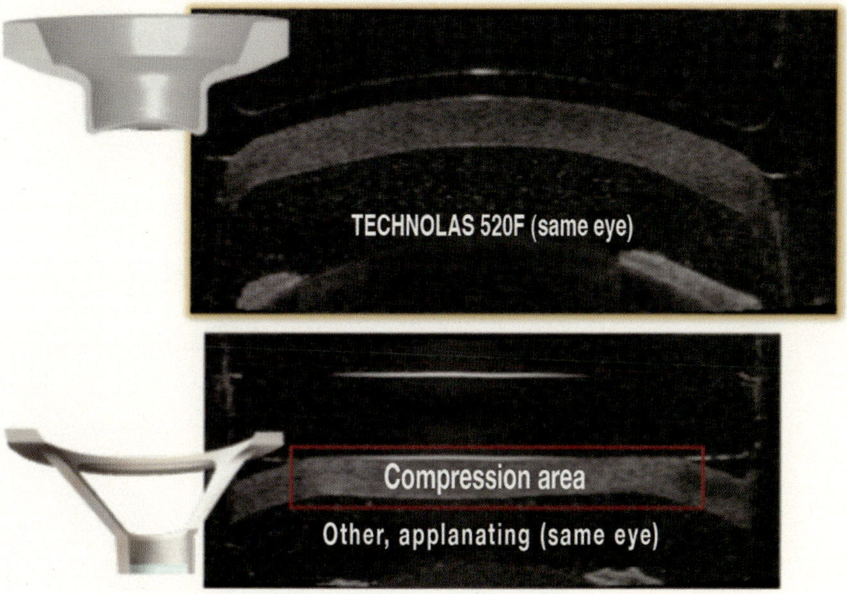

Fig. 18.3 Comparison of the curved PI vs. PI that utilizes applanation

deformation is kept at a minimum (see Figs. 18.3 and 18.4).

Using this approach produces truly curved cuts while improving patient comfort during the procedure. An evaluation of the mean IOP after suction was applied in flap procedures found a mean of IOP of 45 mmHg with the TPV FS laser vs. 71 mmHg with the Intralase laser [2].

The docking procedure typically takes about 10 s once the surgeon has performed a number of cases to become comfortable with the technique. Centration can be based, for example, on the center of the pupil; however the system's software also allows for further adjusting the centration in the procedure planning software. Once the docking is completed, the computer controlled and monitored suction system will automatically stop the procedure if a suction break is detected. The surgeon can start over again, depending on the individual clinical situation.

Imaging System

The TECHNOLAS laser uses an online, real-time OCT imaging system to enable the precise 3D identification and location of the anterior segment (see Fig. 18.5). The OCT imaging is "live," as it is continuously taken and displayed throughout the entire procedure in order to provide additional control and reassurance for the surgeon.

The visualized anatomical landmarks include the anterior and posterior surface of the cornea, as well as anterior and posterior views of the capsule. Appropriate safety distances to the relevant tissue areas are established using the surgical planning software.

In addition, the Graphical User Interface (GUI) of the Femto-Cataract procedure has been developed based on the needs of cataract surgery, and provides the surgeon with visual control of and direct interaction with the imaging data for procedure planning before surgery, as well as for real-time visualization during the cataract procedure [3]. The dimensions of the laser treatments can be adjusted by the surgeon to suit the needs of the individual patient (e.g., diameter of anterior capsulotomy vs. type of IOL used).

Clinical Capabilities

The Femto-Cataract software on the Technolas laser is designed to perform the key steps in the

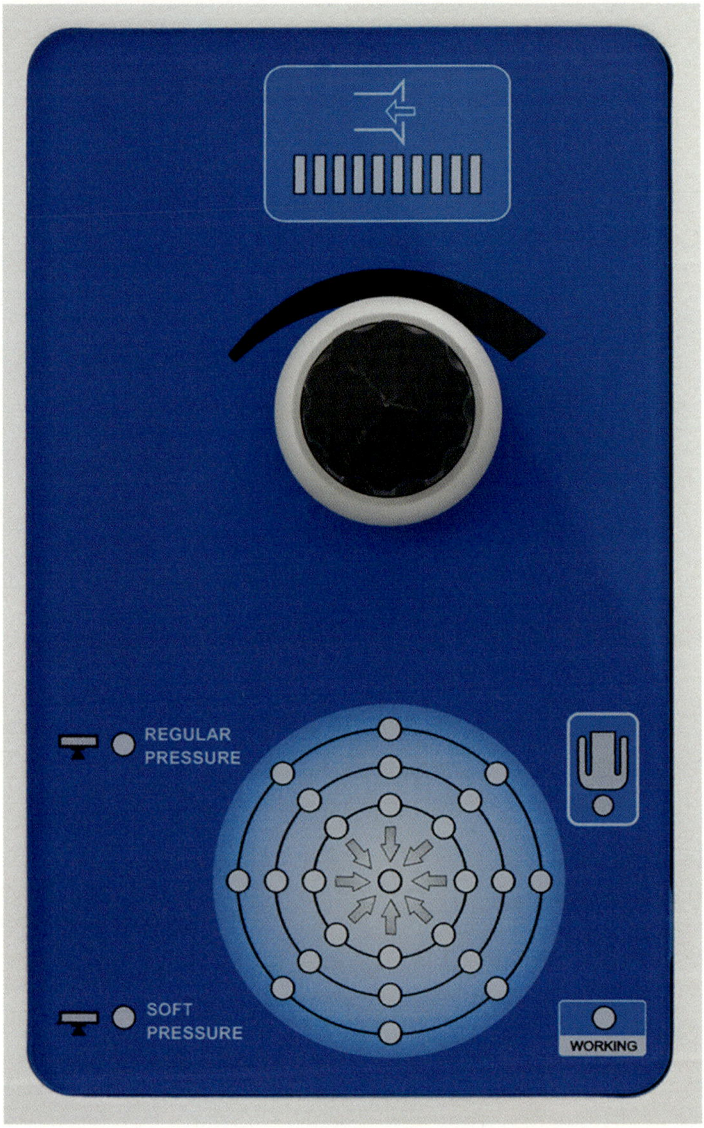

Fig. 18.4 Intelligent Pressure Control for the docking interface

cataract procedure: lens fragmentation, capsulorhexis, corneal incisions, and arcuate incisions which can be used for correction of astigmatism [4].

Fragmentation

Dependent on the cataract grade a specific lens fragmentation pattern is applied to the eye. For all grades (grades 1–5), clinical experience to date has yielded an average reduction of effective phaco time (EPT) (see Fig. 18.6). In addition to the reduction of ultrasonic power, nucleus disassembly was simplified by cracking the hardened nucleus with FS laser pulses [5].

In the 500+ cases performed to date by Dr. Reddy, the laser has been used on all types of cataracts, including intumescent white cataracts and pediatric cataracts. In his initial cases, Dr. Reddy employed his standard chopping technique following laser fragmentation. However, he quickly discovered that chopping was not necessary, even with +5 cataracts, and that it was more effective to divide the cataract into four quadrants and then use minimal phaco power to remove the fragments. In later cases, he used cross and circle patterns during the fragmentation procedure, which helped to further reduce the effective phaco time (EPT).

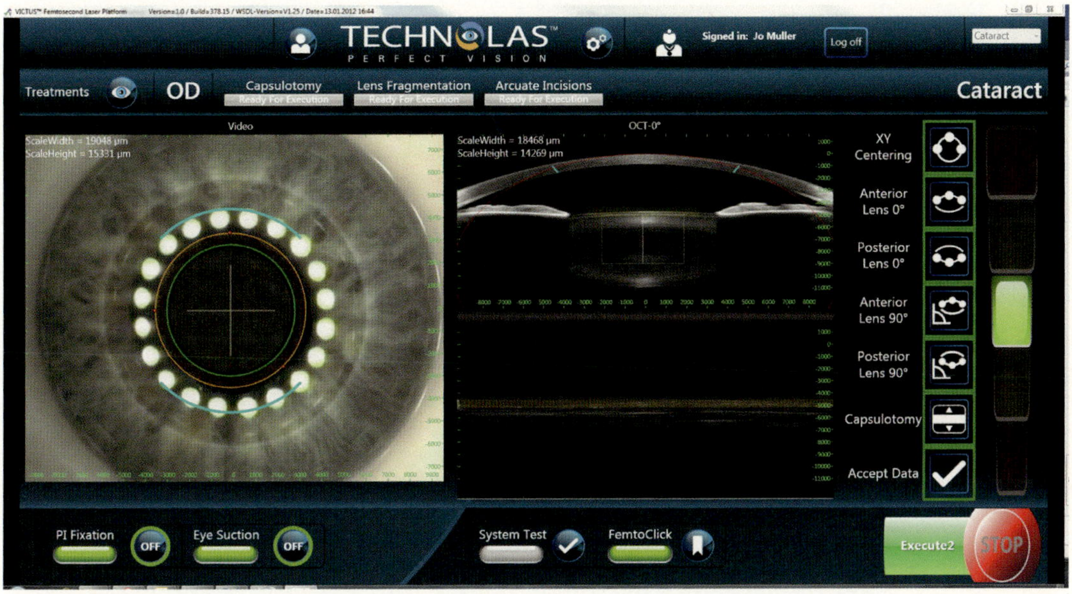

Fig. 18.5 Real-time OCT imaging provides surgeons with a 3D view of the anterior segment

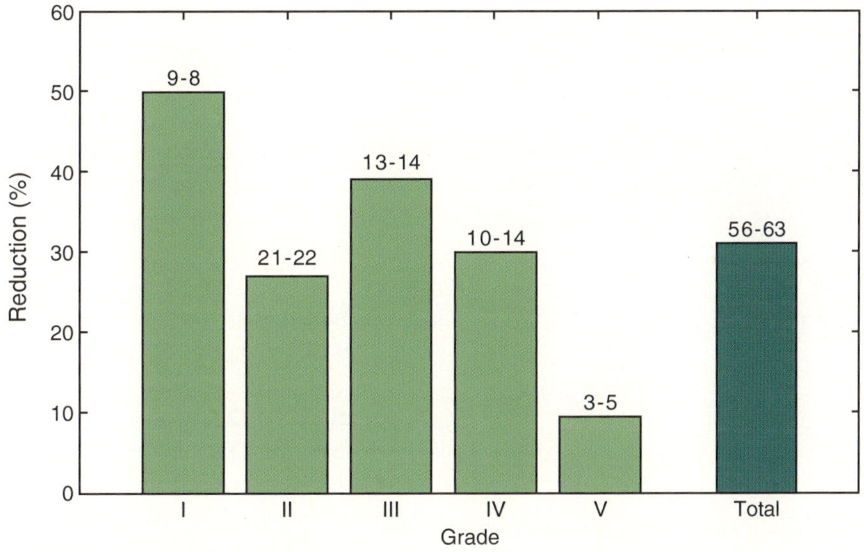

Fig. 18.6 Reduction in phaco power required for different cataract grades following lens fragmentation with the TECHNOLAS Femto-Cataract Procedure

To date, cross cuts, rings and quadrant ring cuts have been used to fragment the nuclei. Preliminary results indicate that radial cut patterns appear to be the most effective during fragmentation. In addition, FS laser during nucleus fragmentation was also found to help with the dissection of the nucleus and the cortex (see Figs. 18.7a–d and 18.8). Further evaluations on laser fragmentation are ongoing.

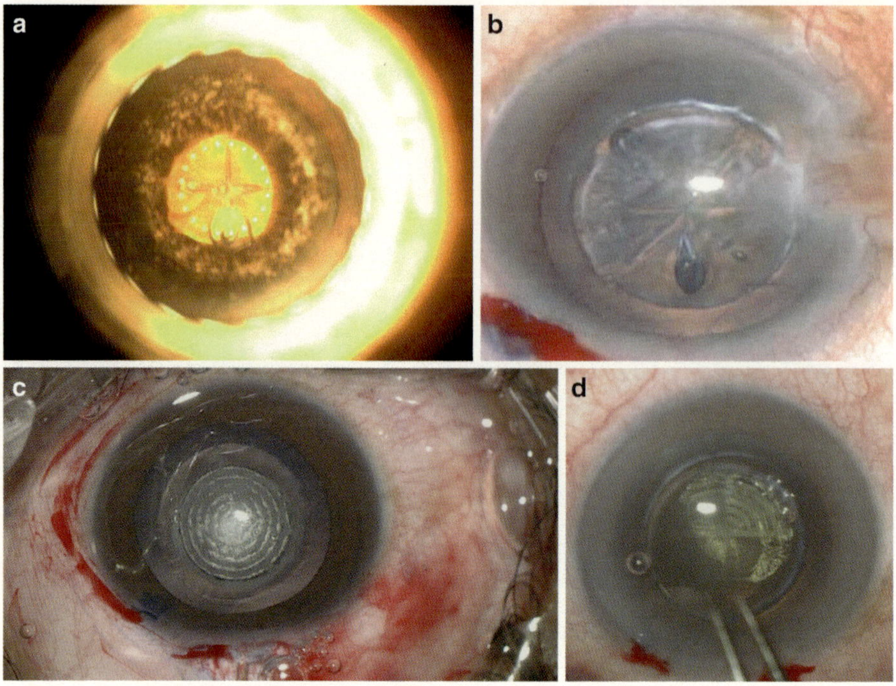

Fig. 18.7 (**a–d**) Cataract following laser fragmentation using a number of lens fragmentation patterns. Visible are the cuts plus the gas dissection of the nucleus and cortex

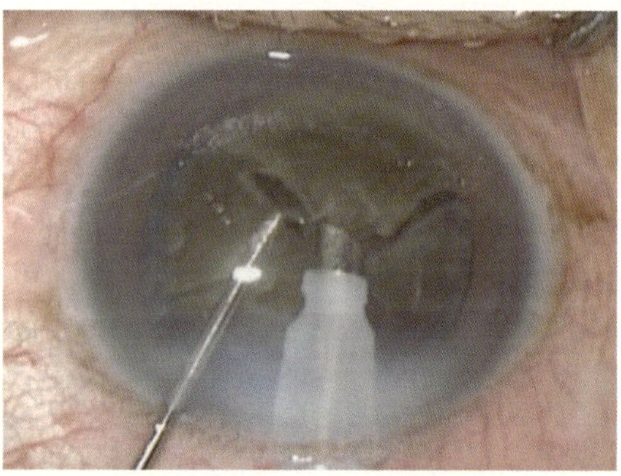

Fig. 18.8 Quadrant removal. Initial studies show that the lens fragments require minimal effective phaco time following laser treatment

Laser Capsulotomy

Particularly when premium IOLs are involved, the need for a perfectly sized and shaped capsulotomy is of great importance. As cataract surgeons well know, it can also be the most challenging step in a cataract surgery case. With the TPV Femto-Cataract software, the experience to date has been that it creates a perfect capsulotomy every time—making the surgeon's job much safer and more effective. In particular, Dr. Reddy has found that the laser is able to safely and effectively create anterior capsulotomies—even in the most challenging eyes—those with white, intumescent cataracts, as well as in pediatric eyes.

Clinical Study Design

To evaluate the TPV Femto-Cataract procedure's effectiveness in creating an anterior capsulotomy, a prospective, multi-surgeon study was performed at Dr. Reddy's center in India (Maxivision Eye Care Centre in Hyderabad). The study compared capsulotomies created by the TECHNOLAS FS Laser with those created manually using a 26-g bent needle. Besides four Maxivision team surgeons, two international surgeons also participated in the Femto-Cataract procedure evaluation: Gerd U. Auffarth, University of Heidelberg, Germany and Luis A. Ruiz from the Centro Oftalmologico, Bogota, Colombia.

There were 31 eyes included in each group. In the FS laser group, the mean patient age was 60 ± 10 years (range, 34–80). The mean cataract grade was 2.6 ± 1.1 (grades 1–5, white/brown cataracts). In the manual group, the mean age was 63 ± 13 year (range, 42–90) and the mean cataract grade was 2.5 ± 1.1 (grades 1–5, white cataracts).

Clinical Study Results

There were no complications encountered during capsulotomy creation in either group. In the laser group, the creation of the capsulotomy was quick, safe and effective with easy removal of the rhexis (see Fig. 18.9a–e). Visual inspection showed that the rhexis in the laser group were more circular compared to the manual group [4] (see Fig. 18.10).

Analysis of the capsulotomy diameter, centration and circularity involved the removal and staining of the rhexis with trypan blue. The samples were placed along a scale and photographed. Software analysis of the photographs was then used to evaluate the outcomes, where an ellipse was fitted to the photos of the extracted tissue samples to calculate the average, minimal and maximal diameters (see Fig. 18.11a, b). Circularity (ε) was calculated from d_{min} and d_{max}, where $\varepsilon = d_{min}/d_{max}$. Diameter ($\emptyset$) was calculated using $\emptyset_{intended}/\emptyset_{measured}$.

Deviation from centration (ΔR) was calculated using $\Delta R = \text{Pupil}_{\text{centre-of-mass}} - \text{Rhexis}_{\text{centre-of-mass}}$ (see Fig. 18.12).

The centration was superior in the FS group, with a deviation from perfect centration of 95 ± 37 μm compared to 160 ± 90 μm in the manual group. This difference was statistically significant. There was also a statistically significant difference in the circularity of the capsulotomies between the laser and manual groups. The circularity achieved in the laser group was 0.97 ± 0.01 compared to 0.93 ± 0.04 in the manual group (1.0 indicates a perfect circle). Surgeons performing the manual procedures were very experienced cataract surgeons. In both groups, the intended diameter of the capsulotomy was 5.5 mm. In the laser group, there was very little deviation from the intended size. Table 18.1 summarizes the results seen in this study [6].

A significant difference is shown both for the average value (μ), indicating higher accuracy, and also for the standard deviation (σ), indicating higher reproducibility of the outcomes.

Incisions

The TECHNOLAS femto laser product has already in the past demonstrated its strong capabilities for performing corneal cuts with personalized three-dimensional shapes (e.g., with its keratoplasty applications in the therapeutic software module of the laser). Thus, the design of specific corneal incisions for cataract surgery can build on this broad experience, further strengthening the Femto-Cataract treatment capabilities on the TPV laser. Also, a software module for performing precise and highly customizable arcuate incisions already is an established standard with the laser device, as it has been available commercially for many years on the TECHNOLAS laser (see Fig. 18.13).

Ergonomics

The TECHNOLAS Femtosecond Workstation features a new ergonomic, surgeon-friendly design. The system comes with its own bed, which is joystick controlled and can be adjusted in three dimensions, or it can be used in conjunction with the bed from the TECHNOLAS excimer laser if it is part of a laser suite. In addition, the Graphical User Interface (GUI) has been completely redesigned to make it more user friendly for cataract surgeons. These changes include providing for user visual control and direct interaction with the imaging data while planning the procedure, as well as for monitoring while the laser is carrying out the various steps of the cataract surgery procedure.

The latest version of the laser, known as the VICTUS™ Femtosecond Laser Platform (Bausch + Lomb/Technolas Perfect Vision), received CE mark approval in December 2011.

510(k) clearances are currently in the process and the company expects to receive respective approvals soon.

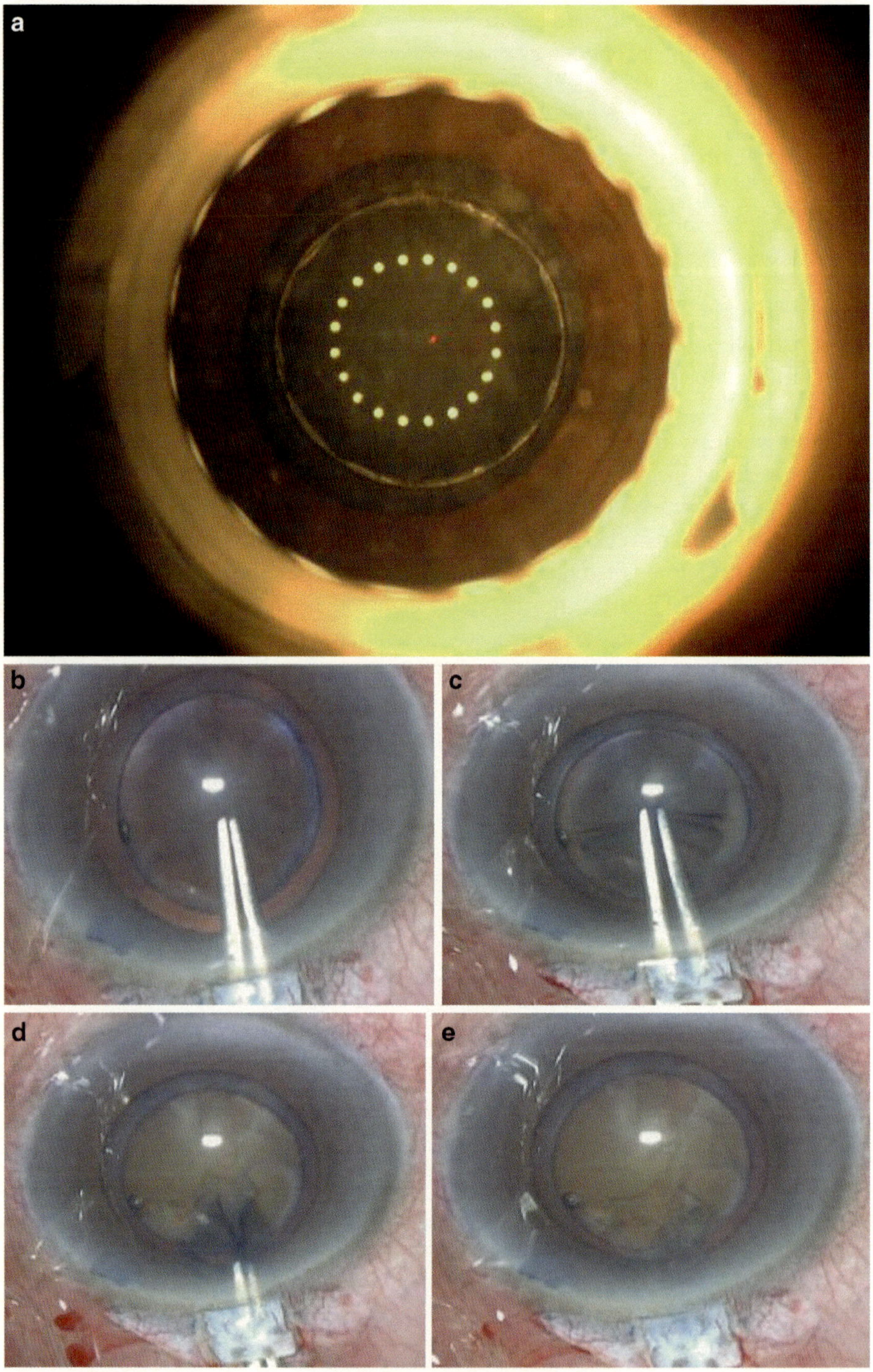

Fig. 18.9 (**a**) Capsulotomy creation with the TECHNOLAS Femto-Cataract procedure software. (**b–e**) Removal of the rhexis is easy to accomplish

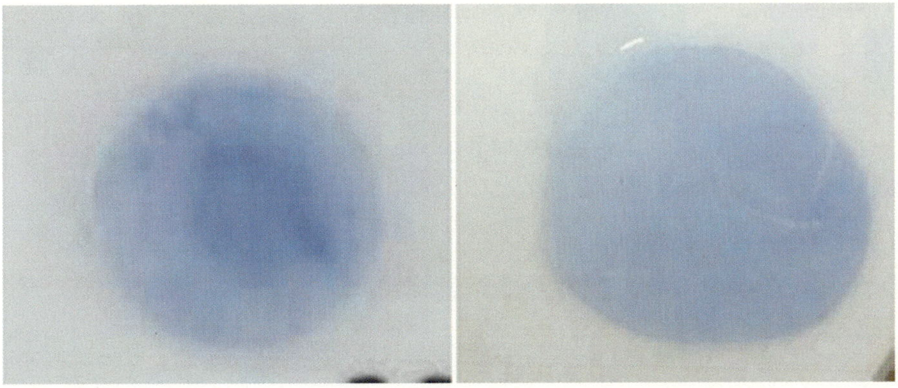

Fig. 18.10 (*Left*) Rhexis removed from capsulotomy created with the TECHNOLAS laser shows an almost perfect circle compared to a rhexis removed following creation of a capsulotomy using a 26-g bent needle (*right*)

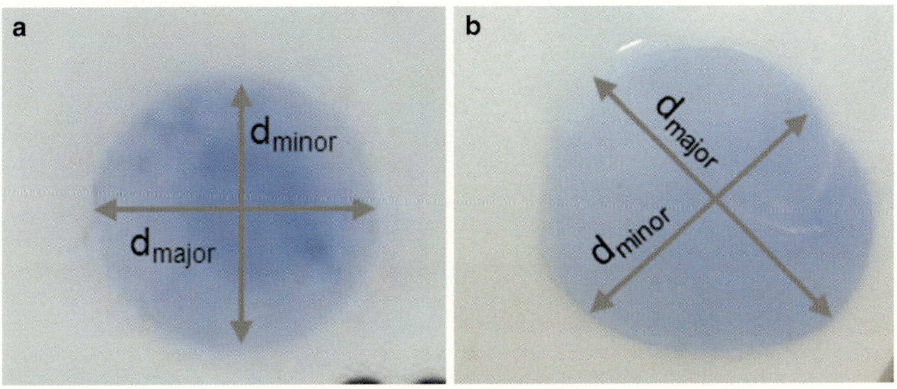

Fig. 18.11 (**a** and **b**) Principle for measuring circularity and diameter of the capsulotomy

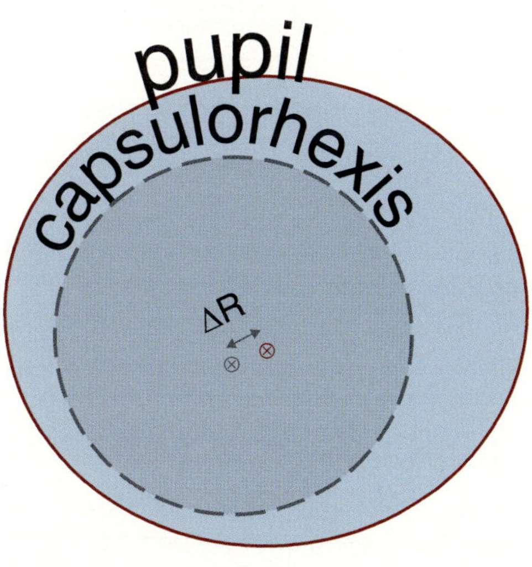

Fig. 18.12 Schematic to show the principle of measuring centration of the capsulotomy

System Benefits

The most significant advantage that the TECHNOLAS Femtosecond Workstation has over other FS lasers on the market is its versatility. As mentioned earlier, not only can this system perform the Femto-Cataract procedure, but it is also capable of correcting presbyopia (INTRACOR), as well as corneal and more refractive procedures with the therapeutic and LASIK flap software modules. It is this versatility that makes the TECHNOLAS Femtosecond Workstation the most cost effective option for surgeons considering the purchase of a FS laser.

Table 18.1 Summary of anterior capsulotomy clinical study results

Parameter	Laser (mm)	Manual	μ Significant difference	σ Significant difference
Diameter, $\varnothing$	5.5 ± 0.12	N/A	N/A	N/A
Circularity, ε	0.97 ± 0.01	0.93 ± 0.04	P 0.001	P 0.001
Decentration, ΔR (μm)	95 ± 37	160 ± 90	P 0.001	P 0.001

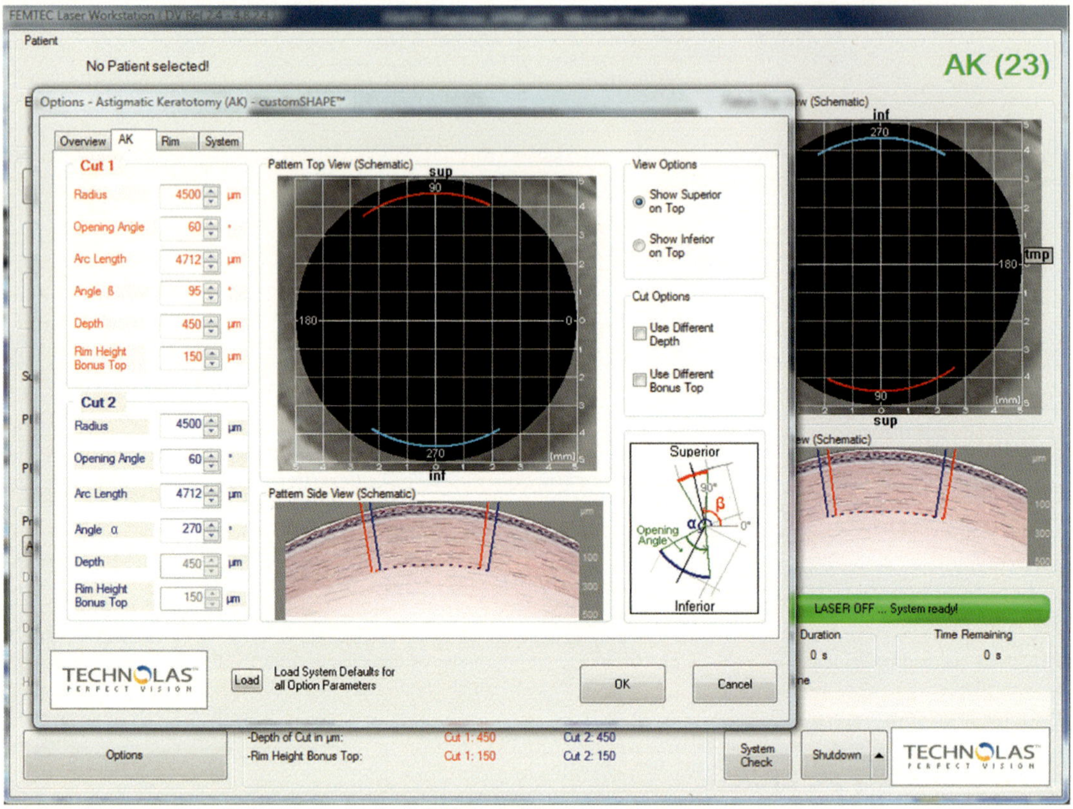

Fig. 18.13 CUSTOMSHAPE module with highly customizable arcuate incisions, as commercially available on the TECHNOLAS FS laser for many years. Incisions can be tailored according to surgeon's preferred nomogram

Compelling Reasons to Acquire TPV's Femto-Cataract Technology

1. *Safety*. We believe that one of the most important reasons why surgeons consider the TECHNOLAS Femtosecond Workstation and the Femto-Cataract procedure is safety. Between the steps of capsulotomy and fragmentation, our experience to date finds that no complications have been encountered in more than 500+ cases.
2. *Reproducible results*. For all steps, the performance of the Femto-Cataract procedure on the Technolas laser has been highly reproducible with only minimal variation in creation of the anterior capsulotomy or in the fragmentation of the cataract—no matter the density or type.
3. *Accuracy* is the third reason why we believe surgeons should consider Femto-Cataract

procedure with the Technolas laser—when it comes to the creation of the capsulotomy, the centration, diameter, and circularity are spot on and make the surgeon's job much safer and efficient.

4. *Real-time, live OCT images are being obtained during the procedure*, which is also a tremendous benefit and allows the surgeon to not only accurately plan the procedure but also view the procedure and make adjustments, if necessary. This allows for a high level of personalization as an added benefit.
5. *The docking procedure*. The curved PI in combination with the TECHNOLAS Intelligent Pressure Control provides for globe fixation which keeps corneal distortion to a minimum—a very important point when one wants to ensure accurate laser treatment within the anterior segment. Patients are also more comfortable when high pressure is not applied to the eye during the surgical procedure.
6. *Precision of the Femto-Cataract procedure's software on the Technolas laser*. With laser treatment times on the order of only 15 s it is also a fast and efficient procedure, and we have found that the procedure has had a minimal impact on added time to a typical cataract case.
7. *Patient preference*. Experience to date has found that patients are excited to have their cataracts removed using a novel and safe laser technology. They believe that a laser offers more precision over other more conventional technologies.
8. *The transition to using the Femto-Cataract procedure on the Technolas laser is very easy*. For a busy cataract surgeon, reducing the worry of key steps has been very easy.

Future Developments

As a renowned innovator in the field of laser surgery, Technolas Perfect Vision will continue to innovate and bring novel applications and new features to its versatile FS laser workstation. This respective development is driven in close collaboration with its users, to make the FS laser treatment experience uniquely satisfying for surgeon and patient as well. The company believes that FS laser technology will further broaden its footprint in ophthalmic surgery, making the femto laser an indispensable tool for the modern ophthalmic surgeon.

Company Contact Information

Technolas Perfect Vision GmbH
Messerschmittstr. 1 + 3
80992 München
Germany
www.technolaspv.com

References

1. Technolas 520F product brochure. Munich, Germany: Technolas Perfect Vision; 2011.
2. Fichte CM, Endl MJ, Elmer TR. US surgeon experience—TECHNOLAS 520F. In: TPV Symposium presentation by Dr Endl, ASCRS; 2011.
3. Technolas Perfect Vision. Company data on file.
4. Auffarth GU. Clinical evaluation into the safety and efficacy of femtosecond laser cataract surgery procedure. ESCRS 2011, free paper.
5. Reddy KP. Clinical evaluation of femtosecond laser cataract surgery procedure in Indian eyes. ESCRS 2011, free paper.
6. Auffarth GU, Reddy KP, Ruiz LA. Preliminary clinical results of the Femto-Cataract procedure using the VICTUS Femtosecond Laser Platform: White Paper. 2011 Technolas Perfect Vision.

The Future of ReLACS and Femtosecond Laser Ocular Surgery

19

Ronald R. Krueger, Jean-Marie A. Parel, Krystel R. Huxlin, Wayne H. Knox, and Kristian Hohla

Introduction

When speaking about the future, there is always a tradeoff between imaginative speculation and a natural forecasting of trends and events. As this is one of the first books published on this subject, much of the material in this book is new. One might consider it speculation to say that femtosecond (FS) laser technology will have a dramatic impact and be fully embraced by the field. If that statement were made 10 years ago, it would be speculation. The fact is that FS laser technology has already had a dramatic impact on refractive corneal surgery over these past 10 years, and it is now poised to see a similar dramatic impact on refractive cataract surgery. Although refractive laser assisted cataract surgery (ReLACS) is only just beginning, it is a reality, and hence it is not unreasonable to say that its impact in the field is more than just speculation, but rather a natural forecasting of the trends and events we have seen thus far. What are those events and trends?

1. FS lasers have been used in corneal refractive surgery for nearly a decade, and although they started out slow, with many overestimating their success in the first 2 years, it is fair to say that we have underestimated their success over these past 10 years, as 70% of LASIK flaps in the USA are currently made with this technology, and there are now five FS laser platforms on the market, specifically for corneal refractive surgery, with a sixth one, using nanosecond technology, on the way.
2. Commercialization of image-guided FS lasers for cataract surgery sprung up simultaneously through the independent efforts of three separate US based companies, each of which then proceeded to gain US FDA and European CE Mark approvals.
3. One of these femto-laser cataract companies was purchased by the largest provider of commercial ophthalmic products worldwide, even before a single laser was sold.
4. More than a hundred of these lasers have been sold to ophthalmic surgeons for clinical use in the USA with more internationally.

R.R. Krueger, M.D., M.S.E. (✉)
Cole Eye Institute, Dept of Refractive Surgery, Cleveland Clinic Lerner College of Medicine, Cleveland, OH, 44106, USA
e-mail: ronrkrueger@aol.com

J.A. Parel, Ph.D., Ing.E.T.S.-G., F.A.R.V.O.
Ophthalmic Biophysics Center, Bascom Palmer Eye Institute, University of Miami School of Medicine, 1638 NW 10 Avenue, Miami, FL 33136, USA

K.R. Huxlin, Ph.D.
Flaum Eye Institute, University of Rochester, 601 Elmwood Ave, Box 314, Rochester, NY 14642, USA

W.H. Knox, Ph.D.
The Institute of Optics and Center for Visual Sciences, University of Rochester, 275 Hutchison Road, Rochester, NY 14627, USA

K. Hohla, Ph.D.
Technolas Perfect Vision GmbH, Munich, Bavaria, Germany

R.R. Krueger et al. (eds.), *Textbook of Refractive Laser Assisted Cataract Surgery (ReLACS)*, DOI 10.1007/978-1-4614-1010-2_19,

5. The topic of refractive laser assisted cataract surgery (ReLACS) is the dominant topic at many major ophthalmic meetings.

So, as we forecast the future, it appears that we will see great success of this technology with broad sweeping use of image-guided laser capsulotomy, laser fragmentation and laser corneal incisions. But what else does the future hold? The following sections outline both natural forecasting of trends as well as a certain level of speculation for the use of this technology, at least from our limited, yet informed perspective.

Corneal and Combined Corneal/ Cataract Laser Procedures

With five corneal refractive FS laser platforms currently being used for LASIK and other corneal based incisions, why would the future of ReLACS be in the area of corneal laser procedures? After all, the corneal laser technologies are there for the corneal procedures, so why suggest that the cataract laser technologies will have a role in the cornea as well.

One reason is the fact that the cataract laser technologies already have a role in corneal incisions; in both transcorneal self-sealing wounds (Chap. 9) and intrastromal corneal relaxing incisions (Chap. 10). These are naturally included with the cataract laser technologies, because they are essential in the steps of cataract surgery, and hence, a corneal component is necessary with the cataract based lasers.

The second reason is because of the enhanced technologies available with the cataract lasers that facilitate improvement in precision of corneal incisions. Both image-guided laser delivery and a liquid immersion interface in laser docking add to the precision.

Immersion Corneal Optics and Image-Guided Surgery

When both OptiMedica and LensAR began designing and building their laser systems, they found that flat and curved contact applanation created folds in the cornea which impacted the passage of laser light to deeper structures. In addition, they also found that contact applanation impacted the orientation of laser pulses within the cornea. In response, each company independently chose liquid immersion as a form of laser docking, which provides no compression or distortion of the cornea and no significant rise in intraocular pressure. This added a significant advantage over the corneal cutting provided by the cornea-only FS lasers, which each use either flat or curved contact applanation. Although these lasers can effectively treat any laser pattern in the cornea, the deeper laser treatments are most limited by the folds/wrinkling of the posterior stroma with applanation. Liquid immersion optics significantly improves the uniformity of laser pulse placement, which improves accuracy and precision in creating the desired corneal shape. It also provides a less reflective and scattering interface for a more refined focus of laser light intrastromally and intraocularly.

With each of the cataract lasers systems, imaging plays a critical role in defining the structures within the eye and establishing safety margins of treatment. With both ocular coherence tomography (OCT) and 3D confocal structured illumination (3D CSI), confocal or coaxial imaging with laser delivery allows for precise placement of laser pulses with targeted precision. This targeted precision together with the uniformity of corneal shape achieved with fluid immersion allow for unprecedented shaping of both deep and superficial corneal structures, and opens up a whole new category of cornea laser procedures that can be pursued with this technology. The following sections outline these new and/or improved capabilities.

Femto-laser Anterior Lamellar Keratoplasty (FALK)

FS laser lamellar keratoplasty can be easily performed with anterior stromal scars or opacities if the lamellar plane of dissection is limited to the anterior half of the cornea. Several publications of this technique have been reported for anterior

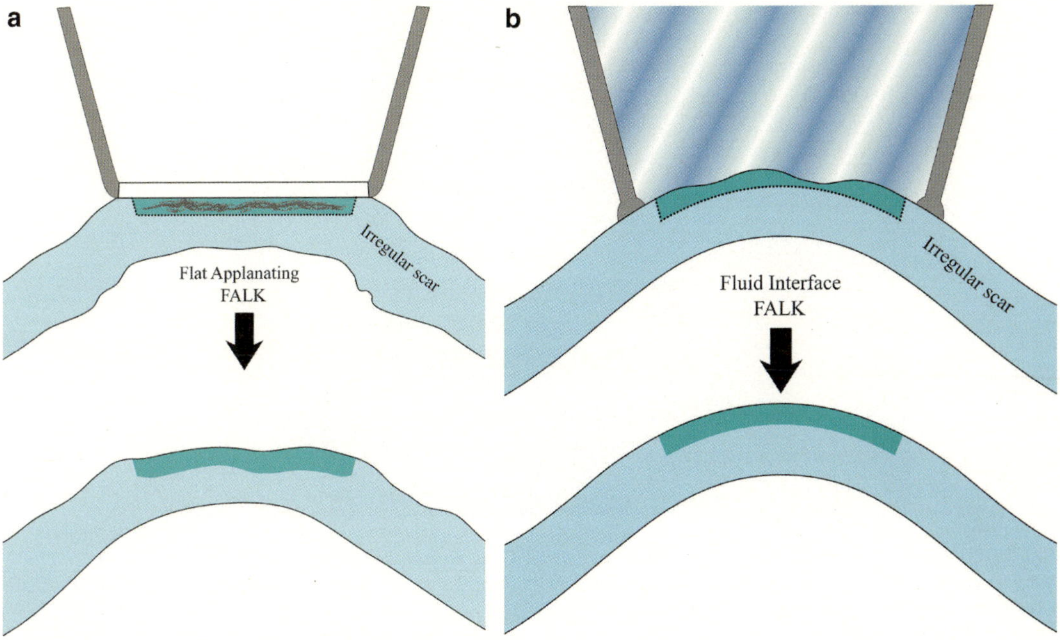

Fig. 19.1 (**a** and **b**) Graphic illustration of the cornea, revealing FS laser anterior keratoplasty (FALK) of an irregular corneal scar. (**a**) The flat applanation of the surface leads to translation of the irregularity to the deeper laser created layer. (**b**) The fluid immersion interface avoids compression of the cornea, and together with image guidance, allows for a uniform laser dissection of the irregular scar

pathologies, and overall there is good restoration to the corneal clarity and corneal shape with this procedure [1]. This, however, is not without a level of residual refractive error, often with irregular astigmatism, due to the transmission of preexisting irregularities from the scar to the deeper dissected lamellar plane (see Fig. 19.1a). This often results in the need for subsequent laser vision correction (PRK/PTK) in an effort to restore the refraction and irregularity, and even this is with a mixed visual outcome. Several patients that have received PRK with mitomycin C after a FS laser lamellar keratoplasty, by the author (RRK), have developed subepithelial haze in response to the laser enhancement (see Fig. 19.2), and with loss of best spectacle corrected vision. Here the potential benefit of the precise FS laser lamellar dissection is lost by transmission of the irregularity to the deeper dissected layer, due to the corneal applanation, and the resulting irregular astigmatism and/or post-excimer laser haze and scarring.

With the noncontact fluid immersion interface and image-guided surgery offered by two of the new cataract laser systems, the transmission of an irregularity from the scar is something that can be fully avoided, because the plane of laser dissection can follow the natural lamellar layers of the cornea in both the donor and recipient corneas (see Fig. 19.1b). Although this has not yet been documented, it does forecast a future capability of these new lasers, which would augment the reported corneal incisions associated with ReLACS.

Femto-laser Deep Anterior Lamellar Keratoplasty (DALK)

Once attempts are made at using a FS laser to perform anterior lamellar keratoplasty in the deep corneal layers, as with DALK [2, 3], the folds and wrinklings of the posterior stroma with contact applanation (flat applanation greater than curved contact docking) destroy the uniformity of laser delivery, making this procedure more difficult to pursue. Consequently, the depth of laser placement must be limited to avoid perforation. Additionally,

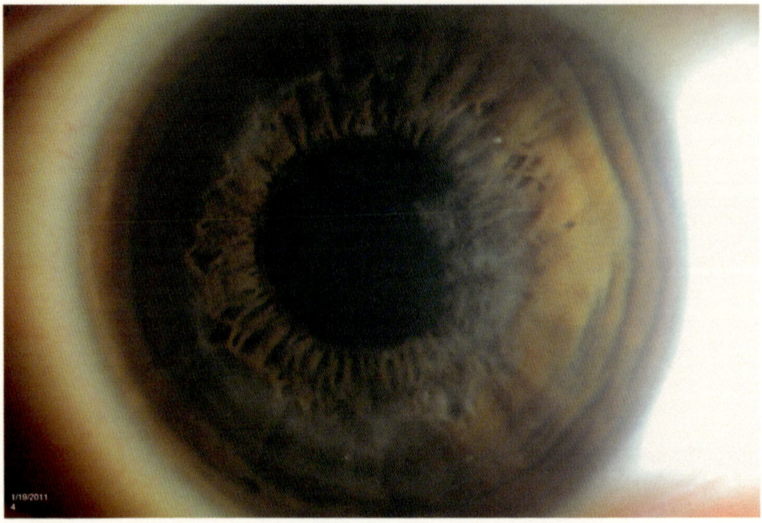

Fig. 19.2 Subepithelial corneal haze with loss of best spectacle corrected visual acuity (BSCVA) after excimer laser photorefractive keratectomy (PRK) with mitomycin C in an eye in which a FS laser anterior keratoplasty (FALK) was performed using a flat applanating laser interface

the absence of OCT or 3D CSI imaging and laser targeting limits the precision for laser dissection at the level of Descemet's layer, so that a residual layer of corneal stroma often remains. Even the big bubble technique that strives to dissect the deepest stroma off of Descemet's layer with air cleaving dissection, often does not achieve a clean bubble dissection because of the remaining residual layer of posterior stroma.

Now, with the help of image-guided surgery, as well as the fluid immersion interface, big bubble dissection at the level of Descemet's layer should be much more reproducible, making the DALK procedure much easier and less time and effort consuming for corneal surgeons. The chance of corneal perforation, necessitating the conversion to a penetrating keratoplasty, should also be infrequent, because of the image-guided placement of laser pulses, that can precisely localize and avoid Descemet's membrane while still targeting the posterior most corneal stroma (see Fig. 19.3a).

Femto-laser DSAEK and DLEK

The rather crude, yet effective, methods for shaping a posterior lamellar donor lenticule for Descemet's stripping automated endothelial keratoplasty (DSAEK) using a deeply set microkeratome has had a profoundly positive effect on keratoplasty techniques and outcomes among corneal surgeons [4, 5]. The efficacy of DSAEK, above and beyond that of deep lamellar endothelial keratoplasty (DLEK), could be even more elegantly performed if the donor lenticule were precisely shaped with a FS laser. Once again, the shape of a FS laser created lenticule would be optimized if it were image-guided to follow the contour of the posterior corneal surface, and in order to do this, a fluid immersion interface would be needed to eliminate the possibility of corneal compression folds that might distort the uniformly created posterior lenticule shape.

Beyond the idea of precisely shaping a DSAEK lenticule, it might also be possible to shape the recipient cornea in exactly the same way as the donor, allowing a tongue in groove fit in what could be called, a "FS laser DLEK procedure." DLEK, which was first popularized by Dr. Mark Terry, required hand dissection of the recipient lamellar surface as a preparation for transplantation of the posterior donor lenticule [6]. It was ultimately replaced by DSAEK, in popularity and quality of outcomes, because of the smooth posterior surface after Descemet's layer was removed. However, unlike DLEK, the smooth surface also

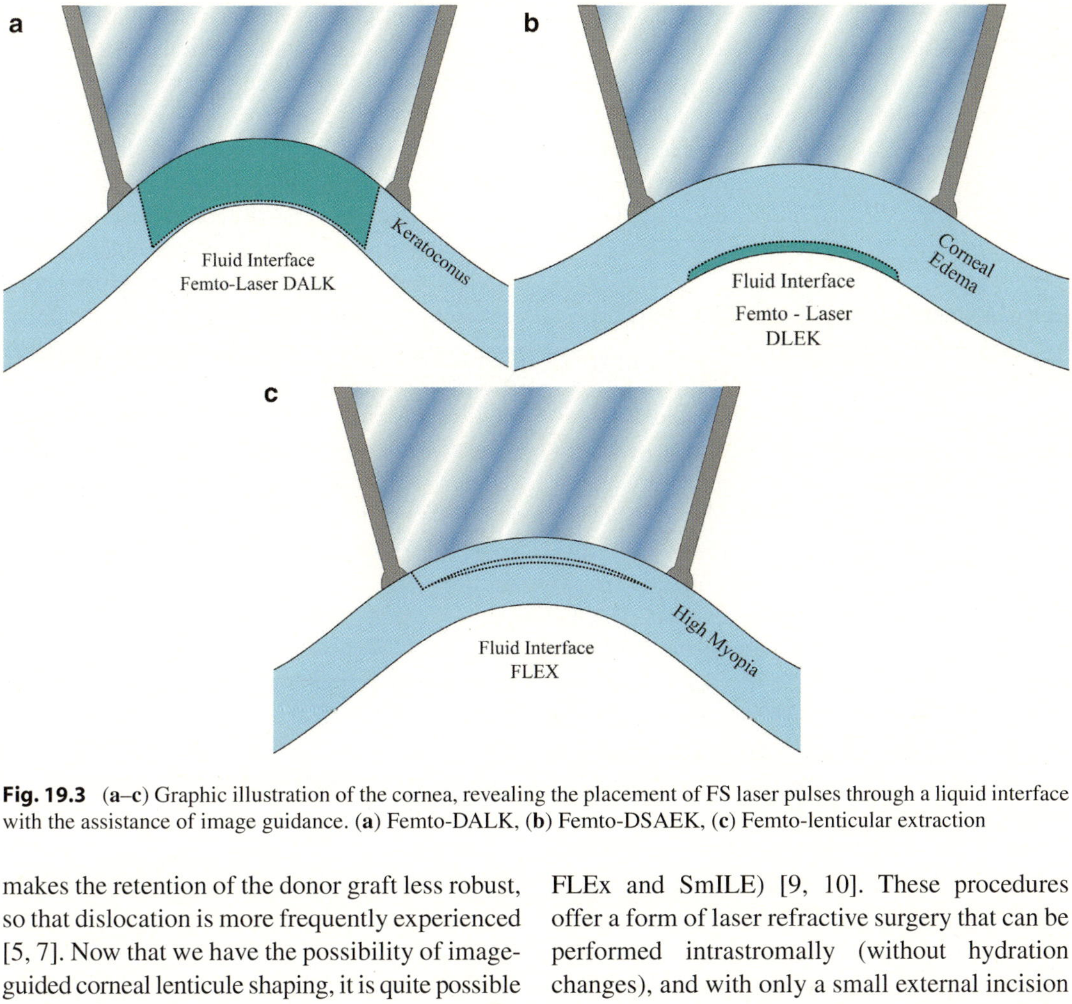

Fig. 19.3 (**a–c**) Graphic illustration of the cornea, revealing the placement of FS laser pulses through a liquid interface with the assistance of image guidance. (**a**) Femto-DALK, (**b**) Femto-DSAEK, (**c**) Femto-lenticular extraction

makes the retention of the donor graft less robust, so that dislocation is more frequently experienced [5, 7]. Now that we have the possibility of image-guided corneal lenticule shaping, it is quite possible that DLEK could give an improved outcome when both the donor and recipient corneas are prepared similarly. Figure 19.3b shows the graphic illustration of a FS laser created posterior lenticule using image guidance and a liquid interface to avoid tissue deformation.

Femto-laser Lenticular Extraction

In the late 1990s, the author (RRK) published the concept and early clinical data of corneal lenticular extraction with the use of an ultrashort pulse (picosecond) laser [8]. Although the outcomes were crude and less predictable than excimer laser in situ keratomileusis (LASIK), it was the precursor to the modern day FS laser refractive lenticular extraction (ReLEx) procedures (both FLEx and SmILE) [9, 10]. These procedures offer a form of laser refractive surgery that can be performed intrastromally (without hydration changes), and with only a small external incision (less biomechanical change). These unique refinements make ReLEx a procedure that has a great potential for minimizing the variability in refractive outcomes, seen with LASIK today.

Although FS lenticular extraction (FLEx) has been successfully implemented as a substitute procedure for LASIK, its modification, small incision lenticular extraction (SmILE), has the greatest potential for minimizing both the hydration changes and biomechanical changes associated with LASIK [10]. The techniques of ReLEx currently use a curved contact applanation docking system, which lightly compresses the cornea. With the femto-laser cataract systems, both image-guided surgery and liquid immersion offers an even greater improvement to the precise refractive profiles currently experienced with ReLEx. The bubble expansion with sequential pulse placement compresses and deforms the corneal tissue against the contact applanation, while liquid immersion would avoid such compression (see Fig. 19.3c). The refractive precision of ReLEx has the potential for improvement as femto-lasers, such as those being offered with refractive laser assisted cataract surgery, are further improved.

Femto-laser Pockets for Inlays and Intrastromal Cross-linking

With the previously mentioned corneal procedures, the need for refractive precision seems to outweigh the comparative benefit of image-guided surgery and liquid immersion in pocket formation. However, when the pocket is created for the placement of a presbyopic refractive inlay, the need for precise centration becomes of critical importance [11]. With each of the commercially investigated refractive inlays, centration is one of the most limiting factors toward achieving an ideal outcome. Methods for achieving accurate centration are diverse and not universally reliable. With image-guided surgery, the location of the corneal apex, and corneal intercept of the center of the entrance pupil are now identifiable, especially with the visualization and compensation of tilt during the alignment process. Good centration and accurate placement may enhance with the outcomes of intrastromal inlays, and may also be useful in the intrastromal injection of riboflavin for selective corneal cross-linking.

Combined Femto-laser Corneal/Cataract Procedures

With each of the corneal procedures that could be enhanced with image guidance and liquid immersion, the additional benefit of simultaneous laser cataract surgery together with these procedures opens up an elegance to combined cataract procedures that has not yet been experienced. In the case of a superficial corneal scar and cataract, a combination of FALK and cataract extraction could be pursued. With keratoconus and cataract, a combination of cross-linking and cataract extraction might be pursued in milder cases, while DALK and cataract extraction might be pursued for more advanced cases. In the case of Fuch's corneal dystrophy and cataract, a DSAEK or DLEK could be pursued with the cataract extraction. Finally, with presbyopia and cataract, in the absence of a presbyopia correcting IOL, negatively aspheric refractive lenticular extraction (ReLEx) could be pursued or, perhaps more preferably, a well centered corneal pocket for a presbyopic inlay. Although simultaneously performing these procedures might not be optimal or even considered awkward, the possibility of refractive laser assisted cataract surgery in combination with FS laser assisted corneal procedure does offer an attractive level of precision surgery that might encompass part of the future of this technology.

Lens Densitometry for Customized Laser Fragmentation

Imaging and Quantification for Lens Densitometry

Like optical coherence tomography (OCT), Scheimpflug tomography has become a popular imaging technique for evaluation both the anterior and posterior corneal curvature. Additionally, both OCT and Scheimpflug tomography have been utilized for evaluating the anatomy of deeper structures in the anterior chamber, including the crystalline lens. Although OCT shows a greater level of reflection for denser structures, Scheimpflug is particularly useful in qualitatively and quantitatively assessing the density and level of opacity of ocular structures, especially the crystalline lens [12]. This is called lens densitometry, and it can be particularly useful in quantitating the level of lens opacity.

The 3D-confocal structured illumination (3D-CSI) technology of LensAR (Winter Park, FL) utilizes a confocal laser imaging technique that is optically captured at a Scheimpflug angle and is optically enhanced with a form of structured illumination that scans less reflective structures

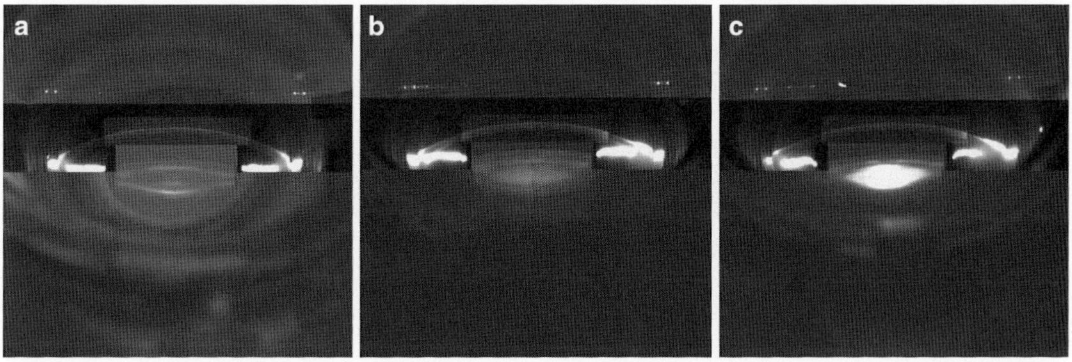

Fig. 19.4 Lens densitometry using 3D confocal structured illumination (3D CSI), revealing multiple densities of lens nuclei varying from LOCS III grades 1, 3, and 5

(posterior capsule) more than highly reflective structures (anterior corneal surface). Lens densitometry is also possible with this technology, similar to that experienced with Scheimpflug tomography, and it nicely shows the graded density of nuclei from LOCS III grades 1–5 (see Fig. 19.4).

Laser Adjustment of Lens Densitometry

Because lenses with greater density are harder and more difficult to separate with laser photodisruption, adjusting the laser energy during FS laser nucleus fragmentation would be helpful in reaching a therapeutic value, while minimizing the total amount of laser energy entering the eye. Excessive laser energy can scatter within the eye, and should be minimized to maintain safety. The therapeutic level of laser energy for fragmentation is ~10 mJ for most FS laser cataract technologies. Obviously, this value is too high for softer nuclei and too low for denser nuclei and hence should be adjusted to deliver the optimal level for lens fragmentation. At present, none of the ReLACS technologies use greater laser energy for denser nuclei, and for several systems, nuclei harder than LOCS III grade 4 are not possible to treat. Using lens densitometry to quantitatively access the level of hardness and adjusting the laser energy to match this density would be a future improvement to this technology.

Densitometry-Guided Laser Lens Fragmentation

Beyond the qualitative and quantitative assessment of lens densitometry and manual adjustment of therapeutic laser energy for fragmentation, a closed loop system could be designed in the future to assess the lens density and then automatically adjust the laser energy for optimal fragmentation. Since laser energy is currently not being adjusted for denser nuclei, this would be a more advanced capability that would likely be offered in later generation FS laser cataract surgical systems.

Phaco Ersatz: Capsular Refilling for Accommodation Restoration

The Search for Presbyopia Correcting Cataract Surgery

The concept of a cataract as a dysfunctional lens, due to lens opacity, brings attention to the other major dysfunction of the lens, the loss of accommodation. Historically, replacing the dysfunctional lens with an intraocular lens implant only takes care of the first dysfunction. It has been the quest of modern day cataract surgery to not only remove the opacity and neutralize the refractive error, but also to correct the presbyopia with specialized premium channel IOLs. Both multifocal and pseudo-accommodating IOL designs have been proposed and commercialized, but these are still associated with limitations of function and/or distracting side effects. What is ideally required is a lens substitute that not only restores clarity and refractive emmetropia, but also restores the accommodative function that is lost with removal of the natural crystalline lens.

Although such a lens substitute does not yet exist, attempts have been made to design pseudo-accommodative lenses with sufficient accommodative function to sufficiently restore the full range of visual function. Single optic accommodating IOLs have at best ~1.00 D of effect [13], while dual optics accommodating IOLs, such as the Abbott Medical Optics Synchrony lens, can achieve ~3.00 D [14]. Other novel accommodating lens designs have been proposed, by changing the lens curvature (NuLens) for a greater accommodative effect [15]. Unfortunately, some of these novel lens designs will also require a larger incision size, and in the quest to restore accommodative function, surgeons are also seeking to further reduce the incision size to reduce astigmatism and make the procedure less externally invasive. For this, the concept of capsular refilling with an injectable polymer has the greatest potential advantage. It requires the smallest possible incision (<1 mm), and also can achieve the most natural restoration of lens accommodation with ~7.00 D of refractive effect (see Fig. 19.5) [16].

Technology of Capsular Refilling

In approaching this concept, it is important to differentiate the two techniques that are being investigated: (1) direct refilling of the capsular bag and (2) the endocapsular balloon. The former has a longer history of more than 50 years of development, while the latter is a newer concept that may have a greater potential for commercialization. In both techniques, the stiff, senile lens nucleus is replaced with a soft, synthetic material. The premise of the two techniques is that accommodation will be restored if the content of the capsular bag has an elastic modulus similar to that of the newborn's crystalline cells, about 600 Pa. For these techniques to work the capsule must remain as intact as possible, and therefore, surgery must be made through a very small capsule opening, a mini-capsulotomy or mini-capsulorhexis [17]. To avoid visual distortion of the retinal image and weakening of the fragile, zonular ligaments, the mini-capsulorhexis is made at the

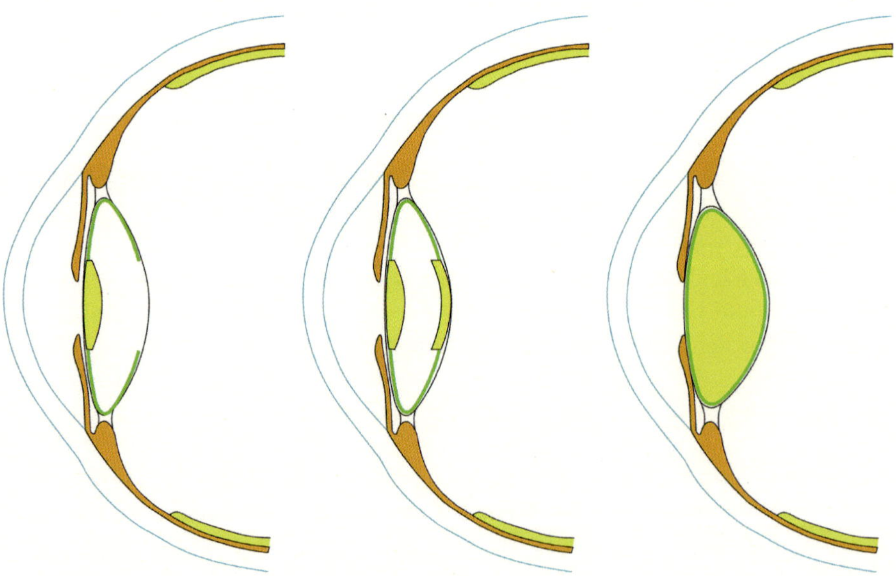

Fig. 19.5 Single optics, dual optics and capsular refilling optics, achieving ~1.00, ~3.00, and ~7.00 D of accommodation (figure provided courtesy of Adrian Glasser, PhD)

periphery of the anterior capsule. Removal of lens substance and epithelial cells and implantation of the synthetic lens material is performed through the mini-capsulorhexis. Access to the crystalline lens is obtained via a small (<2 mm wide) corneal or cornea-limbal incision to minimize loss of the anterior chamber contents and postoperative corneal astigmatism.

Lens Capsule Refilling

Julius Kessler introduced direct refilling of the capsular bag in the late 1950s. He showed feasibility in Eye Bank eyes [18] as well as rabbit eyes [19], and demonstrated the prolificacy of the rabbit in regenerating its lens substance [20]. Agarwal reproduced Kessler's techniques in the rabbit and attempted to assess accommodation in young primates [21–24]. Although they lacked modern microsurgical instrumentation, and had to rely on "off-the-shelf" industrial polymers that had inadequate physical properties, the work of these pioneers is extraordinary, in the scope, ingenuity, and quality of their studies. Phaco-Ersatz (cataract surgery designed to preserve and restore accommodation) was introduced in 1981 (see Fig. 19.6), applying modern day technologies to the concept of lens refilling [25]. After demonstrating feasibility in cadaver eyes [26] and safety in rabbits, the preservation of accommodation was shown in young owl monkeys [27] with a later restoration of accommodation in senile rhesus monkeys [28]

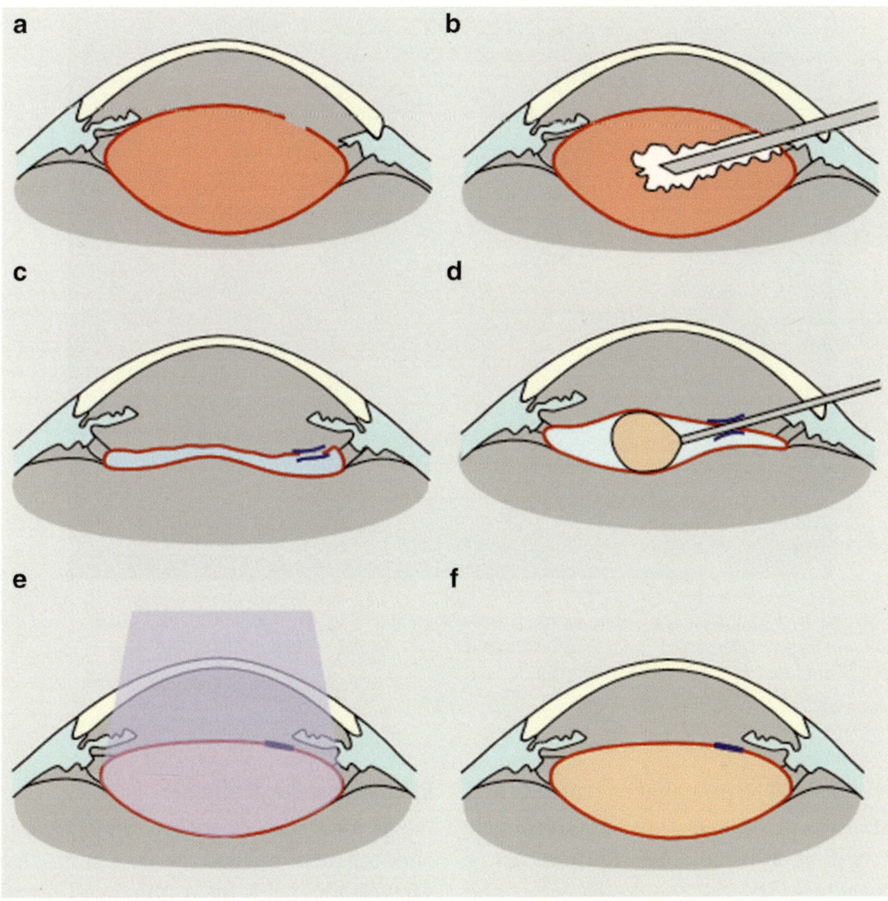

Fig. 19.6 (**a**–**f**) Phaco-Ersatz procedure done through two clear cornea incisions of 1.8 mm. (**a**) Mini-capsulorhexis at lens periphery; (**b**) bimanual phacoemulsification of nucleus with 0.7 mm titanium tip; (**c**) evacuation of lens capsule and insertion of mini capsulorhexis valve; (**d**) injection of the siloxane polymer; (**e**) polymer photo-cross-linking using external source; (**f**) synthetic crystalline lens

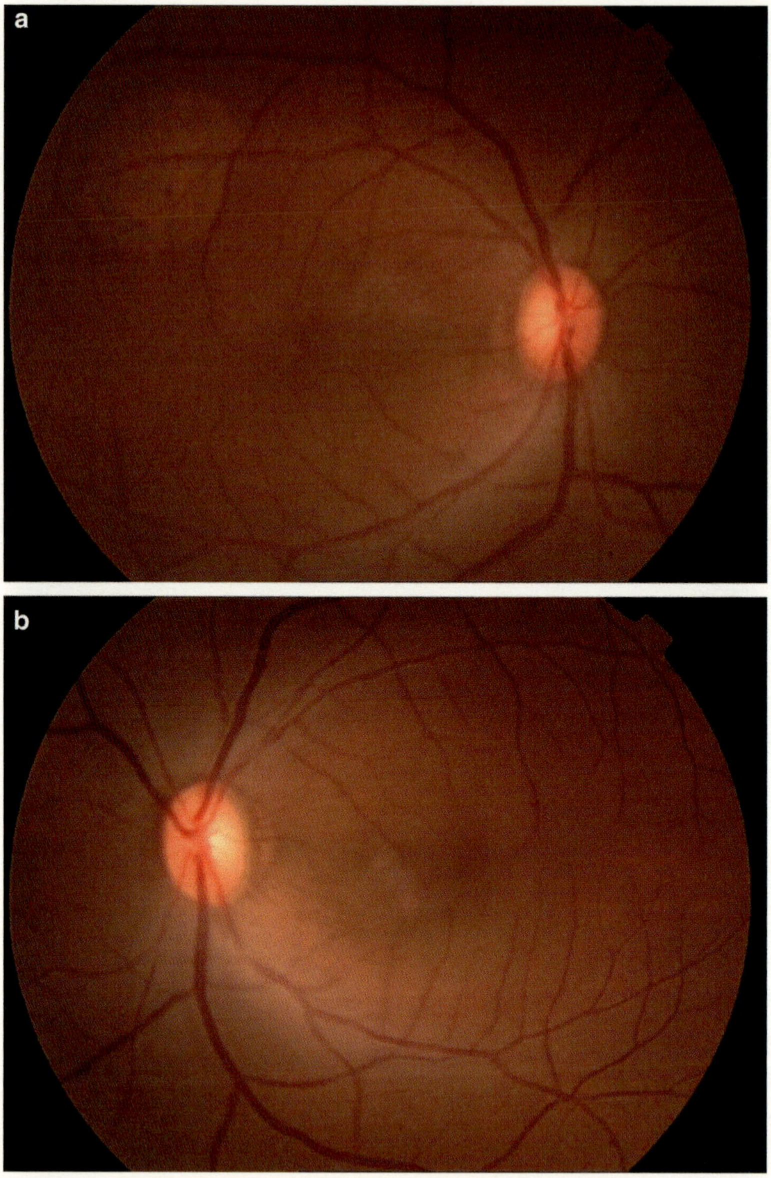

Fig. 19.7 (**a** and **b**) Fundus images of a monkey post Phaco-Ersatz. (**a**) Refilled lens, (**b**) natural contralateral eye (control). Stimulated accommodation amplitude was greater than 10 D in both eyes. Courtesy of Les Donovan OD, BHVI, Sydney, Australia

(see Fig. 19.7a, b). The potential of lens refilling shown possible in human eyes by Barraquer [29], as well as further investigation using various polymers [30–35], eventually led to the more recent demonstration of long term restoration of accommodation in non-human primates [16].

Endocapsular Balloon

Nishi and Hara were the first to implant an endocapsular balloon in the early 1990s [36]. They conceived of a thin-wall cross-linked polydimethylsiloxane (PDMS) balloon having the dimension of the crystalline lens and a thin umbilical tube located at the periphery. The balloon was to be implanted in its collapsed form through a small, 1.2 mm capsulorhexis, and insufflated with a PDMS fluid injected via the umbilical tube, which was then easily sealed and cut off close to the capsule surface. Following feasibility and biocompatibility studies in the rabbit [37], Nishi showed preservation of accommodation in a small series of young primates [38, 39].

Capsular Microvalve

Unfortunately, Nishi also observed a decline in accommodative amplitude from 9.00 to 1.00 D within the first year. The decrease in amplitude was attributed partially to lens epithelial cell fibrosis, which encapsulated the balloon, but also to a change in the balloon's physical properties, leading to permeation and oozing of the PDMS fluid through the balloon wall and capsulorhexis opening into the anterior chamber [40]. He determined that containment of the injected material and control of the lens shape were two important parameters to be managed [41]. Nishi et al. then created a self-sealing capsulotomy filling plug, which he adapted from the valve-device designed to pump air into bicycle tire tubes. The valve was created by sandwiching the capsulorhexis edge between two washers using a medical grade silastic adhesive. Once the polymeric fluid filled the evacuated capsular bag, and was sealed, it was cross-linked in situ, over several hours, becoming a soft pliable gel.

After having shown safety and biocompatibility in the rabbit model [42], Nishi et al. demonstrated the restoration of accommodation in senile primates [43]. To avoid postoperative iris inflammation caused by the protruding washer outer disk and tube stump, Nishi had to perform a sectorial iridectomy in all the animals receiving either a balloon or the sealing washer with direct capsular refilling.

Limitations of Capsular Refilling

The barriers to the success of both direct capsular filling and the endocapsular balloon are many. They include:

(a) Challenging to manually perform a peripheral capsulorhexis of <1 mm at a predefined distance from the lens apex.
(b) Lack of ultrasonic phacoemulsification system for removal of the lens content via a 1 or 1.2 mm capsulorhexis.
(c) Unwanted postoperative lens epithelium cell (LEC) proliferation and subsequent fibrosis and opacification of the posterior capsule (PCO) that obscures the visual axis.
(d) Preventing leakage of the injected polymer.
(e) Inability to intraoperatively control the volume of polymer injected for simultaneously achieving an emmetropic outcome, while maximizing the restored accommodation.

Challenging Mini-capsulotomy

If the delicate tearing of a 1 mm capsulorhexis is nearly impossible to perform in a reproducible manner, then the advent of femto-laser capsulotomy provides a specific solution to this limitation. Whether a 1 or 6 mm capsulotomy is required, the image-guided laser is able to deliver the precise size, shape and orientation to the capsular opening, which would more easily facilitate the placement of a capsular microvalve for sealing the opening during surgery.

Lack of Phaco System for Lens Removal Through a Mini-capsulotomy

Once again, where conventional technology is limited in the delivery of ultrasonic energy for chopping and emulsifying of hard nuclei through a 1 mm capsular opening, the FS laser is a specific solution that allows for pretreatment and fragmentation of the lens, so that mild emulsification and simple aspiration is all that may be required to extract the lens substance from its capsular bag. Here is yet another specific solution is offered by the FS laser to overcome the limitation of lens removal through a nearly intact capsular bag.

Lens Epithelial Cell (LEC) Proliferation

Several authors have experimentally demonstrated the tendency for LEC proliferation in animal models. Meanwhile, Kessler in rabbits [20], Agarwal in monkeys [22], and later Parel have all attempted to prevent the proliferation by using aqueous solutions containing antimitotics (methotrexate, mitomycin C, and 5-fluouracil) [44], by using di-hematoporphyrin-ether photodynamic therapy (DHE-PDT) [45], and by using hypoosmotic solutions, acetic acid, EDTA, and toxins [44, 46]. Unfortunately, none of these agents really worked well, partly because of problems encountered with leakage into the anterior chamber, leading to postoperative inflammation and toxicity to the delicate intraocular tissues, specially to the corneal endothelium, uvea and retina.

With the addition of the FS laser for creating small (~1 mm) capsulotomies of precise size, shape, and location, the use of a capsular microvalve ensures adequate containment of the injectable agents that would cause inflammation. In this way, the FS laser assists in minimizing the negative impact of lens epithelial cell proliferation.

Preventing Leakage of Injected Polymer

As mentioned above, the capsular mini-valve helps to prevent leakage of polymer into the anterior chamber [44, 47]. This is further secured by postcuring of the injected polymer [34, 47]. A further removal of risk is achieved by the precise diameter and shape of the image-guided FS laser capsulotomy. The precise size and circularity of the capsular opening allows for a snug fit of the capsular mini-valve, preventing any leakage of polymer into the anterior chamber.

Inability to Control the Volume of Polymer Injected

Another concern is that capsular bag refilling leads to ametropia, mainly hyperopia, in animal eyes [47]. The main reason for this inadequate refractive power of the new lens is related to the insufficient index of refraction of the injected polymer, and lack of gradient index, as seen within the natural crystalline lens [48, 49]. This can be remedied by formulating polymers having a higher refractive index and implementing adjustability to the compounds being injected [50].

Underfilling and overfilling of the polymer can also lead to ametropia, which can be improved upon by monitoring and modeling the amount injected to achieve refractive emmetropia, with sufficient accommodative amplitude [51, 52]. In this regard, the use of long range SD-OCT to assess the real time accommodation in vivo [53] and mathematical methods for extracting the lens geometrical parameters [54] have been implemented with some success. In the future, intraoperative OCT [55, 56] will enable surgeons to better measure the patient's crystalline lens volume before removal, and titrate the refilling of the capsular bag during the surgical procedure. With the new developments of image-guided ReLACS, the imaging component in these devices would be of value in monitoring the endpoint of capsular refilling.

The above mentioned limitations, once overcome, have successfully preserved and restored accommodation in young and senile primates, using lens-refilling techniques. Further development of ex vivo and in vivo models are being used to rapidly screen the efficacy of antiproliferating agents on lens epithelium. The development of new anti-LEC agents [57] is promising.

One potential limitation that has not yet been adequately studied is change in optical profile and retinal image quality with accommodation using lens refilling [35]. Replacing a presbyopic, but perfectly transparent human crystalline lens with a synthetic accommodating lens requires assurance that vision will be restored to at least the same preoperative level (20/20), and with a success rate that equates to at least the 96% level experienced with present day cataract surgery [58].

ReLACS Contribution to Capsular Refilling

The potential benefit of ReLACS to the concept of capsular refilling (Phaco-Ersatz) has been well outlined for creating the microcapsulotomy that can be precisely fitted and sealed with the microcapsular valve (MCV). Equally as important, the lens pretreatment with image-guided lens fragmentation, that will allow for easy removal of the lens nucleus in the setting of endocapsular extraction. In addition, the small shaped corneal incisions for bimanual lens removal and astigmatic corrections make the goals of capsular refilling more easily achievable.

The FS laser solves problems that could not be accomplished by micromechanical engineering with conventional instruments. FS-capsulotomies are more precise and more uniform than those done manually and their strength has been shown to be equal if not superior to manual capsulorhexis [45]. Moreover, the possibility to fragment the lens in very small pieces [46] will allow the use of a submillimeter cannula to safely empty the bag, simplifying lens refilling surgery.

Intralenticular Photodisruption for Accommodation Restoration

The Search for Non-invasive Presbyopia Correcting Lens Surgery

Presbyopia is defined by the progressive loss of accommodation and subsequently reduced ability to achieve a near focus when distance-corrected. The loss of accommodation that leads to presbyopia is a component of the dysfunctional lens that eventually leads to cataract formation. Therefore, a non-invasive solution for preventing or delaying this dysfunction, could have a beneficial effect on not only maintaining accommodative function, but also in delaying the onset of cataract formation. At present, nearly all proposed surgical solutions for presbyopia either involve the cornea for enhancing its asphericity and depth of focus, or with lens replacement for the implantation of presbyopia correcting intraocular lenses. Both of these categorical solutions have compromises, because they do not restore the true accommodation of the natural crystalline lens. Since the mechanisms of accommodation and presbyopia are complex, an adequate understanding of how they actually work is the first step towards the development of an effective restorative procedure.

The most widely accepted theory proposed by Helmholtz [59] and confirmed by more recent studies in primates [60], states that the movement of the equatorial edge of the lens is away from the sclera during accommodation and toward the sclera during disaccommodation. To accommodate, a contraction of the ciliary muscle releases the resting tension on the zonular fibers. It releases the equatorial tension on the lens capsule and allows the elasticity of the lens proteins and capsule to change its shape. This causes a decrease in the circumferential lens diameter and increases the curvature of the anterior and posterior lens surfaces. When the ciliary muscle relaxes (ceasing the accommodative effort), it moves toward the sclera, pulling the zonular fibers and increasing the tension on the lens equator. This is responsible for a flattening of the lens and a decrease in the anterior and posterior lens curvature. According to this theory, the age-related loss of lens elasticity is one of the most important components of the progressive age-related loss of accommodation.

Decreased ciliary muscle activity and lens geometry were also suggested as possible causes of presbyopia. However, these suggestions have not been confirmed in experimental studies. In fact, an increase in human ciliary muscle contraction has been found [61], which may occur as a response to an increased resistance in lens deformation (caused by the loss of elasticity). Classical experimental studies by Fisher in 1971 showed an age-related decrease in lens elasticity [62]. This was then validated and further defined by Glasser, showing a decrease in lens deformation in an experimental model of accommodation where older lenses showed less optical changes than younger lenses when subjected to the same magnitude of stretching [63]. Although scleral modifying surgical procedures are also being investigated for restoring accommodation, changes within the lens contribute most significantly to the loss of accommodation, and this is the ultimate target to pursue.

Based on this information, the main focus of accommodation restoration procedures should, then, be on the lens. With laser surgery in ophthalmology becoming widely successful in multiple applications, a non-invasive laser procedure for treating presbyopia, preserving the natural crystalline lens, should be considered. FS laser technology is revolutionizing ophthalmic surgery by its capability of delivering ultrashort laser pulses to a tightly localized focal point without interacting with the surrounding transparent ocular tissues or causing collateral damage. This laser and its internal focusing capability should, then, be able to precisely treat the crystalline lens in a non-invasive procedure and, when safely and effectively proven, would have the potential to break old paradigms regarding the internal surgical manipulation of the crystalline lens. This concept of laser lens modulation for accommodation restoration was first proposed by Myers and Krueger in 1998 [64].

The History of LensAR

In 1994, Vogel et al. compared the effect of a picosecond laser versus a nanosecond laser on the crystalline lens. Using neodymium:yttrium–aluminum–garnet (Nd:YAG) lasers, they noticed that a decreased laser pulse duration allowed for the use of less energy and consequently reduced the collateral damage induced by localized thermal and large cavitation bubble effects [65].

In 2001, Krueger et al., using only the nanosecond laser, were able to prove increased flexibility in an aging lens after a laser treatment [66]. In this study, freshly excised cadaver lenses were removed and tested with the method proposed by Fisher. In the first part of the study, an age-dependent decrease in the polar strain (elasticity) was observed. Then, Nd:YAG laser pulses were applied in a central annular pattern within the lenses and they were tested again and compared with their pair as a control. The results showed that each lasered lens had statistically significantly greater rotational deformation when compared to their unlasered pair. Some of the older lasered lenses showed deformation values comparable to lenses 20 years younger (Fig. 19.8) [66], suggesting that laser photodisruption within the lens was able to enhance its accommodative potential.

In 2005, Krueger et al. sought to demonstrate the safety of such a procedure with a short pulse, lower energy, laser source, and published an experimental study using titanium sapphire FS laser pulses applied to six living rabbit eyes [67] (using the contra lateral eye as a control). This study showed that ultrashort laser pulses of low energy (1 μJ/pulse) could be delivered transcorneally in living eyes and used to microdisrupt the mid-periphery of the lens without causing any cataractous damage to adjacent lens fibers. Optical quality studies assessing light scatter showed no difference between the laser-treated eyes and their untreated controls. Ultrastructurally, the rabbit eyes showed a 0.5-μm electron-dense border layer with adjacent normal lens architecture.

After laser treatment, all lenses displayed a tightly packed array of intralenticular bubbles, which resolved within the first day or two. Those results were confirmed in 2007 by Gerten et al., in another experimental study on porcine lenses [68].

Methods for Ex Vivo Testing of Accommodation

In order to investigate the elasticity of the lens, several different methods have been proposed. It is important to objectively evaluate the true effect of FS laser lentotomy for accommodation restoration, so that the procedure's efficacy and best treatment pattern can be established. The following in vitro methods have been proposed and utilized in experimentation:

1. *Rotational deformation*: Introduced by Fisher in 1971 [62], this method puts the crystalline lens on top of a rotating cylinder to simulate the force of zonular traction. The changes in the lens thickness based on the rotational speed are measured to define the deformability of the tissue. Note the method of Fig. 19.8.
2. *Zonular stretching* [69]: After dissecting out the ciliary muscle with overlying sclera and zonular fibers with the attached lens, and positioning this complex into a stretching device, accommodative measurements are made by recording the changing curvature of the lens and by focusing rays of laser light through the crystalline lens in a fluid-filled chamber and observing their aberration profile with stretching.
3. *Lens compression* [70]: The crystalline lens is placed into a mechanically compressive device "Squidger," which tests the relative lens resistance to displacement with gradient steps of compressive force.

All of these methods are invasive and can only be used ex vivo. Despite their relative importance in validating procedures for restoring accommodation,

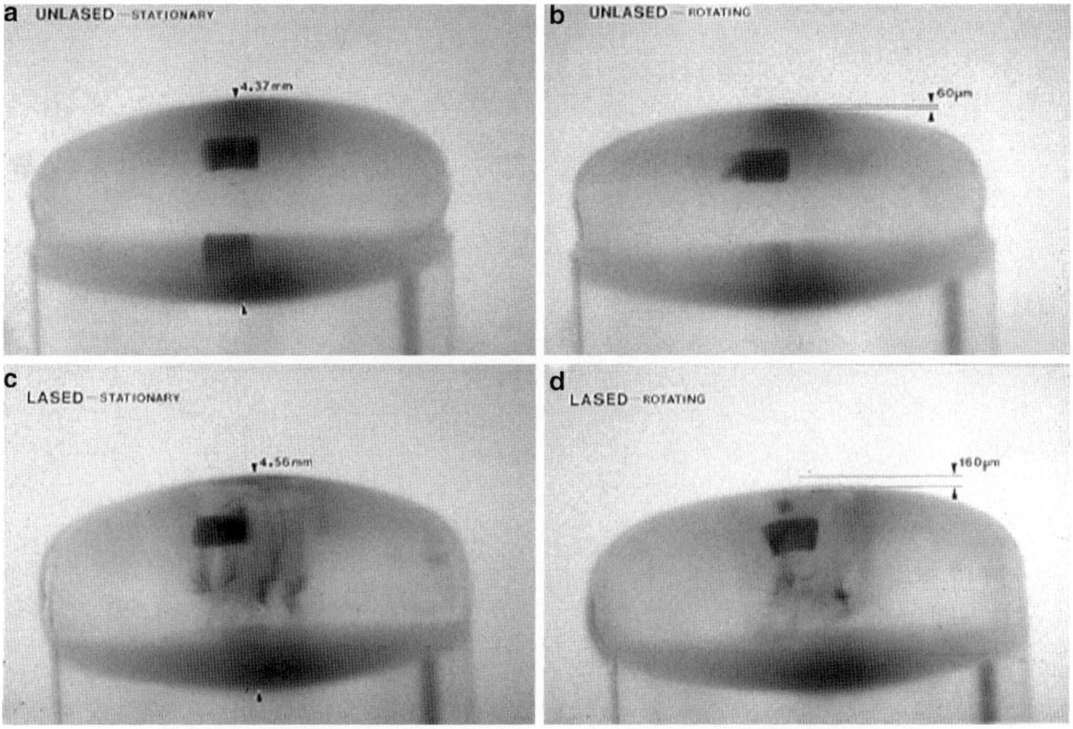

Fig. 19.8 Rotational deformation (**a** and **b**, **c** and **d**), leading to statistically significant increases in age dependent polar strain in cadaver eyes treated with laser (**c** and **d**) relative to their contralateral unlasered control lens (**a** and **b**). Here the polar strain (60 µm) of a 54-year-old lens (**b**) behaves like a 35-year-old lens (160 µm) when treated with the laser (**d**). Credit to Elsevier?

none of them is ideal and completely representative of the clinical process. A non-invasive, accurate and reproducible in vivo test is needed to aid in the quest of restoring accommodation.

Models for Laser Lens Treatment

The human crystalline lens is a very complex structure that continually evolves throughout life. A complex, finite element model based on the microanatomy and physiologic function of the lens fibers within the lens is needed to assess the impact of specific intralenticular laser microincisions on the lens flexibility in order to optimize the sliding and deformation of lens fibers and hence improve accommodation.

In 2006, Kuszak and colleagues [71] reported the development of a finite element analysis (FEA) model of the human crystalline lens that most closely mirrored scanning and transmission electron microscopic images of lens ultrastructure (see Fig. 19.9a, b). It was based on the systematic change in embryologic, juvenile and adult ultrastructure of the lens with consideration of lens suture development and interfiber digitations. This model provided the framework for the initial development of laser treatment algorithms within the lens.

A variety of different laser pulse patterns were tested in the computer-generated model, including treatments both within and sparing the center of the lens. The most intuitive and best-working algorithms tested in the computer generated FEA model were "concentric shells," "incisions along lens sutures" and "concentric cylinders." In an effort to minimize the potential for visual dysphotopsia, ablation algorithms sparing the center was preferred, and for minimizing of the density of pulses (and bubbles) within the lens, an anterior and posterior "waffle" pattern was applied, following the fiber orientation along concentric shells within the mid-periphery of the lens (Fig. 19.10a, b).

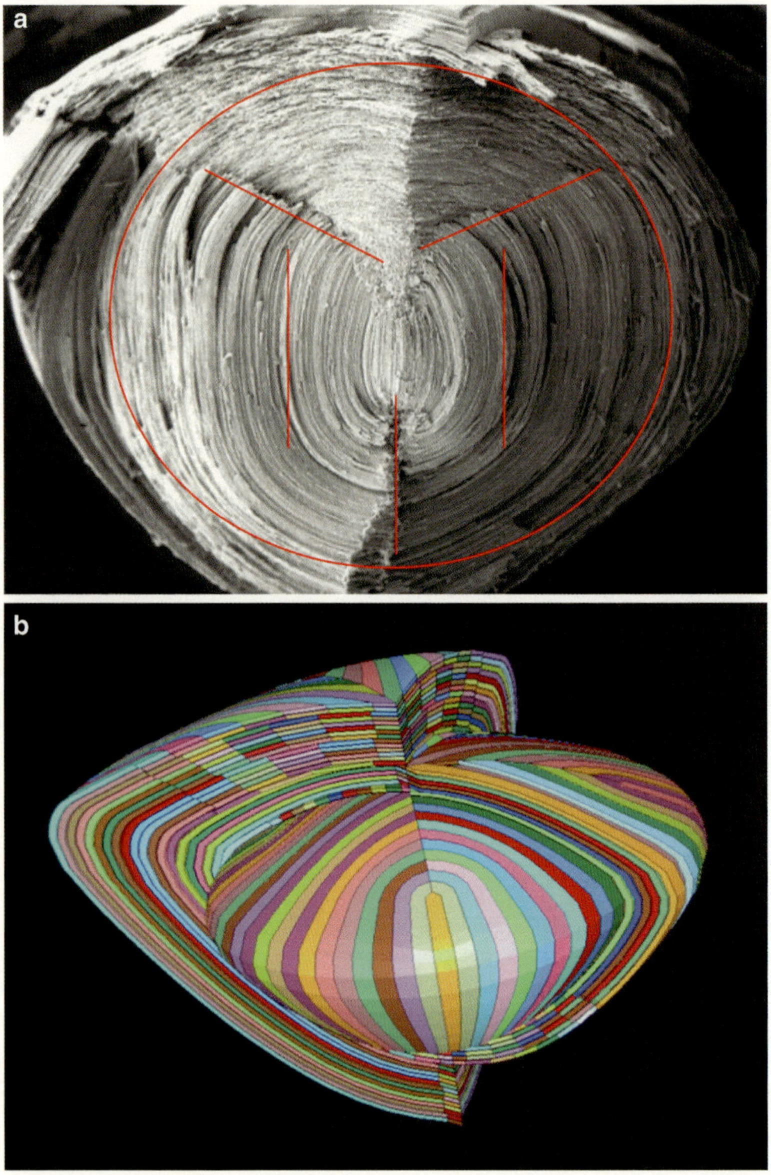

Fig. 19.9 (**a**) Scanning electron microscopy of a human crystalline lens, revealing a detailed ultrastructural network of lens fibers and overlapping sutures. (**b**) Finite element analysis (FEA) model of the human crystalline lens that most closely represents the lens ultrastructure

Early Clinical Investigation in Subjects Prior to Refractive Cataract Surgery

After initial experiments in vitro and animal safety studies in vivo, the next step was to initiate a clinical study to prove its safety and then effect. Although the earliest clinical studies were started with Dr. Ramon Naranjo Tackman in Mexico City as early as 2008, the first series of patients following a clinical protocol were performed with Dr. Harvey Uy in the Philippines. Over the past 1–2 years, two series of 5 subject and then 11 subjects were unilaterally treated after meeting the following criteria: (1) age between 45 and 60 years, (2) previously electing to undergo refractive cataract surgery, (3) best spectacle corrected visual acuity (BSCVA) of 20/40 or better, and (4) a cataract assessed at no greater than grade 2

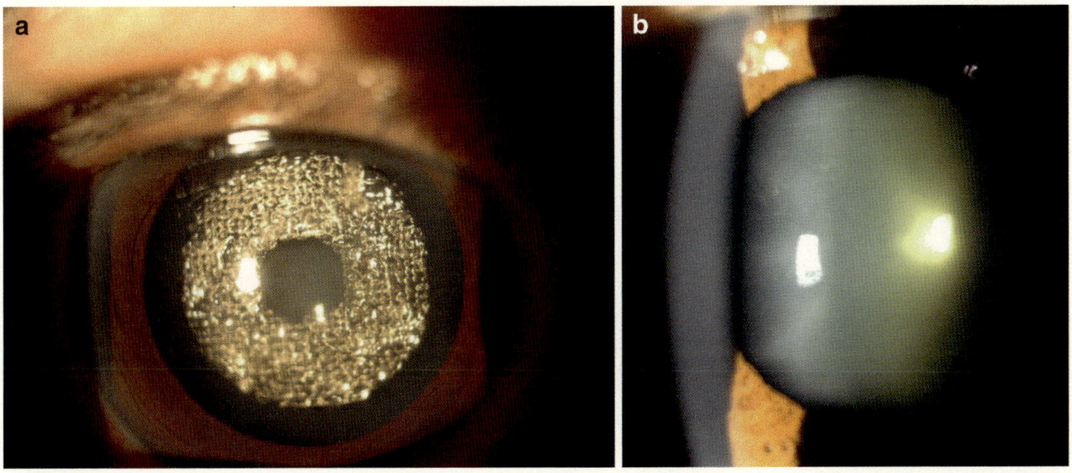

Fig. 19.10 (**a**) Center sparing laser treatment in a "waffle pattern" with remaining intralenticular bubbles immediately after application. (**b**) Center sparing "waffle pattern" seen 1 week later, revealing small pinpoint opacities at site of laser pulsing with no evidence of progressive cataract

Table 19.1 Investigational cohort of clinical eyes treated with the LensAR Laser System for accommodation restoration

Number and percentage of cases showing an improvement over baseline			
	1-Week, *n* (%)	2-Weeks, *n* (%)	1-Month, *n* (%)
Objective accommodation	20 (33.3%)	13 (22.8%)	10 (19.2%)
Subjective accommodation	35 (53%)	33 (51.6%)	35 (55.6%)
Best distance-corrected near VA	28 (37.3%)	35 (48.6%)	29 (40.8%)

The number and percentage of eye demonstrating objective accommodation, subjective accommodation, and improvement in BDCNVA are recorded at 1 week, 2 weeks, and 1 month after the laser surgery

(unpublished data). The reason for choosing eyes with a lesser grade nuclear cataract and better BSCVA is because these eyes would most closely represent those of a typical presbyopic patient who would be seeking this procedure, and also to avoid fractures within the lens, being frequently seen in the fragmentation of denser nuclei during ReLACS. Only one of each patient's eyes was treated, in order to minimize the risk of visual morbidity, and the subject had the option to proceed with refractive cataract surgery after 1 month or to delay lens extraction, in which case they would be followed for up to 36 months.

Three alternative algorithms selected from the computer-generated model were evaluated and applied in a randomized fashion. In all of the models, the central optical pathway of the lens was spared. The accommodative and visual effect of the treatment was assessed by objective accommodation (Grand Seiko autorefractor), subjective push down near point of accommodation and logMAR best distance-corrected near visual acuity.

Immediately after this nonexternally invasive procedure, it was possible to visualize the intralenticular bubbles (Fig. 19.10a), which fade over the first day or two, leaving only faint, pinpoint opacities (Fig. 19.10b). No intraoperative complications were reported, and the early postoperative results showed no progressive cataract formation. Overall, 80 eyes have been treated and analyzed at 1 week, 2 weeks and 1 month follow up and the percentage improvement in the three indicies of accommodation are shown in Table 19.1.

Here we see that 1/3 of the study eyes at 1 week and only 20% at 1 month show signs of improvement in objective accommodation after treatment with the various patterns. For subjective accommodation, this improves a little to over 50% improvement at both 1 week and 1 month after laser application. Finally, for the logMAR best distance corrected near visual acuity (BDCNVA), the improvement was experienced in ~40% of eyes at both 1 week and 1 month.

In order to understand the magnitude of these improvements, the change in objective accommodation was a mean (SD) of 0.44 D (±0.31), with a maximum of 1.25 D at 1 week and 0.76 D (±0.42), with a maximum of 1.50 D at 1 month. This modest objective improvement may, in part, be limited by the diameter of capture of the Grand Seiko autorefractor in light of the central sparing diameter of laser pulsing. The change in subjective accommodation was a mean (SD) of 0.66 D (±0.84), with a maximum of 3.62 D at 1 week, and 0.72 D (±0.68), with a maximum of 2.33 D at 1 month. Here, the mean change is similar to the objective accommodation, but the maximum is considerably higher. Finally, the LogMAR best distance corrected near visual acuity (BDCNVA) was a mean (SD) of 6 letters (±5), with a maximum of 23 letters (five lines) at 1 week, and a mean (SD) of 7 letters (±6), with a maximum of 31 letters (six lines) at 1 month. The relatively small percentage of eyes showing a change in accommodation/near vision, and this modest amount of change, suggests a level of unpredictability that warrants further investigation of additional patterns to determine a more efficacious laser profile. The recruitment and testing of additional clinical subjects is anticipated in the coming months.

Refractive Index Modification of the Cornea and Lens

Laser Refractive Surgery without Ablation FS laser pulses can cause a number of different effects in materials. Of particular interest for ophthalmology are effects in transparent materials such as polymers and ocular tissues. An example of a desirable effect is the capacity to change the refractive index of an optical material within a prescribed three-dimensional region. This would allow us to precisely change the refractive properties of the optical device. For instance, one could write a refractive index modification into an IOL before or even after it has been inserted. Furthermore, if it were possible to directly write a refractive index modification into the human cornea or lens, this could eliminate the need for eyeglasses or contact lenses. Obviously, for such applications, it would be necessary to change the refractive properties of the material in a predictable fashion without creating undesirable effects such as optical scattering, halos, rainbow effect, induced absorption or in the case of ocular tissues, a significant wound healing response. Using FS laser pulses above a given material's damage threshold causes cutting, physical modifications of the material, cellular disruption and cell death (if the material is biological). However, recent work shows great promise for this approach by showing that it may be possible to non-invasively change the refractive index of transparent materials like hydrogels as well as live tissues such as the cornea and lens.

Subthreshold Disruption Modifies the Refractive Index

In the late 1990s, studies of tissue cutting and disruption using trains of high repetition rate pulses showed that it was possible to induce mainly refractive index modifications if one remained below the bulk damage threshold of the material [72–74]. Indeed, when using high repetition rate trains of FS pulses (30–100 MHz and greater), it is possible to locally deposit energy on a time-scale that is faster than the thermal diffusion time. This localized energy deposition can alter the material's properties so that below a certain energy threshold (Threshold 1 in Fig. 19.11), there is no detectable refractive index change, while above this first threshold, a refractive index change is induced.

Generally, when using FS light pulses in transparent materials, the absorption of light will only occur at the focus point, and it will be dominated by a two- or higher-order, multi-photon process. This process requires a certain minimum intensity to reach the first threshold for index change.

Above this first threshold, the refractive index is increased, generally, by a localized material densification process. For hydrogels, this may be the result of a polymer phase transition wherein hydrophilic materials are locally altered to become more hydrophobic. The local expulsion of water causes a local densification of the polymer, which in turn increases the index of refraction. Refractive index change continues to increase as additional laser energy is applied (yellow region in Fig. 19.11), up to a sharp threshold (Threshold II in Fig. 19.11). In hydrogels, once Threshold II is reached, additional deposition of laser energy causes the material to burn and blacken [76], a behavior that is also observed in cornea and lens [77].

In hydrogels, the magnitude of refractive index change attainable at a given scanning speed can be strongly enhanced by doping the material with a two-photon absorbing dye [78] (Fig. 19.12).

As shown in Fig. 19.12, significant index changes can be induced below the damage threshold by carefully controlling scanning speed and other laser parameters. Moreover, the induced refractive index changes appear permanent, with no significant degradation over a period of at least 2.5 years.

Recently, it was shown that a cylindrical lens structure with as much as +1.0 D of astigmatism could be written in Akreos polymer [79]. In related research, Bille and colleagues have developed a co-doped polymer system capable of sustaining refractive index modifications [80]. Hampp and colleagues also recently reported on the development of yet a different polymer compound system [81] intended for refractive modifications of IOLs [82]. It is exciting to contemplate the possibility of a fully customizable refractive technology that could correct aberrations in an already-implanted IOL, while being reversible and adjustable in future operations.

Investigation and Refinement of Refractive Index Modification

In 2008, Ding and colleagues showed that it was possible to use relatively safe, near-infrared laser pulses to write refractive index changes into corneal and lens slices [77], and in 2010, Nagy et al. [83] showed that enhancement of two-photon absorption could be applied to living corneas (Fig. 19.13a) in a manner similar to that used for hydrogel polymers.

Whereas refractive index writing speeds in cornea or lens could be enhanced by doping the tissue with common dyes like fluorescein, such doping may be undesirable clinically. This has led

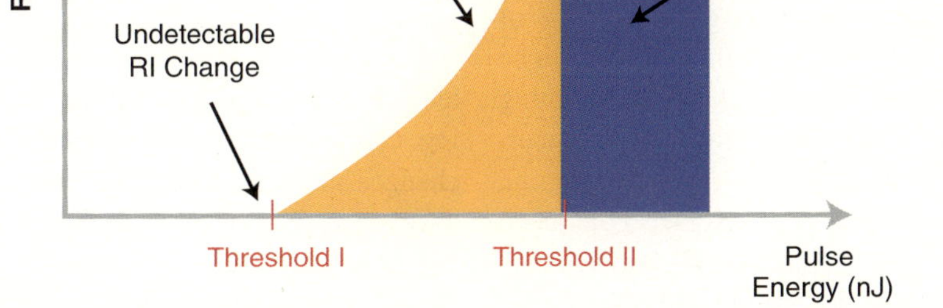

Fig. 19.11 Schematic picture of refractive index and gross material changes attained as a function of laser pulse energy. Modified from Ding et al. [75]

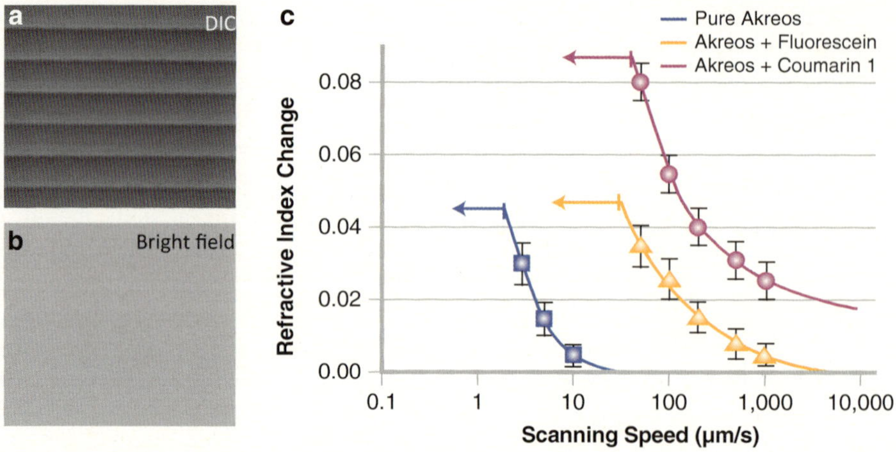

Fig. 19.12 (**a**) Differential Interference Contrast (DIC) photograph of diffraction grating written in Akreos polymer; (**b**) corresponding bright field microscope photograph showing no visible damage (which would appear as *dark brown lines* or *spots*); (**c**) plot of refractive index change as a function of laser scanning speed for native Akreos hydrogel polymer (*black symbols*) and Akreos polymer doped with different two-photon absorbers—Fluorescein (*red symbols*) and Coumarin I (*blue symbols*). *Arrows* indicated areas of damage rather than index changes

to experimental investigations of the efficacy of blue FS light pulses for inducing refractive index changes in both native hydrogels and living ocular tissues. Near-infrared light is safe in the eye and prevents "dazzling" effects in patients. However, in the blue spectral region, there is also a window of transparency and relatively low visual sensitivity in the range 350–400 nm [84]. In that region, there is significant, native, two-photon absorption in the live cornea [85]. As such, one should expect a significant enhancement of refractive index change at this wavelength without the use of doping dyes. The safety of blue light for all parts of the eye needs to be more fully investigated. However, preliminary determinations using 80 mW average power at 400 nm wavelength showed that diffraction gratings consisting of refractive index changes up to almost 0.04 can be written into live cat corneas at higher writing speeds than possible in doped corneas with near-infrared light (Fig. 19.13b) [86]. At low scanning speeds (<5 mm/s), excessive damage is induced including formation of blebs, or gas bubbles, and burns. At higher speeds, grating patterns of pure refractive index change are written into the tissue. The optical quality of such corneal diffraction gratings is high, as evidenced by low scattering between the zero-order and first-order diffraction peaks [86]. This is important, as it ensures maintained transparency of the corneal tissue, a critical property for optimal visual quality.

Future Clinical Applications

The ability to write three-dimensional refractive index modifications into polymers and/or ocular tissues could have a profound impact upon vision care. In the case of polymers, it may be possible to effectively write a lens structure within an IOL either before or after it has been implanted into the eye. This has many advantages for cataract surgery, since follow-up procedures could allow the surgeon to correct ocular aberrations induced by lens misalignment. As for directly writing into living cornea or lens, the longevity of the index changes attained and their effects on tissue biology have not yet been established past 10 days. Finally, while refractive structures with up to +1.0 D astigmatism have been written into Akreos polymers, it should be possible to extend this to ±3.0 D of refractive power in hydrogels as well as in cornea

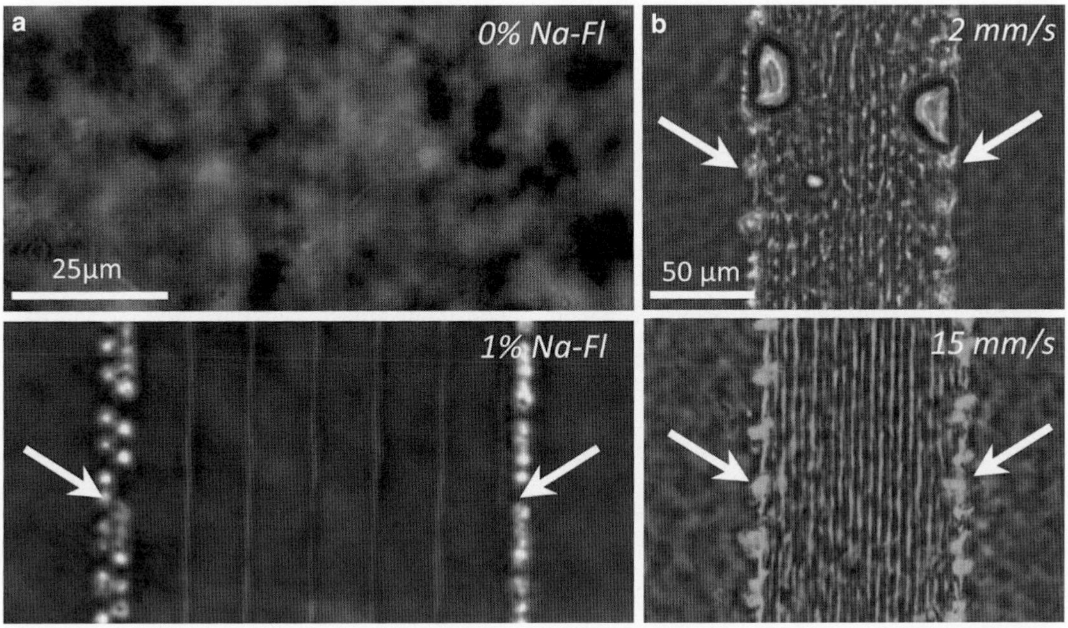

Fig. 19.13 (**a**) Differential interference contract photographs of diffraction gratings written with near infra-red laser pulses into live feline corneal pieces that were either undoped (0% Na–Fl) or doped with 1% sodium fluorescein (1% Na–Fl). The two *outside lines* of each grating were intentionally written at slow speeds to cause damage (bubbles and burns), while the *central lines* were written at 2 mm/s. Note the more distinct *central lines* in the doped corneal piece relative to the undoped piece. This difference in visibility was associated with a greater increase in refractive index in the doped corneal piece. (**b**) Differential interference contrast photographs of diffraction gratings written with blue FS laser pulses at 80 mw average power at 2 and 15 mm/s scanning speeds. Again, flanking damage lines were intentionally created on either side of a grating pattern. However, because of the greater energy content of blue laser light, damage was created in undoped, live corneal pieces at 2 mm/s. Clean, *central lines* of pure refractive index change were achieved at 15 mm/s

and lens tissue using purpose-designed, three-dimensional patterns. Current research is working to optimize such designs to ultimately correct a large range of both lower-order and higher-order optical aberrations in the human eye.

Adaptive Optics Femtosecond Laser Delivery

History of Adaptive Optics

While most ophthalmologists are familiar with wavefront aberrometry, few clinicians know about the details of adaptive optics. Yet, it is this technology that has led to the introduction of wavefront aberrometry into ophthalmology, and is now beginning to fuel its real time dynamic use, as well. So, what is the history of adaptive optics, and how did it contribute to ocular wavefront sensing?

The earliest use of adaptive optics (AO) is in the field of astronomy. Horace Babcock first theorized the use of adaptive optics to overcome atmospheric turbulence as early as 1953 [87]. However, it was not until the early 1990s that technological innovation began to bring this from theory to reality. Around this same time, the Hubble telescope was launched into orbit in an effort to bypass the effects of atmospheric turbulence. Yet in comparison to the modern day Keck telescope, using adaptive optics, the more expensive Hubble telescope in space is not as resolute, demonstrating the power of adaptive optics [88].

It is this successful refinement of astronomical imaging that has piqued the interest of physiologic optical scientists. In 1994, Liang and Bille saw the potential in this technology for measuring and correcting the aberrations in the eye, publishing the first article on the ocular use of adaptive optics [89]. The era of ocular wavefront sensing then began, experiencing its natural growth in refractive surgery, because with the early rise of LASIK surgery, there was also a rise in visual symptoms among those who saw 20/20 after surgery, but were dissatisfied. The reason for their dissatisfaction was the creation of laser-induced aberrations [90]. Wavefront detection then gave rise to wavefront-guided LASIK, in an effort to customize the outcomes of laser vision correction [91]. In both detection and surgical treatment, ocular wavefront sensing utilized the principles of adaptive optics in a static manner, but it is the dynamic measurement and real time optical correction of aberrations that is now only beginning to experience its clinical application in retinal imaging and visual simulation [92, 93].

Adaptive Optics Retinal Imaging

Just as the astronomer desires to see the stars with great clarity, the retina specialist desires to see the details of the retina beyond what is possible with the optics of the naked eye. Adaptive optics retina imaging is now possible, with imaging capabilities for resolving individual photoreceptors (cones and rods) and micro-capillaries in both early diseased eyes and normal eyes (Fig. 19.14). This same resolution for imaging the retinal details can be used to better focus light rays into the eye, as well.

Adaptive Optics Refinement of Light Delivery and Lasers

It is the progress of this technology beyond that of real time, dynamic detection and optical correction (imaging) that brings it into the realm of adaptive optics laser delivery. The delivery of light rays into the eye for stimulating individual photoreceptors (microperimetry) [94] is the first step toward adaptive optics delivery of an actual laser for the treatment of intraocular structures with the resolution of the retina photoreceptors. The AO delivery has the potential for not only receiving aberration-free images from the eye, but of aberration-free laser surgery inside the eye, as well.

In simulating and demonstrating this concept, Hansen and coauthors have been focusing FS laser pulses through adaptive optics in order to refine the focal spot shape through a turbid media [95]. They were able to design a model eye composed of a plano-convex lens, representing the cornea and lens, photopaper as the retina and a low quality optical material 2-hydroxyethyl-methacrylate (HEMA) as the turbid media of the vitreous. In experiments, they were able to show that the threshold for visible bubbling of photopaper when applying a FS laser through the model eye was 2.2 μJ, and this was reduced to 1.2 μJ when adaptive optics was applied (Fig. 19.15a). Similarly, the threshold for developing a hole in the photopaper was not possible at the highest tested energy of 3.0 μJ, but when applying adaptive optics, the threshold was noted at 2.0 μJ (Fig. 19.15b). Thus, the intraocular delivery of FS lasers can be refined with the use of adaptive optics, leading to lower therapeutic energies for greater laser safety.

Although this has implications for the future of laser cataract surgery, the extraction of the crystalline lens may not require a much lower energy than what currently exists, since laser fragmentation is relatively safe with the current laser platforms. This, however, is not the case with modifications of the crystalline lens for accommodation restoration or refractive index change, since greater optical refinement of the laser spot size, shape and energy would increase its efficiency, while minimizing its potential side effects. The refinement of FS laser delivery with adaptive optics has implications in the crystalline lens and beyond.

Beyond Cataract and Lens Applications

Adaptive Optics Vitreolysis and Retinal Surgery

While the subject of this book is ReLACS and FS laser refractive lens surgery, there are other ocular and intraocular structures that can be treated with clinical benefit using the internal focusing of a FS

Fig. 19.14 Adaptive optics retinal imaging, revealing individual cones, rods, and micro-capillaries in a normal retina (courtesy of Imagine Eyes, Orsay, France)

laser. In our previous example of AO FS laser delivery through a turbid media (HEMA) [95], the reduction of laser energy in treating photopaper in a model eye, suggests that clinical treatment of the retina and vitreous would also benefit from this technology. This is especially true since the retina and vitreous are much deeper structures inside the eye, than the cornea and lens, hence the focusing optics must be of lower numerical aperture, and refinement is necessary in order to reduce the potential for peripheral side effects and collateral laser damage. The micro-cutting action of FS laser pulses can be particularly useful in separating structures under tension. The lysis of vitreous traction seen in both vitreo-macular interface disorders [96] (macular holes, vitreomacular traction syndrome, epiretinal membranes, etc.) and diabetic retinopathy [97] (macular edema and tractional detachments, etc.) might be possible with adaptive optics delivery of FS laser pulses. Laser retinotomy might also be possible for complex vitreoretinal surgeries.

The Femto-laser Scalpel in Ophthalmology

The non-invasive nature of intraocular laser delivery makes it extremely attractive for a host of clinical disorders. In the treatment of glaucoma, ab interno ablation of the trabecular meshwork allows for a less invasive outflow of aqueous humor from the eye [98]. FS laser pulses could theoretically be delivered through a gonio lens to specifically open obstructed channels. Scleral treatment with FS laser pulses might allow for creative, new alternatives for glaucoma filtration and other wall of the eye procedures. Focusing the FS laser over the extraocular muscles could potentially weaken strongly contracting EOM's by performing partial myotomies, which could correct strabismus non-invasively. There is a host of possible solutions to clinical problems that might be addressed by the use of FS lasers in eye surgery. In its own unique way, the laser is fast becoming the new scalpel in eye surgery. The future is bright, and we await the full realization of how versatile the ophthalmic use of the FS laser will become in the years ahead.

Beyond Image-Guided Femtosecond Lasers as We Know Them Today

As a final consideration of the future of refractive cataract surgery, we should consider not only the clinical procedures that are likely to arise from this new technology, but also the way the technical machinery will improve in the future, making this technology even more attractive for the cataract surgeon. Current imaging, FS lasers and interfacing are likely to improve in the future, and with this there will be an even more user friendly system for the clinician. In this regard, one of our authors, Kristian Hohla, PhD, gives a veteran engineer, entrepreneur and executive officer perspective of what we will see in the ReLACS surgery laser of the future.

Better Imaging

As mentioned in the beginning of this chapter, it will be a natural next step that the imaging technology integrated for the purpose of ReLACS will also begin to service its anatomic and topology data to other FS laser treatments, like keratoplasty,

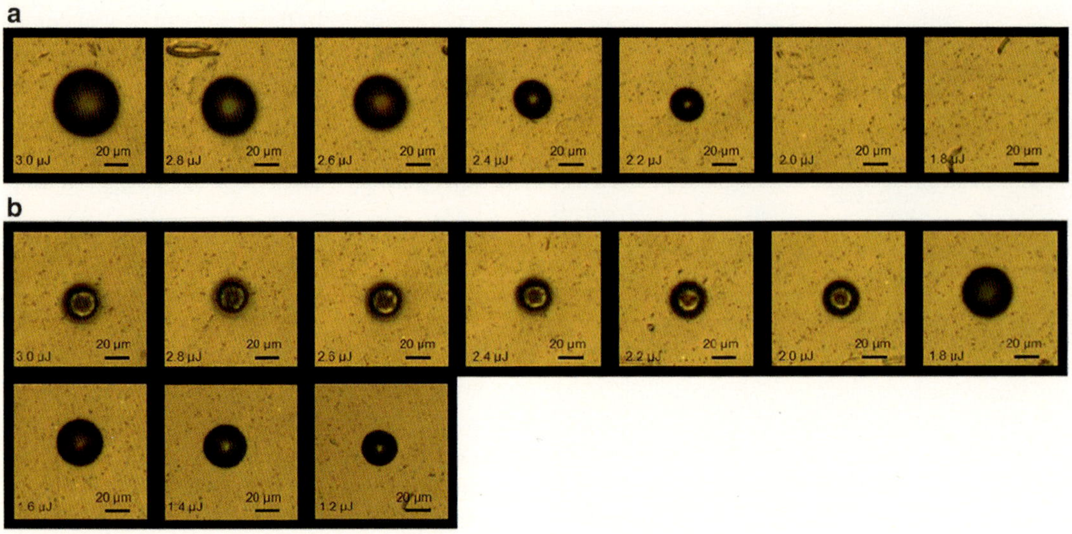

Fig. 19.15 (**a** and **b**) Adaptive optics refinement of FS laser focal spot shape through a turbid media (HEMA) in a model eye with photopaper representing the retina. (**a**) The threshold for visible bubbling of the photopaper was reduced from 2.2 to 1.2 µJ with adaptive optics, (**b**) the threshold for creating a hole was not possible at 3.0 µJ, but reduced to 2.0 µJ with adaptive optics (figure Courtesy of SPIE)

flap cuts, or corneal presbyopia treatments. Furthermore, newer, even more advanced imaging technologies will emerge and will be integrated in the FS lasers of the future. We may even be able to measure biomechanical and/or biological tissue responses to the laser treatment on a lamellar or even cellular level in the future.

Better Femtosecond Lasers

We also anticipate being able to use the improvements that have been experienced with industrial lasers to improve the reliability and reduce the cost of our lasers, as well as to make them smaller, lighter and more mobile. In parallel with that development we may see a further increase in the technical capabilities, like a faster pulse repetition rate and lower energies. However, there will likely be limits in energy per time delivered to the eye, beyond which a clinical application will no longer be acceptable, as for example, collateral thermal effects might occur.

Laser physicists have already driven the frontiers of research laser systems into regimes with pulse durations shorter than femtoseconds. However, the value of extremely short pulses for ophthalmic surgery most likely will be limited. Also, the technical efforts for handling extremely short pulses on the order of only a few femtoseconds become basically prohibitive. Laser pulses so short in time show an extremely wide bandwidth in the wavelength regime, on the order of several hundred nanometers. Thus, this laser light is no longer monochromatic, but occupies a broad wavelength band. In this situation dispersion needs to be considered, when passing such short laser pulses through application systems optics, as the different wavelengths travel at different speeds through the glass of lenses. Dynamic scanning of such a laser beam then even increases the technological challenges of such significant dispersion, which in principle could be handled, but with high technical efforts.

Better Interfacing

We can also legitimately expect that the ophthalmic FS lasers of the future will become more "intelligent." They will combine the input from various diagnostic systems into even more elaborate treatment plans, and many steps of the laser surgery will feature highly automated components. However, the surgeon still will have the last say. Future ophthalmic FS lasers will also link more deeply into the clinic's technical and data environment, optimizing patient flow and making the treatment experience as seamless as possible. Advances in computer technology will bring the man–machine interaction to new frontiers, with novel user interfaces and modes of interaction different from the keyboards and touch screens in use today.

Another aspect of man–machine interfacing is the interface between the laser system and the patient. Here, we will see a steady stream of new developments in patient interfaces (PI), making the patient experience as comfortable as possible, and the respective handling for the surgeon will experience improvements by automation steps. Tracker-based contact-free treatments, like we know them from refractive excimer procedures, might materialize in the future, but the technological challenges regarding the speed and precision of the required tracking and scanning systems is extremely high [99].

Better Cutting Tool

The non-thermal nature and the unique mechanisms of FS laser–tissue interaction make it ideal for also reaching deeper into the eye, for other therapeutic applications. For the future, we may for example look at how we can apply our ultrashort pulsed "light knife" technology to treatments for glaucoma and retinal diseases. While today primarily FS lasers emitting around 1 μm wavelength are in use, lasers supporting new realms of treatments may use totally different wavelength windows of the eye, depending on what type of tissue is to be treated. Even sclera can be treated with FS laser light of proper wavelength.

Summary

The clinical utilization of FS lasers is already incredibly active and competitive with nearly ten different companies currently working on FS and ultrashort laser technology for use in ophthalmology. The arrival of the femto laser applications for cataract surgery completely changed the playing field, initiated by Alcon's entry when it purchased LenSx (Chap. 15). However, we also believe that this creates an opportunity for mid-sized companies, like Technolas Perfect Vision (Chap. 18), considering the wider range of treatments available, as well as their partnership with Bausch & Lomb. Finally, companies such as LensAR (Chap. 16) and OptiMedica (Chap. 17) have their place by offering their own technological approaches, such as fluid optics interfacing or alternative means of imaging. Beyond these, more systems will follow (i.e., Ziemer, AMO, etc.), and these will likely be included in the subject of the next book.

In conclusion, FS technology in ophthalmic surgery is a game changer, nothing less than a revolution. And it does not stop where it is today, but will continue to shape and immensely change the picture of modern ophthalmology.

Key Points

1. The steady progression of FS lasers into the mainstream of refractive surgery, with applications in corneal and now cataract surgery, leverages this technology as the new scalpel in ophthalmic surgery.
2. The significant addition of immersion optics and image guidance in femto-laser surgery offers new precision to various corneal procedures, including anterior and posterior lamellar transplants, refractive lenticular extraction and intrastromal lamellar pockets for precision inlays and selective cross-linking.
3. Advancements in image guidance offers quantification of lens density, which may lead to real-time feedback for customized densitometry-guided laser lens fragmentation or lens tissue alteration.
4. FS laser lens fragmentation makes it possible to disrupt a dense nucleus for extraction through a small capsulotomy, which furthers the possibility of capsular refilling procedures as a future technique for lens replacement surgery with accommodation restoration.
5. FS laser photodisruption of the crystalline lens is being proposed as a method for

accommodation restoration in presbyopic lenses. Image-guided surgery and fluid optics will facilitate its delivery.

6. FS laser delivery may go beyond the lens to deeper ocular structures, such as the vitreous cavity for vitreolysis. Adaptive optics is being proposed as a means of refining the beam for safe and precise intraocular tissue cutting. This is why the FS laser is being considered as a laser scalpel for use in ocular surgery.
7. The technology of FS lasers, imaging and delivery will only improve with time and lead to better laser cutting tools. Although expensive now, FS laser cutting tools will become cheaper and more versatile over time, and provide a revolutionary change in ophthalmic surgery.

Acknowledgments We would like to acknowledge and thank Brien Holden and his team, as well as Fabrice Manns, Esdras Arrieta, and the team at the Ophthalmic Biophysics Center at the University of Miami for their contribution toward the section on capsular refilling.

References

1. Shousha MA, Yoo SH, Kymionis GD, Ide T, Feuer W, Karp CL, O'Brien TP, Culbertson WW, Alfonso E. Long-term results of femtosecond laser-assisted sutureless anterior lamellar keratoplasty. Ophthalmology. 2011;118(2):315–23.
2. Buzzonetti L, Laborante A, Petrocelli G. Standardized big-bubble technique in deep anterior lamellar keratoplasty assisted by the femtosecond laser. J Cataract Refract Surg. 2010;36(10):1631–6.
3. Price Jr FW, Price MO, Grandin JC, Kwon R. Deep anterior lamellar keratoplasty with femtosecond-laser zigzag incisions. J Cataract Refract Surg. 2009;35(5):804–8.
4. Gorovoy MS. Descemet-stripping automated endothelial keratoplasty. Cornea. 2006;25(8):886–9.
5. Meisler DM, Dupps Jr WJ, Covert DJ, Koenig SB. Use of an air-fluid exchange system to promote graft adhesion during Descemet's stripping automated endothelial keratoplasty. J Cataract Refract Surg. 2007;33(5):770–2.
6. Terry MA, Ousley PJ. Small-incision deep lamellar endothelial keratoplasty (DLEK): six-month results in the first prospective clinical study. Cornea. 2005;24(1):59–65.
7. Terry MA, Hoar KL, Wall J, Ousley P. Histology of dislocations in endothelial keratoplasty (DSEK and DLEK): a laboratory-based, surgical solution to dislocation in 100 consecutive DSEK cases. Cornea. 2006;25(8):926–32.
8. Krueger RR, Juhasz T, Gualano A, Marchi V. The picosecond laser for nonmechanical laser in situ keratomileusis. J Refract Surg. 1998;14(4):467–9.
9. Sekundo W, Kunert K, Russmann C, Gille A, Bissmann W, Stobrawa G, Sticker M, Bischoff M, Blum M. First efficacy and safety study of femtosecond lenticule extraction for the correction of myopia: six-month results. J Cataract Refract Surg. 2008;34(9):1513–20.
10. Shah R, Shah S, Sengupta S. Results of small incision lenticule extraction: all-in-one femtosecond laser refractive surgery. J Cataract Refract Surg. 2011;37(1):127–37.
11. Seyeddain O, Riha W, Hohensinn M, Nix G, Dexl AK, Grabner G. Refractive surgical correction of presbyopia with the AcuFocus small aperture corneal inlay: two-year follow-up. J Refract Surg. 2010;26(10):707–15.
12. Kirkwood BJ, Hendicott PL, Read SA, Pesudovs K. Repeatability and validity of lens densitometry measured with Scheimpflug imaging. J Cataract Refract Surg. 2009;35(7):1210–5.
13. Macsai MS, Padnick-Silver L, Fontes BM. Visual outcomes after accommodating intraocular lens implantation. J Cataract Refract Surg. 2006;32(4):628–33.
14. Ossma IL, Galvis A, Vargas LG, Trager MJ, Vagefi MR, McLeod SD. Synchrony dual-optic accommodating intraocular lens. Part 2: Pilot clinical evaluation. J Cataract Refract Surg. 2007;33(1):47–52.
15. Alió JL, Ben-nun J, Rodríguez-Prats JL, Plaza AB. Visual and accommodative outcomes 1 year after implantation of an accommodating intraocular lens based on a new concept. J Cataract Refract Surg. 2009;35(10):1671–8.
16. Koopmans SA, Terwee T, Glasser A, Wendt M, Vilupuru AS, van Kooten TG, Norrby S, Haitjema HJ, Kooijman AC. Accommodative lens refilling in rhesus monkeys. Invest Ophthalmol Vis Sci. 2006;47(7):2976–84.
17. Tahi H, Hamaoui M, Parel J-M, Fantes F. A technique for small peripheral capsulorhexis. J Cataract Refractive Surg. 1999;25:744–7.
18. Kessler J. Experiments in refilling the lens. Arch Ophthalmol. 1964;71:412–7.
19. Kessler J. Refilling the rabbit lens. Further experiments. Arch Ophthalmol. 1966;76(4):596–8.
20. Kessler J. Lens refilling and regrowth of lens substance in the rabbit eye. Ann Ophthalmol. 1975;7(8):1059–62.
21. Agarwal LP, Angra SK, Khosla PK, Tandon HD. Lens regeneration in mammals: I. Rabbits (after extracapsular extraction). Orient Arch Ophthalmol. 1964;2:1–17.
22. Agarwal LP, Angra SK, Khosla PK, Tandon HD. Lens regeneration in mammals: II. Monkeys (after extracapsular extraction). Orient Arch Ophthalmol. 1964;2:47–59.
23. Agarwal LP, Angra SK, Tandon HD. Lens regeneration in mammals: III. Rabbits (after intracapsular extraction). Orient Arch Ophthalmol. 1964;2:95–100.
24. Agarwal LP, Narsimhan EC, Mohan M. Experimental lens refilling. Orient Arch Ophthalmol. 1967;5:205–12.

25. Parel JM, Treffers WF, Gelender H, Norton EWD. Phaco-Ersatz: a new approach to cataract surgery. Ophthalmology. 1981;88(9 Suppl):95.
26. Parel JM, Gelender H, Trefers WF, Norton EWD. Phaco-Ersatz: cataract surgery designed to preserve accommodation. Graefe's Arch Clin Exp Ophthalmol. 1986;224:165–73.
27. Haefliger E, Parel J-M, Fantes F, Norton EWD, Anderson D, Forster RK, Hernandez E, Feuer WJ. Accommodation of an endocapsular silicone lens (Phaco-Ersatz) in the non-human primate. Ophthalmology. 1987;94:471–7.
28. Haefliger E, Parel J-M. Accommodation of an endocapsular silicone lens (Phaco-Ersatz) in the old rhesus monkey. Refract Corneal Surg. 1994;10:550–5.
29. Barraquer J. Lentilles intraoculaires 1949–1994. Phaco-Ersatz 2001. An Inst Barraquer. 1993–1994;24:27–36.
30. Gindi JJ, Wan WL, Schanzlin DJ. Endocapsular cataract surgery: I. Surgical technique. Cataract. 1985;2:6–10.
31. Lucke K, Hettlich HJ, Kreiner CF. A method of lens extraction for the injection of liquid intraocular lenses. Ger J Ophthalmol. 1992;1(5):342–5.
32. Hettlich HJ, Lucke K, Kreiner CF. Light-induced endocapsular polymerization of injectable lens refilling materials. Ger J Ophthalmol. 1992;1(5):346–9.
33. Hettlich HJ, Lucke K, Asiyo-Vogel MN, Schulte M, Vogel A. Lens refilling and endocapsular polymerization of an injectable intraocular lens: in vitro and in vivo study of potential risks and benefits. J Cataract Refract Surg. 1994;20:115–23.
34. Hettlich HJ, Lucke K, Asiyo-Vogel M, Vogel A. Experimental studies of the risks of endocapsular polymerization of injectable intraocular lenses. Ophthalmologe. 1995;92(3):329–34.
35. Hettlich HJ, Asiyo-Vogel M. Experimental experiences with balloon-shaped capsular sac implantation with reference to accommodation outcome in intraocular lenses. Ophthalmologe. 1996;93(1):73–5.
36. Nishi O, Hara T, Sakka Y, Hayashi H, Nakamae K, Yamada Y. Refilling the lens with inflatable endocapsular balloon. Dev Ophthalmol. 1991;22:122–5.
37. Nishi O, Hara T, Hara T, Sakka Y, Hayashi F, Nakamae K, Yamada Y. Refilling the lens with a inflatable endocapsular balloon: surgical procedure in animal eyes. Graefe's Arch Clin Exp Ophthalmol. 1992;230:47–55.
38. Nishi O, Nakai Y, Yamada Y, Mizumoto Y. Amplitudes of accommodation of primate lenses refilled with two types of inflatable endocapsular balloons. Arch Ophthalmol. 1993;111(12):1677–84.
39. Sakka Y, Hara T, Yamada Y, Hara T, Hayashi F. Accommodation in primate eyes after implantation of refilled endocapsular balloon. Am J Ophthalmol. 1996;121:210–2.
40. Hara T, Sakka Y, Sakanishi K, Yamamda Y, Nakamae K, Hayashi F. Complications associated with endocapsular balloon implantation in rabbit eyes. Cataract Refract Surg. 1994;20:507–12.
41. Nishi O, Nishi K, Mano C, Ichihara M, Honda T. Controlling the capsular shape in lens refilling. Arch Ophthalmol. 1997;115(4):507–10.
42. Nishi O, Nishi K, Mano C, Ichihara M, Honda T. Lens refilling with injectable silicone in rabbit eyes. J Cataract Refract Surg. 1998;24(7):975–82.
43. Nishi O, Nishi K. Accommodation amplitude after lens refilling with injectable silicone by sealing the capsule with a plug in primates. Arch Ophthalmol. 1998;116(10):1358–61.
44. Fernandez V, Fragoso MA, Lamar P, Orozco MA, Dubovy S, Willcox M, Parel J-M. Efficiency of various drugs in the prevention of Posterior Capsular Opacification (PCO). J Refract Cataract Surg. 2004;30(12):2598–605.
45. Takesue Y, Mui MM, Hachiya T, Parel J-M. Comparative photodynamic effect of Rose Bengal, Erytrocin B and DHE on lens epithelial cells. In: Parel J-M, Ren Q, editors. Ophthalmic technologies III. Proc SPIE 1993;1877:323–7.
46. Behar-Cohen F, David T, D'Hermies F, Pouliquen YM, Buechler Y, Nova MP, Houston LL, Courtois Y. In vivo inhibition of lens regrowth by fibroblast growth factor 2-saporin. Invest Ophthalmol Vis Sci. 1995;36:2434–48.
47. Hao X, Jeffery JL, Wilkie JS, Meijs GF, Clayton A, Watling JD, Ho A, Fernandez V, Acosta C, Yamamoto H, Aly MG, Parel J-M, Hughes TC. Functionalised polysiloxanes as injectable, in situ curable accommodating intraocular lens. Biomaterials. 2010;31(32):8153–63.
48. Borja D, Siedlecki D, de Castro A, Uhlhorn S, Ortiz S, Arrieta E, Parel JM, Marcos S, Manns F. Distortions of the posterior surface in optical coherence tomography images of the isolated crystalline lens: effect of the lens index gradient. Biomed Opt Exp. 2010;1(5):1331–40.
49. Manns F, Maceo B, Ho A, Parel J-M. Contribution of the refractive index gradient to the spherical aberration of the human crystalline lens. ARVO. Invest Ophthalmol Vis Sci. 2011;52 [E-Abstract 3406].
50. Olson R, Mamalis N, Haugen B. A light adjustable lens with injectable optics. Curr Opin Ophthalmol. 2006;17(1):72–9.
51. Urs R, Manns F, Ho A, Borja D, Amelinckx A, Smith J, Jain R, Augusteyn R, Parel J-M. Shape of the isolated ex-vivo human crystalline lens. Vis Res. 2009;49(1):74–83.
52. Urs R, Ho A, Manns F, Parel J-M. Age-dependent Fourier model of the shape of the isolated ex-vivo human crystalline lens. Vis Res. 2010;50(11):1041–7.
53. Ruggeri M, Uhlhorn S, De Freitas C, Manns F, Parel J-M. Real-time imaging of accommodation using extended depth spectral domain OCT. ARVO. Invest Ophthalmol Vis Sci. 2011;52 [E-Abstract 3402].
54. Kim E, Uhlhorn SR, Erhmann K, Borja D, Parel J-M. Semi-automated analysis of ex vivo accommodation simulated OCT crystalline lens image. J Biomed Opt. 2011;16(5):056003.
55. Binder S, Falkner-Radler CI, Hauger C, Phd HM, Glittenberg C. Feasibility of intrasurgical spectral-domain optical coherence tomography. Retina. 2011 Jan 26 [Epub ahead of print].

56. Ehlers JP, Tao YK, Farsiu S, Maldonado R, Izatt JA, Toth CA. Integration of a spectral domain optical coherence tomography system into a surgical microscope for intraoperative imaging. Invest Ophthalmol Vis Sci. 2011;52(6):3153–9.
57. Koopmans SA, Terwee T, van Kooten TG. Prevention of capsular opacification after accommodative lens refilling surgery in rabbits. Biomaterials. 2011;32(25):5743–55.
58. Parrish II RK. Bascom palmer eye institute atlas of ophthalmology. Philadelphia, PA: Current Medicine; 1999.
59. Von Helmholtz H. Mechanism of accommodation. In: Southall JPC, editor. Helmholtz's treatise on physiological optics (trans: Southall in 1924, original German in 1909); 1962.
60. Glasser A, Kaufman PL. The mechanism of accommodation in primates. Ophthalmology. 1999;106(5):863–72.
61. Strenk S, Semmlow J, DeMarco J. Age-related changes in human ciliary muscle and lens: a magnetic resonance imaging study. Invest Ophthalmol Vis Sci. 1999;40:1162–9.
62. Fisher RF. The elastic constants of the human lens. J Physiol. 1971;212(1):147–80.
63. Glasser A, Campbell MC. Presbyopia and the optical changes in the human crystalline lens with age. Vis Res. 1998;38(2):209–29.
64. Myers R, Krueger RR. Novel approaches to correction of presbyopia with laser modification of the crystalline lens. J Refract Surg. 1998;14:136–9.
65. Vogel A, Busch S, Jungnickel K, Birngruber R. Mechanisms of intraocular photodisruption with picosecond and nanosecond laser pulses. Lasers Surg Med. 1994;15(1):32–43.
66. Krueger RR, Sun XK, Stroh J, Myers R. Experimental increase in accommodative potential after neodymium: yttrium-aluminum-garnet laser photodisruption of paired cadaver lenses. Ophthalmology. 2001;108(11):2122–9.
67. Krueger RR, Kuszak J, Lubatschowski H, et al. First safety study of femtosecond laser photodisruption in animal lenses: tissue morphology and cataractogenesis. J Cataract Refract Surg. 2005;31(12):2386–94.
68. Gerten G, Ripken T, Breitenfeld P, et al. In vitro and in vivo investigations on the treatment of presbyopia using femtosecond lasers. Der Ophthalmologe: Zeitschrift der Deutschen Ophthalmologischen Gesellschaft. 2007;104(1):40–6.
69. Pierscionek BK. Age-related response of human lenses to stretching forces. Exp Eye Res. 1995;60(3):325–32.
70. Glasser A, Campbell MC. Biometric, optical and physical changes in the isolated human crystalline lens with age in relation to presbyopia. Vis Res. 1999;39(11):1991–2015.
71. Kuszak JR, Mazurkiewicz M, Zoltoski R. Computer modeling of secondary fiber development and growth: I. Nonprimate lenses. Mol Vis. 2006;12:251–70.
72. Vogel A, Noack J, Huttman G, Paltauf G. Mechanisms of femtosecond laser nanosurgery of cells and tissues. Appl Phys B. 2005;81:1015–47.
73. Loesel FH, Niemz MH, Bille JF, Juhasz T. Laser-induced optical breakdown on hard and soft tissue and its dependence on the pulse duration: experiment and model. IEEE J Quant Electron. 1996;32:1717–22.
74. Giguere D, Olivie G, Vidal F, et al. Laser ablation threshold dependence on pulse duration for fused silica and corneal tissues: experiments and modeling. J Opt Soc Am A. 2007;24:1562–8.
75. Ding L, Blackwell R, Künzler JF, Knox WH. Large refractive index change in silicone-based and non-silicone-based hydrogel polymers induced by femtosecond laser micro-machining. Opt Exp. 2006;14: 11901–9.
76. Ding L, Cancado LG, Novotny L, et al. Micro-Raman spectroscopy of refractive index microstructures in silicone-based hydrogel polymers created by high-repetition-rate femtosecond laser micromachining. J Opt Soc Am B. 2009;26:595–602.
77. Ding L, Knox WH, Bühren J, Nagy LJ, Huxlin KR. Intra-tissue Refractive Index Shaping (IRIS) of the cornea and lens using a low-pulse-energy femtosecond laser oscillator. Invest Ophthalmol Vis Sci. 2008;49:5332–9.
78. Ding L, Jani D, Linhardt J, et al. Large enhancement of femtosecond laser micromachining speed in dye-doped hydrogel polymers. Opt Exp. 2008;16: 21914–21.
79. Knox WH, Huxlin KR. Writing 3D refractive index modifications in ophthalmic polymer & ocular tissue—a novel means of altering refraction & biomechanics with minimal cellular damage. Engineering the Eye III. Benasque, Spain; 2011.
80. Sahler R, Bille JF, Zhou S, Aguilera R, Schanzlin DJ. Non-invasive in-situ power adjustment of intraocular lenses by refractive index shaping. Ft. Lauderdale, FL: ARVO; 2011.
81. Kim H-C, Härtner S, Hampp N. Single- and two-photon absorption induced photocleavage of dimeric coumarin linkers: Therapeutic versus passive photocleavage in ophthalmologic applications. J Photochem Photobiol A: Chem. 2008;197:239–44.
82. Hampp N. IOLs controlled by 2-photon processes. Engineering the Eye III. Benasque, Spain; 2011.
83. Nagy LJ, Ding L, Xu L, Knox WH, Huxlin KR. Potentiation of femtosecond laser Intratissue Refractive Index Shaping (IRIS) in the living cornea with sodium fluorescein. Invest Ophthalmol Vis Sci. 2010;51:850–6.
84. Li DY, Borkman RF. Photodamage to calf lenses in vitro by excimer laser radiation at 308, 337, and 350 nm. Invest Ophthalmol Vis Sci. 1990;31:2180–4.
85. Vogel A, Capon MR, Asiyo-Vogel MN, Birngruber R. Intraocular photodisruption with picosecond and nanosecond laser pulses: tissue effects in cornea, lens, and retina. Invest Ophthalmol Vis Sci. 1994;35:3032–44.
86. Xu L, Knox WH, DeMagistris M, Wang N, Huxlin KH. Non-invasive Intra-tissue Refractive Index Shaping (IRIS) of the cornea with blue femtosecond laser light. Invest Ophthalmol Vis Sci. 2011;52(11):8148–55.

87. Babcock HW. Adaptive optics revisited. Science. 1990;249:253–7.
88. Lorenz RD. Planetary science: the weather on Titan. Science. 2000;290:467–8.
89. Liang J, Grimm B, Goelz S, Bille JF. Objective measurement of wave aberrations of the human eye with the use of a Hartmann-Shack wave-front sensor. J Opt Soc Am A Opt Image Sci Vis. 1994;11:1949–57.
90. Hong X, Thibos LN. Longitudinal evaluation of optical aberrations following laser in situ keratomileusis surgery. J Refract Surg. 2000;16:S647–50.
91. Mrochen M, Kaemmerer M, Seiler T. Wavefront-guided laser in situ keratomileusis: early results in three eyes. J Refract Surg. 2000;16(2):116–21.
92. Roorda A. Applications of adaptive optics scanning laser ophthalmoscopy. Optom Vis Sci. 2010;87:260–8.
93. Rocha KM, Vabre L, Chateau N, Krueger RR. Enhanced visual acuity and image perception following correction of highly aberrated eyes using an adaptive optics visual simulator. J Refractive Surg. 2010;26(1):52–6.
94. Chen Y, Ratnam K, Sundquist SM, Lujan B, Awaquari R, Gudiseva VH, Roorda A, Duncan JL. Cone photoreceptor abnormalities correlate with vision loss in patients with Starguardt disease. Invest Ophthalmol Vis Sci. 2011;52:3281–92.
95. Hansen A, Ripken T, Heisterkamp A. Focal spot shaping for femtosecond laser pulse photodisruption through turbid media Trans SPIE, 2011.
96. Shechtman DL, Dunbar MT. The expanding spectrum of vitreomacular traction. Optometry. 2009;80:681–7.
97. Karatas M, Ramirez JA, Ophir A. Diabetic vitreopapillary traction and macular oedema. Eye (Lond). 2005;19:676–8.
98. Chai D, Chaudhary G, Mikula E, Sun H, Juhasz T. 3D finite element model of aqueous outflow to predict the effect of femtosecond laser created partial thickness drainage channels. Lasers Surg Med. 2008;40:188–95.
99. Tam J, Roorda A. Speed quantification and tracking of moving objects in adaptive optics scanning laser ophthalmoscopy. J Biomed Opt. 2011;16:036002.

Index

DOI 10.1007/978-1-4614-1010-2, © Springer Science+Business Media, LLC 2013

L

M

Printed by Printforce, the Netherlands